MASTERI

MACMILLAN MASTER SERIES

Banking
Basic Management
Biology
British Politics
Business Communication
Chemistry
COBOL Programming
Commerce
Computer Programming
Computers
Data Processing
Economics
Electronics
English Grammar
English Language
English Literature
French
German
Hairdressing
Italian
Keyboarding
Marketing
Mathematics
Modern British History
Modern World History
Nutrition
Office Practice
Pascal Programming
Physics
Principles of Accounts
Social Welfare
Spanish
Statistics
Study Skills
Typewriting Skills
Word Processing

OTHER BOOKS BY THE SAME AUTHOR

Mastering Biology
Multiple Choice Questions in Biology and Human Biology
Multiple Choice Questions in Food and Nutrition
An Introduction to the Biological Aspects of Nursing Science
Shopping Science
Introductory Science for Catering, Cooking and Homecraft Students
Experimental Science for Catering and Homecraft Students

MASTERING NUTRITION

O. F. G. KILGOUR

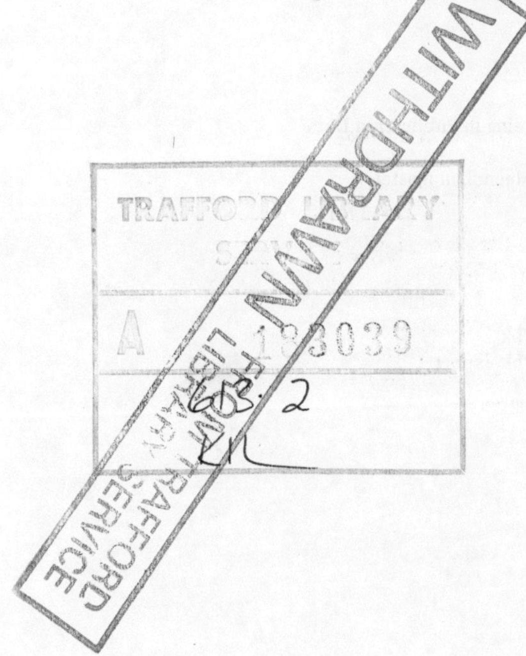

M
MACMILLAN

First published 1985 by
MACMILLAN EDUCATION LTD
Houndmills, Basingstoke, Hampshire
RG21 2XS and London

Companies and representatives
throughout the world

Typeset in Great Britain by
RDL ARTSET LTD
Sutton, Surrey

Printed in Hong Kong

British Library Cataloguing in Publication Data
Kilgour, O. F. G.
Mastering nutrition.–(Macmillan master series)
1. Nutrition
I. Title
613.2 TX353
ISBN 0-333-35430-3
ISBN 0-333-35431-1 Pbk
ISBN 0-333-35789-2 Pbk export

DEDICATION

TO
REBEKAH RUTH, JANET SUSANNAH,
OWEN ABRAM

CONTENTS

CONTENTS

CONTENTS

CONTENTS

LIST OF TABLES

LIST OF FIGURES

LIST OF PLATES

(Acknowledgement of source in brackets)

INTRODUCTION

This book is a self-contained factual presentation of the theoretical and practical principles of human nutrition through a chemical, physical and biological approach which assumes *no* previous knowledge.

Nutrition and health go together, and the book will interest the general reader who eats to live, and those who produce, prepare, process or are otherwise concerned with food. Parents, school pupils, people preparing meals in the home, farmers, nurses, home economists, caterers, hoteliers and food-processing workers, will find sufficient to meet the needs of various examination syllabuses which have a food and nutrition content.

I have attempted to direct my presentation towards an international understanding of the world problem of nutrition, in feeding a rapidly growing population of more than *four billion* on an inadequate and unequally shared food supply – a world where one in ten of us is underfed and hungry, and two in ten are overfed.

The reader is referred particularly to the author's books published by Heinemann, which complement this volume: *Shopping Science* for a range of experiments on measurement and value for money, food testing and composition; *Introductory Science for Catering, Cookery and Homecraft Students* for further treatment of basic food science; *Multiple Choice Questions in Food and Nutrition* for a range of questions of the multiple choice type, and *Experimental Science for Catering and Homecraft Students* (with Aileen L'Amie) for further experimental work including general procedures for the conduct of practical work in food and nutrition.

O. F. G. K.

ACKNOWLEDGEMENTS

I express my sincere thanks to the following who gave help in preparing the manuscript: Meinwen Parry, B.Sc., M.I.Biol., a teacher of long experience; Dr T. R. W. Cowell, M.B., Ch.B, and Dr C. W. Cowell, M.B., B.S., long-established medical practitioners; Mr R. P. W. Cowell, B.Sc.; Mr F. R. Jones, B.A., the Ven S. Closs Parry, B. A. and my son A. D. Kilgour of New Zealand.

I appreciate the use of reference facilities of the Marine Society, granted me by Dr R. Hope and Miss P. O'Connor.

Generous assistance has been given by industrial and international organisations who provided illustrations acknowledged in the captions, and I appreciate the permission to quote and use reference information from *Population Concern*, an organisation under the auspices of the Family Planning Association of the UK.

My thanks are also due to the following for permission to quote and use reference information from their literature: the Health Education Council, the FAO (Food and Agriculture Organisation) of the United Nations, the WHO (World Health Organisation); Ciba-Geigy Ltd, Switzerland - a private industry that makes a valuable contribution to education - for permission to publish extracts from their Geigy Scientific Tables. Finally, my sincere thanks are given to Mrs V. C. Stirling for preparing the typescript.

GLOSSARY

absorption the uptake of nutrients, water or other substances by the stomach or intestine following digestion

adipose animal fatty tissue

amino-acid the units which form a protein

autolysis the self-destruction of cells by digestive enzymes

available a nutrient in a form in which it is absorbed and used by the body

bacteria unicellular microscopic organisms

basal metabolism the energy needed to keep an individual in a state of physical, mental and digestive rest

blanching a process to inactivate enzymes by treatment with hot water or steam

bland mild-flavoured or smooth soft textured

buffer a substance that resists a change of pH or hydrogen ion concentration

Calorie or kilocalorie former unit of energy measurement equal to 1000 calories or 4.186 kilojoules

carcinogens substances able to induce cancer in healthy living tissue

cartilage a form of white connective tissue attached to the ends of bones; first substance to form in growing bone

collagen a protein forming the main component of cartilage, tendon, bone, and skin. Changed into gelatine by action of hot water in cooking

deficiency disease a disease caused by inadequate intake of a nutrient

dehydration loss of body-water

digestion the breakdown of complex organic foodstuffs by enzymes into simpler soluble substances absorbable by the body tissues

double bond a double link or unsaturated bond between carbon atoms in a carbon chain molecule

emulsification a process of making an emulsion in which small droplets of a liquid are dispersed in another different liquid

empirical formula the simplest type of chemical formula, it does not represent any molecule structure

enzyme a protein compound which catalyses biochemical reactions

epithelium a layer of cells resembling sheets covering and lining the body cavity and intestine

excretion process of removing harmful waste products of metabolism

factor in nutrition any chemical substance found in foods

fortify to add substances (or fortifying agents) usually vitamins or minerals to replace nutrients lost in processing
gastric pertaining to the stomach
gland an organ that forms a specific chemical substance and secretes this either through a tubular duct, or directly, into the blood
gluten a mixture of proteins (gliadin and glutelin) found in wheat flour
heat of combustion the heat energy produced by the complete burning or oxidation of a food or other combustible substance
homeostasis the maintenance of steady conditions around living cells in the human body
hormone a chemical messenger transported from endocrine glands by means of the blood
hydrogenation the addition of hydrogen to an unsaturated substance containing double bonds
hydrolysis a reaction between a substance and water usually in the presence of enzymes to produce simpler substances
hyper- a prefix meaning 'increased' or 'excessive' or 'over'
hypo- a prefix meaning 'below', or 'deficient'
inorganic a group of chemical substances that do not contain the chemical element carbon
ionic ions form when an atom loses or gains an electron
intake refers to the nutrients taken into the body
joule the SI unit of energy, kilojoules and megajoules
lactation the time when milk is secreted in a woman
lymph a straw-coloured liquid present in the lymphatic vessels
molecule the combination of two or more atoms, whether similar or dissimilar, by means of chemical bonds, single or double
non-fat solids the components of milk remaining after water and butter-fat lipids have been removed
nucleic acids acids composed of sugar, phosphate and nitrogenous bases, found in all living cells
nucleoprotein a complex of nucleic acid and a protein
organic chemical substances which are produced by living things and contain the chemical element carbon
osmosis the movement of water from a dilute solution to a more concentrated solution through a membrane, called a *semi-permeable* membrane
oxidation a process which can be defined as adding oxygen, or removing hydrogen or loss of electrons
peptides compounds formed when amino-acids are linked together; two amino-acids form a *dipeptide*, three form a *tripeptide*, many form a *polypeptide*

pH symbol for potential of hydrogen, used to show the degree of acidity or alkalinity of substances

poly- is a prefix meaning much or many

polyunsaturated means the presence in a long chain organic molecule of more than one double, or unsaturated, bonds

proteolytic describes the breakdown of proteins into amino-acids usually by enzymes

reduction a chemical change in which oxygen is removed from, or hydrogen added to compound – the reverse of oxidation. Also can include gain of electrons

secretion production of fluids by cells and their release into their surroundings

saturated a hydrocarbon chain molecule in which all the carbon atoms are linked by single saturated bonds. Applies to saturated lipids from animals

sugar a loose term usually meaning sucrose or cane sugar; can also mean any substance with a sweet taste from the carbohydrate group of compounds

syndrome a medical term for a disease showing a group of symptoms

synthesis the building-up of a substance from simpler substances, the opposite of analysis which is the breakdown of a substance into simpler substances

therapeutic refers to the curing of disease

tissue a group of cells specialised for a particular function

toxin a harmful chemical substance produced by a disease-causing micro-organism and which damages body cells even in very low concentrations

toxicity the quality of a substance which makes it poisonous

unsaturated refers to a hydrocarbon chain molecule in which there are double bonds between carbon atoms. Hydrogen atoms can be added to these double bonds to form saturated single bonds between carbon atoms. Unsaturated lipids are mainly of plant or vegetable origin.

urea(carbamide) the breakdown product of amino-acids; a component of urine

vegetable can mean *either* of plant origin *or* edible plant parts used as food, collectively called vegetables

vegetarian a diet avoiding meat and fish (and sometimes eggs) but not dairy products

vegan diets excluding *all* animal-product foods

CHAPTER 1

INTRODUCING HUMAN NUTRITION

1.1 WHAT IS NUTRITION?

Nutrition is one of the distinguishing characteristics of *living* things, or *organisms*, both plants and animals. The other characteristics distinguishing living from non-living matter are: *respiration* - energy release; *excretion* - waste removal; *irritability* - response to stimulus; *movement*, *growth* and *reproduction* - the continuity of life.

fig 1.1 *single cell from mouth lining*

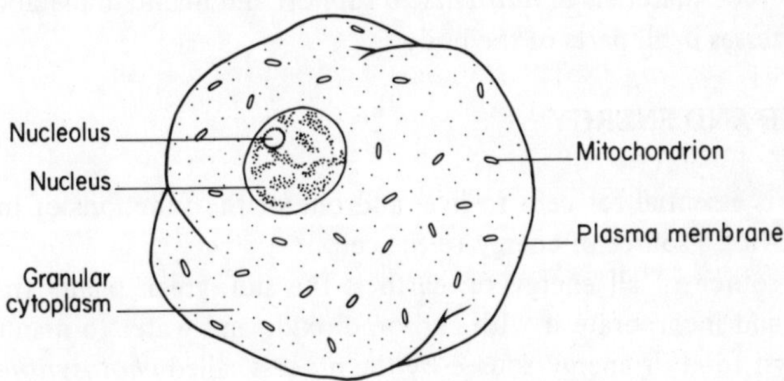

Cells

Living things consist of cells, the structural and functional unit. Simple organisms, bacteria and yeasts, are *unicellular*, whilst higher organisms, including human beings, are *multicellular*, the cells being grouped into tissues, organs and systems (see Section 3.5).

Life and metabolism

Life is the product of all the many chemical processes that occur inside living cells; all these chemical processes are collectively called *metabolism*.

fig 1.2 *multicellular tissue of onion-bulb leaf-scale*

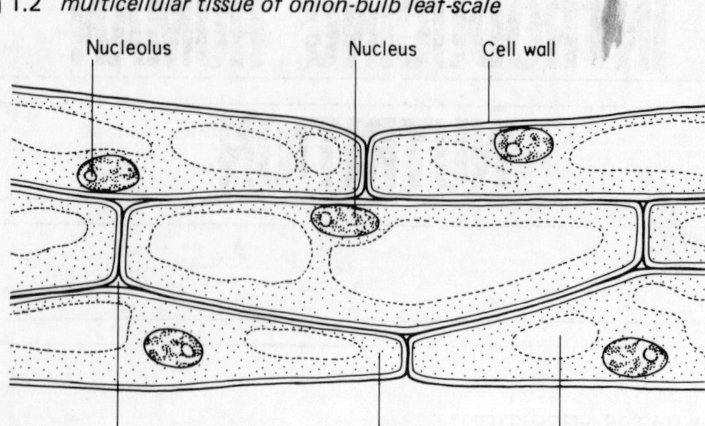

The metabolism of a multicellular human body is the result of the metabolic chemical changes taking place in every component body cell.

Good health is the product of normal orderly metabolism in body cells; ill-health or disease is the product of abnormal or disturbed cell metabolism; death results when cell metabolism stops completely.

Nutrition therefore is a combination of processes by which cells receive and use food materials or *nutrients* to support and maintain metabolism or life processes in all parts of the body.

1.2 LIFE AND ENERGY

Energy is essential for cells to live, and one of the functions of nutrition is to provide a source of energy to the cell.

The source of all energy on earth is the sun, green plants trap solar energy and incorporate it with carbon dioxide and water to manufacture their own food or energy source by the process called *photosynthesis* (see Section 3.8).

Green plant cell nutrition is an example of a type of metabolism called *anabolism* or cell chemical reactions building up by synthesis complex *organic* compounds from simpler chemical substances, using solar energy.

The important products of green plant nutrition by *photosynthesis* are the food nutrients *carbohydrates*, *proteins* and *lipids* or fats. These in turn are used by the plant cells for:

1. Energy supply for metabolism to take place,
2. Construction, repair and maintenance of new cells and plant growth,
3. Manufacture of metabolism control and regulator substances.

Animal cell nutrition depends entirely on the provision of ready-made organic food nutrients containing energy in foodstuffs photosynthesised by green plants. This is provided *directly* to plant-eating (*herbivorous*) animals, or *indirectly* to *carnivorous* animals feeding on herbivorous animals. The *omnivorous* animals, including human beings, feed on foodstuffs of both plant and animal origin.

The ready-made food nutrients are used by the animal cells for the same purpose as in plant cells – to maintain metabolism, provide energy, construct cell material, and produce regulator substance to control metabolism.

Energy supply

Foodstuffs in plants and animals are *complex* organic chemical substances and must be changed into *simpler* substances by one of the processes of nutrition called *digestion.*

The products of digestion are made to *release* their stored energy by the important cell metabolism process called *respiration* (see Section 5.4).

Respiration is a type of metabolic change called *catabolism* or breakdown of organic substance to provide energy, by-products of this chemical change becoming *excretory* materials.

1.3 HUMAN CELL NUTRITION

Living cells in the human body are surrounded by a liquid called *tissue fluid*, produced by the *blood* (fluid plasma) which links the human gut or alimentary canal with all body cells (Section 81.3).

The tissue fluid provides the living cell with all the substances it needs for metabolism and like; these substances are in a *simple* form, mainly as the end-products of *digestion.* Cell tissue fluid in a healthy human being has a steady or *constant* chemical and physical composition. This in turn provides every cell with an *internal environment* kept constant by various automatic control mechanisms. The steady internal environment is maintained despite any changes occurring outside the body. For example, the *temperature* of tissue fluid is constant at 37°C summer and winter, and the amount of food nutrients is constant during and between light or heavy meals.

This steady internal cell environment is called *homeostasis* and is controlled by various *homeostatic mechanisms.* Good health is related to normal homeostasis; any disturbance in the composition of tissue fluid will lead to body disorders and ill-health.

1.4 HUMAN CELL NUTRIENTS

Nutrients are chemical substances which have a metabolic function inside living cells.

These nutrients are the main chemical components of tissue fluid, and with the exception of oxygen are also components of foodstuffs.

The following are the main *essential* nutrient components of tissue fluid:

1. *carbohydrate* - glucose
2. *proteins* - amino-acids
3. *lipids* or fats and oils
4. *mineral* ions or inorganic components
5. *vitamins*
6. *water* -99 per cent
7. *oxygen*

The following *can* be present in tissue fluid, but are not essential as nutrients in cell metabolism, although they may have a function in metabolism: *Ethanol* or alcohol, and *Organic acids* found mainly in fruits, and *drugs* or components of different medicine preparations.

The average composition of tissue fluid is shown in Table 1.1.

Table 1.1 *average composition of tissue fluid*

Component	*Range* (as %)
Water	97.0 -99.0
Glucose	0.08- 0.13
Amino-acids	0.03- 0.05
Lipids	0.2 - 0.45
Mineral ions	0.3 - 0.36
Oxygen	0.8 - 1.0
Vitamins	*variable*

Macronutrients are those essential nutrients required by the body cell in relatively large amounts and include *oxygen*, *water*, *carbohydrates*, *lipids*, *protein*, *amino-acids*, and certain *mineral ions*: calcium, magnesium, iron, sodium and potassium.

Micronutrients are those essential nutrients required in very small amounts by the living cell and include *vitamins*, and certain mineral ions called *trace elements* such as iodine, copper, fluorine and several others.

1.5 FUNCTION OF CELL NUTRIENTS

The nutrient components of the tissue fluid pass through the *cell membrane* into the cell by special cell transport methods called *diffusion*, *osmosis* and *active transport* (see Section 2.7).

Within the cell certain nutrients take part as *metabolites* in different processes of cell metabolism. A nutrient may have more than one function as indicated as follows:

Energy supply

Energy supply is by the catabolic breakdown of the carbohydrate glucose during *respiration* using *oxygen* (see Section 5.4). Protein, amino-acids and lipids are also sources of energy.

Cell construction, repair and maintenance

New body cells are continuously being formed in the *growing* foetus and in children, whilst most old cells must be replaced and damaged cells repaired.

New cell material is made by synthesis or anabolism mainly from substances provided by *proteins* and certain *mineral ions*, together with *water* which forms over 60 per cent of the body structure.

Metabolism regulation

Metabolic changes, like chemical reactions in test-tubes, can proceed rapidly or slowly. The *rate* of a chemical change can be affected by *temperature* and also by the effect of metabolism regulators such as *hormones*, *enzymes* made from *proteins*, or by certain *vitamins* and *mineral ions.*

Body protection

Disease-causing microbes can stimulate certain cells to make protective antibodies from *proteins*: these provide natural protection from further infection with the *same* disease. *Drugs* and components of medicines can affect homeostasis causing ill-health; certain *protein* substances detoxify these substances and render them harmless.

Lactation

All kinds of nutrients are needed to produce *milk* during the breast-feeding of babies (see Section 9.14). The milk-producing cells must have a good supply of tissue fluid for healthy milk formation.

1.6 WHAT IS A FOOD?

A *food* for human beings is a substance which can contribute to the nutrient composition of tissue fluid and participate in cell metabolism.

Milk is almost a complete food in being able to provide nearly all nutrients as components of tissue fluid.

Curry and *mustard* powders, although unpalatable, have most nutrients excepting vitamins, which could contribute to the tissue-fluid nutrient composition (see Appendix A)

A food may have a *non-nutritive component* in addition to its nutrient component. Some non-nutritive components which do not enter into the composition of tissue fluid or participate as metabolites, include *flavours* (synthetic and natural), *essential oils*, mineral *hydrocarbon* oils, *colour* pigments and dyes, and a range of non-nutritive *additives*.

Dietary fibre is a non-nutritive natural component of many foods of plant origin, it is *not* digested in the gut and does not contribute to the composition of tissue fluid. It serves a *dietary purpose* in maintaining the gut function (see Sections 9.3 and 9.4)

Foods are mainly *mixtures* of nutrients and non-nutritive substances present in *variable* amount (see Sections 6.1 and 6.2). Very few foods are *single* nutrients, with the exception of lard (100 per cent lipid) refined cane sugar (100 per cent carbohydrate) rock salt (100 per cent sodium chloride) and refined wheat flour gluten (100 per cent protein).

The composition of foods is listed in various published *food composition tables* which show the amounts of different nutrients (including water) present in a wide range of foods (see Appendix A).

1.7 SCIENCE OF HUMAN NUTRITION

Human nutrition is a *science* or collection of knowledge showing the relationship between *food* and the *health* of human beings. It covers a wide field of knowledge and is closely related to other sciences such as biology, chemistry, biochemistry, physics, human medicine, anatomy and physiology. The following are the main branches of human nutrition science:

Food science and technology, concerned with the nature, origin, structure and composition of food commodities, together with their production, behaviour in processing, cooking, storage, preservation and packaging. It is an area related to food chemistry, physics, engineering and agriculture.

Food physiology is concerned with processes and functions related to food nutrients in the human body. It is an area concerned with cell chemistry, biochemistry, human physiology and anatomy.

Personal health or the relationship between nutrition and health, and dietary needs throughout life is the area of work concerning dietetics, dentistry and human medicine.

Public and world nutrition is concerned with food in society, the social sciences related to nutrition, world food supplies, populations, war, famine and hunger reflief, and the function of governments and international organisations in world nutrition.

1.8 MEASUREMENT IN HUMAN NUTRITION

Human nutrition is a *qualitative* science concerned with *testing* and *recording*, and *identifying* the nutrients present in foods, the textures, odours, tastes, flavours and appearance of food commodities, and the effects of the presence or absence of nutrients on human growth, etc. It is also a *quantitative* science very much concerned with *measurment* of components in foods, amounts in food servings, the daily intake of nutrients, and quantity in tissue fluid. Doctors, nutritionists and dieticians use qualitative and quantitative *observations* in their work, together with repeated *experiment* to *prove* observed facts. In this way human nutrition scientists over the years have contributed to the wealth of knowledge of nutrition which exists today.

Experimental work is a feature of this book. This work should be done at the time coinciding with the theory as shown in the text, or by reference to experimental work in other texts. A record of experimental work done should be written in a *laboratory notebook*, setting out the work done under the following headings: *title*, *method*, *results* and *conclusion*.

1.9 NUMBERS AND UNITS

A single figure or number is called a *digit*, the digit nought, 0, is called *zero*.

One hundred = 100
One thousand = 1 000
One million = 1 000 000.

Spaces are used in writing large numbers, commas are not used.

Decimals

Numbers *less* than one (or *unity*) are written with a *decimal point* which is placed on the line, . , or above the line, ·, as for example 0·65 or 0.65. A zero is placed in front of the decimal point for numbers less than one – for example, 0.65 – and should *not* be left empty as in .65.

Prefixes and symbols

Prefixes are written as the *first* part of a compound word, for example, *kilo*gramme, or *milli*litre. The prefix is placed in front of the name of a *measuring unit*, for example, gramme or litre.

Symbols are one or two alphabet letters used for writing prefixes and units, for example:

kilogramme = kg (*not* KG)
millilitre = ml (*not* ML)

Notice the use of *small* alphabet letters.

Capital letters are also used in writing symbols, and their particular use must be carefully noted.

The following are the main prefixes, symbols and names for numbers used in human nutrition measurement:

Prefix name	*Symbol*	*Number*	*Meaning*
mega	M (Capital)	1 000 000	one million times.
kilo	k	1 000	one thousand times.
centi	c	$\frac{1}{100}$	one hundredth.
milli	m	$\frac{1}{1\,000}$	one thousandth
micro	μ	$\frac{1}{1\,000\,000}$	one millionth.

Note μ is the symbol for the Greek letter m or μ.

1.10 UNITS OF MEASUREMENT

Length

The international system of units, or SI units, are the units of measurement used in almost every country in the world.

The SI unit of length or height, width, circumference and breadth is called the *metre*, symbol m;

One kilometre, km = 1 000m

Each metre is subdivided into one hundred centimetres, symbol cm. Each centimetre is divided into ten millimetres, symbol mm.

$$1\text{m} = 100\text{cm} = 1\,000\text{mm}$$

Note The measurement 56cm or 56mm is *never* written as 56cms or 56mms using an 's'.

The metre *rule* or measuring *tape* is used for human body measurement, for body height, trunk and limb circumference. The study of human measurements is called *anthropometry*.

Calipers are instruments used for measuring thickness of skin fat layers. The skin is gripped between the calipers, and the thickness of the skin fold is measured [see Plate 9.6].

Area

Area is the measurement of *surface* calculated from width multiplied by breadth.

$$\text{Area} = \text{length} \times \text{breadth}$$

Area is measured in *square* metres, m^2, or square centimetres, cm^2. The raised number ^{2} indicates the square.

Experiment 1.1 *to measure the approximate surface area of the human body*

Procedure

(i) Measure the body height = h cm
(ii) Measure the circumference of the mid-thigh = t cm
(iii) Calculate the *approximate* body surface area from the following relationship:

$$\text{Surface area in } m^2 = \frac{2 \times \text{body height} \times \text{thigh circumference}}{10\,000}$$

Example: Body height 174cm^2

Thigh circumference 48cm^2

$$\text{Surface area} = \frac{2 \times 174 \times 48}{10\,000}$$

$$= 1.67\text{m}^2$$

Conclusion
The human body has an *irregular* shape and its surface area cannot be measured *directly* by simple methods (see Section 5.13).

The importance of human body surface area measurement is referred to in Section 5.13 when it is related to the energy produced by a person at rest in basal metabolism.

Volume
Volume is the amount of *space* occupied by *matter*. The unit of volume measurement is the *litre*, symbol l; this is divided into one thousand *millilitres*, symbol ml.

One litre, 1, = 1 000 ml

An alternative measure to the millilitre is the *cubic centimetre*, symbol cm^3.

Volume is measures by means of measuring jugs and measuring cylinders, whilst *small* volumes are measured using *pipettes* or *burettes*.

Weight or mass
Mass is the quantity of matter in a known *volume* of a substance, it remains the same and is not affected by the force of gravity or pull of the earth.

Weight is the measure of the pull of gravity on a body, it *varies* from place to place on earth, and becomes almost zero out in space. For general purposes mass and weight are considered as being the same.

The unit of measurement of mass is the *kilogramme* (also spelt kilogram), symbol kg; this is divided into one thousand *grammes* (also spelt grams), symbol g.

1 kg = 1 000 g

Body weight is measured on weighing scales, whilst food portions are weighed on *direct reading* balances.

Weights of *less* than one gramme are frequently used in human nutrition measurements for weights of food nutrients, as follows:

One gramme is divided into one thousand *milligrames*, symbol mg:

1 g = 1 000 mg

Each milligramme is divided into one thousand *microgrammes*, symbol μg:

1 mg = 1 000 μg

Similarly

$$1\ g = 1\ 000\ mg = 1\ 000\ 000\ \mu g$$

Minerals and vitamins B_1, B_2, (nicotinic acid) and C are measured in milligrammes, whilst vitamins A, B_{12} (folic acid) and D are measured in microgrammes.

1.11 CALCULATIONS IN NUTRITION

Proportions

This type of calculation is very common in human nutrition and concerns relationships in quantity, number, price and weight, etc.

Calculations are done on the 'multiply and divide' rule.

Example: If 100 g of roasted and salted peanuts contain 49 g of lipid fats, what will a 250 g portion contain?

(i) Set out as follows:

100g peanuts contain 49g lipids

1g peanuts contains $\frac{49}{100}$ g lipids

250g peanuts contain $\frac{250 \times 49}{100}$ g lipids

(ii) $\frac{250 \times 49}{100} = 122.5$ g lipids

(iii) 250g roasted and salted peanuts contain 122.5g lipids.

Summary:

If A contains, or buys, B.

Therefore C will contain or buy $\frac{C \times B}{A}$ (See also Section 12.6)

Percentages

This is a similar calculation to proportions but is related to parts of 100 or per cent, %. Percentage is calculated in a similar way using the 'multiply and divide' rule as follows.

Example: If 2.5kg of whole chicken consists of 800g of bones, what percentage of the chicken is bone?

Set out as follows:

(i) If 2 500 g (2.5 kg) chicken contains 800 g bone.

(ii) Therefore 100 g contains [multiply by 800 and divide by 2 500]

$$= \frac{100 \times 800}{2\,500} = 32$$

Therefore, 32% of the chicken is bone.

Experiment 1.2 *What's in the can*?

(i) Obtain any canned food, fruits or vegetables consisting of a fair amount of liquid content. Find the *gross weight* of the can (i.e weigh the unopened can).

(ii) Open and empty the can contents into a sieve and collect the fluid or *liquor* in a bowl.

(iii) Weigh the empty can and its lid; this will provide the *tare weight*. Subtract the tare weight from the gross weight to obtain the *net weight* of can contents.

$$\text{Gross weight} - \text{Tare weight} = \text{Net weight}$$

(iv) Carefully weight the amount of solid on the sieve and record.

(v) Calculate the *percentage* of solid content of the can from the following:

$$\frac{\text{Weight of solid contents}}{\text{Net weight of contents}} \times 100$$

Construct a *pie diagram* showing the solid and liquor content of a can of vegetables or fruits.

Pie diagrams

A pie diagram is a *circular* diagram with *quantities* shown as occupying different circle sectors or "pie slices" (see Fig 1.3).

fig 1.3 *pie diagram showing distribution of world population*

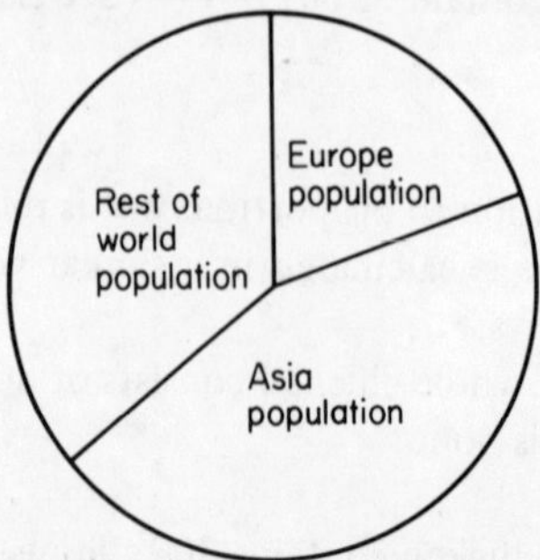

(i) A circle is composed of *360* degrees.
(ii) Sectors and angles of a circle are measured with a *protractor*.
(iii) Calculate number of degrees in a circle sector for a quantity as follows:

$$\frac{\text{quantity}}{\text{total quantity}} \times 360 = \text{degrees for a quantity in a circle sector}$$

(iv) Use the protractor to draw in this sector on a large circle.

Example Duck consists of the following parts: lean meat 41%, lipid fat 23%, bones 24% and giblets 12%.

1. Calculate the number of degrees in a circle sector for 33% lean meat.

$$\frac{\text{quantity}}{\text{total quantity}} \times 360 = \text{circle sector degrees}$$

$$\frac{41}{100} \times 360 = 148$$

Therefore 41% lean meat = 148° of the circle.

2. Repeat calculation for other duck components.

$$\frac{23}{100} \times 360 = 83$$

Therefore 23% lipids = 83° of the circle.

$$\frac{24}{100} \times 360 = 86$$

Therefore 24% bones = 86° of the circle.

$$\frac{12}{100} \times 360 = 43$$

Therefore 12% giblets = 43° of the circle.

3. Draw a large circle and divide into sectors using a protractor using the previously calculated angles for sectors.
4. Label each sector with the component's name and percentage.

Graphs

A graph shows the relationship between one changing quantity and another; for example, the relationship between changing height or weight can be plotted against *time* in years for a person's growth.

Construction of graphs

(i) Use squared paper.
(ii) Draw two lines at right angles to each other as *axes*, the vertical line is called the *y* axis, and the horizontal line the *x* axis.

(iii) A *scale* is decided and marked off along each axis at regular intervals. *Time* in weeks or years, or the steadily increasing quantity is marked on the horizontal x axis. Fluctuating quantities such as height or weight are marked on the vertical y axis.

(iv) *Plot* each quantity with a pencilled dot or small cross.

(v) Connect all plotted points with either a straight or curved line to suit the graph.

fig 1.4 *graph construction*

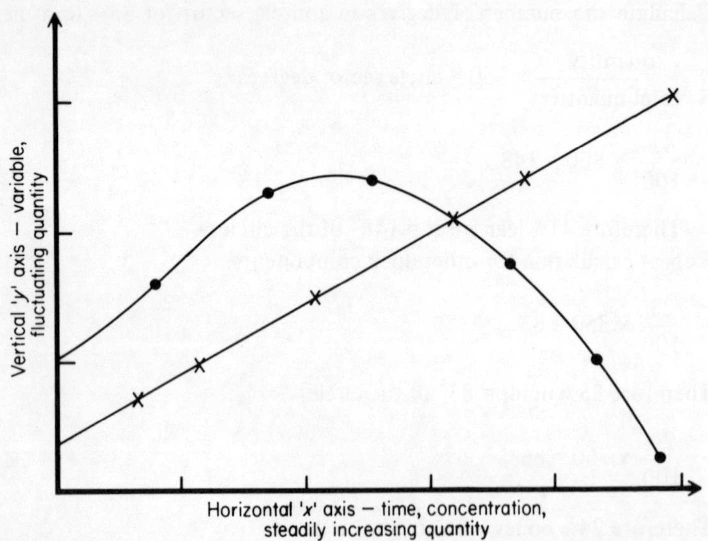

Histograms

This is another graphical diagram for displaying data by means of rectangle or bars. By this method the *distribution* of height and the *frequency* with which a certain height occurs amongst a group of people can be displayed. The range of measurement – height or weight – is shown on the horizontal x axis, whilst the number of people showing this measurement or frequency, is shown on the vertical y axis.

1.12 QUESTIONS

1. Give an account of the nutritional factors which contribute to good physical and mental health.
2. Explain the relationship between a kilogramme, gramme, milligramme and microgramme. Give the correct symbols for each and an example of their use in human nutrition.

3 Explain the meaning of food *synthesis* and food *analysis*.

4 The following gives the composition of certain foods. Construct a pie diagram to display the composition in each case.

Food	*Water* %	*Protein* %	*Fats* %	*Carbohydrate* %
Water biscuit	4.5	10.0	12.5	73.0
Fried fish cake	63.0	11.0	11.0	15.0
Eating apple	85.0	0.5	0	14.5

5 The following figures relate the sweetness of different substances compared with table sugar rated as 100%:

Lactose 16%, maltose 32%, glucose 74%, galactose 32%, fructose 173%, glycerine 70%.

Construct a histogram to display the relative sweetness of these substances.

CHAPTER 2

FOOD, PHYSICS AND CHEMISTRY

2.1 FOOD AS MATTER

Food is *matter*, or a form of *energy* which also has mass and *volume* and occupies *space*. Matter present on earth exists in three physical states, *solid*, *liquid* and *gas*. Food exists mainly as solids and liquids. *Oxygen* which is an important nutrient, exists as a gas.

All food is composed of small component particles called *molecules* or *ions* (see Section 2.10).

(i) *Solid food* - e.g. cane sugar, sucrose - has molecules closely packed together giving it a *definite* shape and volume.

(ii) *Liquid foods*, such as milk, have the molecules spaced further apart, and have a definite volume, but no definite shape, taking up the shape of the container which holds them, e.g. jelly moulds and baking tins.

(iii) Oxygen *gas* has molecules widely apart and consequently has no definite shape, and fills the space which contains it, e.g. the lung or room space.

Physics of food is concerned with those properties of food related to *energy* and different *forms of matter*.

Chemistry of food is concerned with its *composition* and the effects of food components on one another.

Food physics is mainly concerned with physical changes in food substances, whilst food chemistry is concerned with chemical changes or reactions which are alterations in food substances.

The main differences between physical and chemical food changes are summarised in Table 2.1.

Table 2.1 *comparison of chemical and physical changes*

Physical food change	*Chemical food change*
Example: melting and solidification of sucrose.	Example: strong heating and burning of sucrose.
No new chemical substances formed.	New chemical substances formed.
Easy to reverse.	Difficult to reverse.
Small heat change.	Large heat change.
Chemical nature or properties the same.	Chemical properties different.

2.2 CHEMICAL ELEMENTS

All matter and foods are composed of *chemical elements*, of which there are about 100 different kinds forming the earth's living and non-living matter.

Each chemical element is composed of the same component *atoms*, carbon is composed of carbon atoms, whilst iron is composed only of iron atoms.

The important chemical elements in food are listed in two groups, the *non-metal* elements and *metal* elements; each atom of an element is represented by a *symbol* as shown in Table 2.2.

Table 2.2 *Chemical elements of importance in food*

Non-metals		*Metals*	
Element	*Symbol*	*Element*	*Symbol*
Carbon	C	Calcium	Ca
Hydrogen	H	Magnesium	Mg
Oxygen	O	Iron	Fe
Phosphorus	P	Potassium	K
Sulphur	S	Sodium	Na
Nitrogen	N	Copper	Cu
Iodine	I	Cobalt	Co
Chlorine	Cl	Manganese	Mn
Fluorine	F		

2.3 FOOD CHEMICAL COMPOUNDS

Most foods are composed of *chemical compounds* which are formed from *two* or more different chemical elements joined together by *chemical bonds*.

The *molecule* is the smallest part of an element or compound which is able to exist on its own. The molecule is the smallest part of oxygen, water or glucose sugar that can exist alone. Atoms are unable to exist alone.

A chemical formula is a shorthand method for showing *one molecule* of a chemical element or compound. It is written using element *symbols* and *numbers* showing the component atoms present in *one* molecule.

Water, H_2O; the formula shows that one molecule of water consists of *two* hydrogen *atoms* and *one* oxygen *atom*. The following chemical formulae should be known by students of human nutrition: H_2O, water; CO_2, carbon dioxide; O_2, oxygen; H_2, hydrogen; $C_6H_{12}O_6$, glucose; NH_3, ammonia; C_2H_5OH, ethanol; and cane sugar sucrose, $C_{12}H_{22}O_{11}$.

Macromolecules are the very large molecules which compose foods, namely, macromolecules of proteins, polysaccharides and nucleic acids (see Section 4.6) and also the different plastic materials used in food packaging (see Section 10.17).

Chemical composition of a human being

Since a human being is of central importance in human nutrition, the chemical *elements* and *compounds* which occur in the adult body are listed in the following table. The composition of men differs from women as shown in the table; men are composed of *less* lipid or fat, but *more* protein, water and minerals. Similarly the composition of children's bodies alters from birth to childhood (as Table 2.3 shows).

Classes of chemical compounds

Chemical compounds in foods and composing the human body are of *two* main kinds:

(a) Inorganic compounds

These are substances which originate from rocks and mineral or non-living sources, such as chalk or calcium carbonate, and sodium chloride or common salt. They form *mineral ion* components of food and the human body.

(b) Organic compounds

These are compounds made by synthesis in living plants or animals, they are mainly composed of *carbon* and other elements such as hydrogen, oxygen, sulphur, nitrogen and phosphorus.

Table 2.3 *Chemical composition of human body*

Chemical elements		*Chemical compounds*			
Element	*%*	*Compound*	*Men %*	*Women %*	*Children %*
Oxygen	65.0	Water	62	54	60-72
Carbon	18.0	Protein	17	15	11-16
Hydrogen	10.0				
Nitrogen	3.0	Lipids	14	25	14-26
Calcium	1.4	Carbohydrates	1	1	1
Phosphorus	0.7				
Potassium	0.18	Minerals	6	5	5
Sulphur	0.2				
Sodium	0.10				
Chlorine	0.10				
Magnesium	0.045				
Trace elements					
Iron, copper etc.	0.014				

Carbohydrates and lipids or fat are composed of carbon, hydrogen and oxygen, *proteins* consist of carbon, hydrogen oxygen, nitrogen and sometimes phosphorus and sulphur.

Most organic compounds and food substances will char or blacken easily when overheated, similarly some, such as sugar and lard, melt easily. In contrast, inorganic substances do not char and require a high temperature to melt them, for example, chalk and sand.

Experiment 2.1 *to show the chemical elements present in foods.*
A. *Hydrogen (H) and carbon (C) tests*
Procedure

(i) Place a *dry* food sample – for example dried milk powder mixed with an equal amount of dry copper II oxide in a hard glass test tube connected by a cork and delivery tube dipping into clear calcium hydroxide solution, as in figure 2.1.

(ii) Gently heat the mixture and observe how the calcium hydroxide solution turns cloudy, because of *carbon* in the food forming *carbon dioxide. Hydrogen* in the food forms *water* which condenses as droplets in the cooler parts of the test tube.

Fig 2.1 *Testing for the presence of the chemical elements carbon and hydrogen in a dry food sample or organic material*

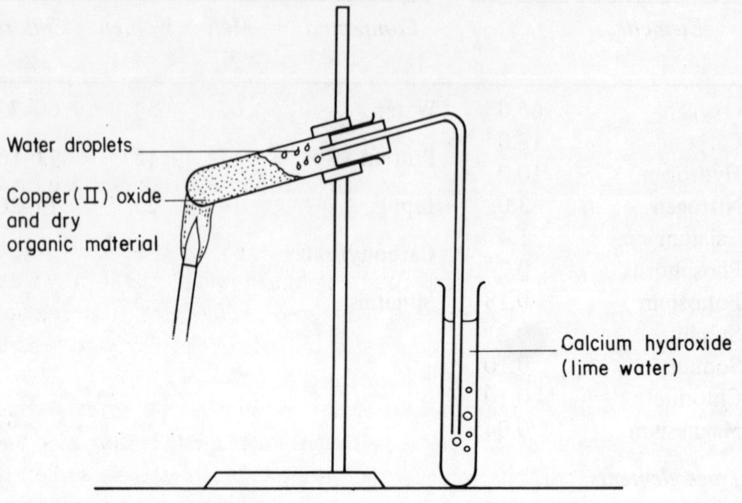

B. *Nitrogen (N) and sulphur (S) tests*
Procedure

(i) Mix equal amounts of *dry* food sample with *soda lime* and heat the mixture in the same apparatus omitting the test tube of calcium hydroxide solution.
(ii) Gently heat the mixture and hold a moist test paper of red litmus or yellow turmeric paper in the fumes issuing from the delivery tube. *Nitrogen* in the food forms *ammonia* causing litmus paper to turn blue and tumeric paper brown.
(iii) Hold a moist lead ethanoate (acetate) paper in the vapour. *Sulphur* in the food forms *hydrogen sulphide* which causes the test paper to turn black.

Oxygen, although present in large amounts in foods, cannot be tested for by simple means such as for C, H, S and N.

2.4 HEAT AND FOOD

Heat is a form of energy, and is the main form for cooking food.

Heat can be measured in units of energy called the *joule*, symbol J; larger units are called kilojoule (kJ) or 1 000 K, and the megajoule (MJ) or 1 000 000 J. The unit was so called after James Joule (1818–89) a physicist. [The former unit was called a small calorie and equalled 4.2 joules approximately. The large calorie or kilocalorie kCal, equalled 1000 small calories].

Heat transfer
Heat travels from a heat source to food by three methods, during the cooking process.

(i) *Radiation* or direct heat transfer; the heat travels as rays or waves called infra-red rays, and does not need any intervening medium to carry the heat.

(ii) *Conduction* is the indirect heat transfer through solids, liquids or gases. Metals are better heat conductors than non-metals such as wood or plastic. Water is a poor heat conductor, whilst air is almost a non-conductor or heat insulator. Heat is indirectly transferred to food by conduction through a metal utensil.

(iii) *Convection* is indirect heat transfer by liquids and gases through bodily movement of their component molecules. In this way heat passes indirectly by convection movement of heat in cooking in water and cooking oils.

Specific heat capacity
This is a measure of the quantity of heat taken up by the same weight of different substances. For example the amount of heat needed to raise the temperature of one kilogramme of a substance by *one* degree Celsius (1 °C) is called its *specific heat capacity*.

The following are specific heat capacities in joules per kg per degree Celsius of different foods.

Food	*J kg °C*
Sugar	1130
Flour	2100
Cooking oil	2100
Butter	2100
Ethanol	2400
Milk	3780
Potato	3800
Water	4200

These values show that equal weights of sugar and cooking oil heat up *more quickly* than corresponding weights of milk and water. Water and milk, however, are *slower* in losing their heat to the food and thus have an advantage in *slow* cooking by boiling and steaming, compared with *faster* cooking by deep frying in oil. Water is therefore a good reservoir of heat for cooking purposes.

Expansion of matter

As a substance gains heat, its molecules *vibrate* with increasing rapidity; this causes the substance to *expand* or increase in volume.

(a) Different *solids* expand differently; for example, metals expand more than non-metals, wood and glass.
(b) Different *liquids* expand differently; for example, mercury and ethanol are liquids used in *thermometers* because they expand more readily than other liquids.
(c) Different *gases* however always expand by the *same* amount for unit rise in temperature.

Thermometers

These are the means to record *temperature* or relative hotness or coldness on some chosen *temperature scale*.

The Celsius scale of temperature has 0°C or *zero* degrees Celsius as its lower fixed point (the temperature of melting ice) and 100°C as its upper fixed point (the temperature of steam from boiling water). The scale was devised by Anders Celsius (1701–44).

Thermostats are instruments for maintaining a constant temperature in ovens etc. The human body has an automatic self-regulating thermostat control located in the base of the brain to maintain a steady temperature of 37°C in the tissue fluid for homeostasis.

Change of state

Substances and many foods can change their physical state by *adding* heat in *heating*, or *withdrawing* heat from them in *cooling*.

The following diagram summarises the main changes of physical state:

$$\text{solid} \underset{\textit{solidification}}{\overset{\textit{fusion or melting}}{\rightleftarrows}} \text{liquid} \underset{\textit{condensation}}{\overset{\textit{boiling or evaporation}}{\rightleftarrows}} \text{gas}$$

The *quantity* of heat needed to bring about a complete physical change of state is called *latent heat*. *Latent heat* of melting or fusion is the heat quantity needed to melt completely one kilogramme of solid into a liquid without causing a change in temperature.

The latent heat for *melting* one kilogramme of ice is 0.334 MJ; this *same* quantity of heat is withdrawn from water to *freeze* it into ice.

The latent heat of *evaporation* for one kilogramme of water is 2.26 MJ; this same amount of heat is given up to cold food when *steam* condenses on it in cooking by steaming food.

Refrigeration is a process of withdrawing heat from food by the *evaporation* of a *refrigerant liquid*. This liquid in its *vapour* form is made to *condense* in a *condenser* outside the refrigerator and give up its heat to the room air, the liquid formed by condensation being *recirculated* within the refrigerator *circuit*.

Pure substances have definite melting and boiling points at which the change of state occurs. Since most foods are mixtures, they do not show definite melting and boiling points. The *pure* foods which do show definite melting and boiling points are pure lard, cooking oils, refined sugar and pure water.

2.5 SOLUTIONS AND MIXTURES OF FOODS

Foods are mostly *mixtures* consisting of two or more different *compounds*, in varying proportions, which can be separated by physical methods. Milk, and orange juice are examples of *mixtures* which can have their components separated by one or more of the following physical methods:

1. *Filtration* is a physical process to separate *insoluble* solids or crystals from a liquid, using a porous filter paper supported in a filter funnel. *Suspensions* are mixtures of *insoluble* solids in a liquid; the solid can be as tiny *granules*, for example starch in cold water.
2. *Solvent extraction* is a means of separating the lipid component from a food using an organic *solvent* and a special apparatus called a Soxhlet extractor. *Essences* are made by extracting certain flavours with *ethanol*. Lipids in foods are extracted by methyl benzene or toluene.
3. A *centrifuge* is an apparatus which can separate by rapid spinning either two *immiscible* liquids such as milk lipids and water, or an insoluble solid and solvent. Milk is separated into cream and skim milk by centrifugal separation.
4. *Distillation* is a means of separating *miscible* liquids which mix freely such as water and ethanol. The mixture is boiled and the vapour condensed in a *condenser*. Milk is concentrated by this method [see Section 7.12]. Steam distillation is achieved by blowing steam through a mixture and the *steam-volatile* component is removed with the steam and condensed. This is used to extract certain essential oils used in food flavours.
5. *Crystallisation* is a method of extraction and purification by the formation of *crystals* prepared by dissolving an impure substance in a minimum of hot solvent to form a *saturated solution* which, on cooling, produces crystals separated from the liquor by filtration or centrifuging. *Slow* cooling forms *large* crystals; *rapid* cooling forms *small* crystals.

Crystallisation occurs in the making of certain sugar confectionery, barley sugar, boiled sweets and fudge.

6. *Chromatography* is a delicate process for separating *closely related* compounds from foods, for example the component amino-acids or added coloured dyes. The process involves the use of solvents and special chromatographic paper.

Concentration of solutions

The *concentration* or *strength* is the *quantity* of a substance in a *definite* quantity of another substance.

The concentration of a nutrient in a food is expressed as grammes, g; milligrammes, mg; or microgrammes, μg, per *100 grammes* of food. 'Concentration' is therefore almost the same as a *percentage*.

Tissue fluid with only a 0.9 per cent concentration of solutes is called a *dilute* solution, compared with single cream with its 21 per cent concentration of lipid components which is a *concentrated* solution.

Relative density (RD)

This is a means of showing how *many times* a substance or solution is heavier or lighter than an *equal volume* of pure water. If a solution is concentrated it will have a high value relative density. Sugar syrup solutions of 30 per cent sugar have an RD of 1.13, whilst an 80 per cent sugar syrup has an RD of 1.41. The relative density of a solution is rapidly measured by means of a *hydrometer*.

2.6 DISPERSION IN FOODS

Foods can be mixtures of different physical states or *phases*, namely a mixture of an *insoluble* liquid oil in water, or of a gas such as air, in a liquid.

An insoluble substance can be dispersed at a *low concentration* as a *disperse phase* in another substance called the dispersion medium or *continuous phase*, to produce a *disperse system*.

$$\text{Disperse system} = \frac{\text{disperse phase}}{\text{low concentration}} + \frac{\text{continuous phase}}{\text{high concentration}}$$

Table 2.4 lists the main types of food dispersion system, with food examples.

The main foods are different dispersions of nutrients, proteins, carbohydrates and lipids in *water*.

Table 2.4 *Main types of food-dispersion systems*

Dispersion system	Phases		Food example
	Disperse	Continuous	
Sol	Solid, liquid	liquid;	
	Cell proteins	cell water	Meat, fish, egg white.
Gels	Liquid;	solid;	Bread, rice pudding, custards,
	water	protein	table jelly and cheese.
Foam	Gas;	liquid;	
	air	milk lipid fat	Whipped cream.
	air	egg white	Whipped egg white.
Solid foam	Gas;	solid;	
	air	protein	Marshmallows, meringues.
	air	milk lipid fat	Ice cream.
Emulsion	Liquid;	liquid;	
(a) water in oil (W/O)	water	butter lipid fat	Butter
	water	hardened vegetable lipid oil	Margarine.
	water	egg protein and lipids	Egg yolk.
(b) Oil in water (O/W)	Liquid;	liquid;	
	butter lipid fat	water	Milk.
	meat lipid fat	water	Gravy and certain cream soups.
	olive oil	vinegar	Mayonnaise.
	various vegetable lipid oils	water	Sauces.

2.7 MOVEMENT IN FOOD SOLUTIONS

Molecules composing *fluids* or liquids and gases, are able to *move* freely. This movement of molecules helps in the natural mixing of fluid mixtures and is important in transport of nutrients in and between *cells*.

1. *Brownian movement* is the movement of particles in the *disperse phase* of sols, gels and other solutions including suspensions. It is seen when a drop of Indian ink or flower pollen is added to water forming a suspension. The suspended particles move because of continuous movement and bombardment by the molecules of the *dispersion medium* or the continuous phase water. It was named after its first observer Robert Brown (1773–1858).

   Brownian movement prevents the *settling* or *sedimentation* of particles in sols and gels.
2. *Diffusion* is the movement of small molecules or ions of substances from a region of *high concentration* to one of *lower concentration*; this continues until the solution is *homogeneous* or the *same* concentration throughout.

   Diffusion occurs in gases, as for example when an aroma of coffee spreads through room air. It is an important process in liquids and explains the movement of digested nutrients from the gut into the blood and from the tissue fluid into the cell and its consequent movements within the cell.

   Soaking certain foods in water may cause the loss of certain soluble nutrients through diffusion or *leaching*.
3. *Osmosis* is the passage of the solvent, *water*, from a dilute or low concentration solution into a *more* concentrated solution, *across a semi-permeable membrane*, as shown in Figure 2.2. The *cell membrane* (see Section 3.3) of living things is also a *semi-permeable* membrane which allows the passage of small molecules of water and some ions, but not the passage of large molecules like proteins, and starches.

Artificial semi-permeable include such membranes as cellophane, and Visking tubing.

Experiment 2.2 *to demonstrate osmosis in potatoes*

Procedure

(i) Cut freshly peeled potatoes into narrow strips 6cm × 1cm of *exactly* equal length using a cork borer.

(ii) Place potato strips in the following solutions of different concentration of glucose: 1%, $2\frac{1}{2}$% and 5%. Place test potato strips in clean water.

(iii) Allow to remain in the solutions for over one hour, then remove

Fig 2.2 *apparatus to demonstrate osmosis using an artificial semi-permeable membrane*

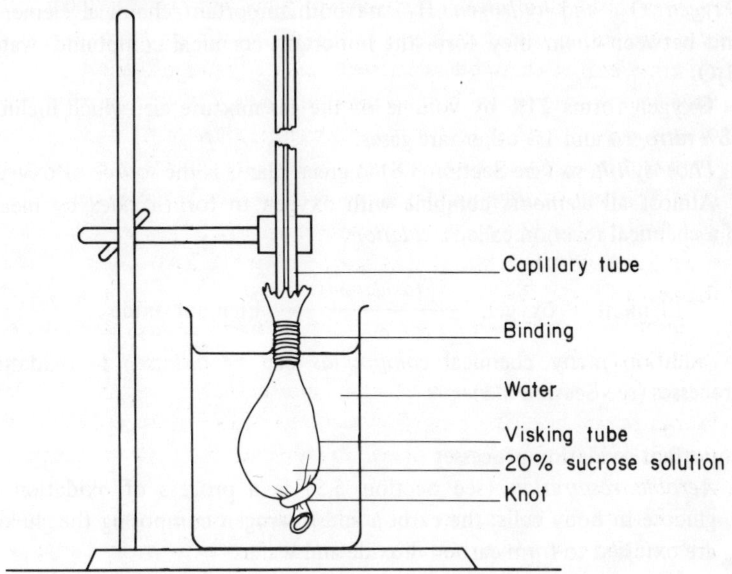

the strips and measure their lengths, and notice their *turgidity* or *flaccidity*.

Osmosis is responsible for water withdrawal causing flaccidity by plasmolysis. Concentrated salt and sugar preserving solutions withdraw water from surface cells of foods and kill microbe cells which may *contaminate* preserved food.

Dehydrated foods and dried fruits are rehydrated by soaking in water, allowing re-entry of water by osmosis.

Tissues fluid water enters the living human body-cells by osmosis.

4. *Active transport* is the movement of substances in and between living cells from regions of *low* to *high* concentration; this is done using cell *energy*. Diffusion and osmosis do not use cell energy.

Dialysis

This is a method of physically separating large macromolecules of proteins and starches (also called *colloids*), from solutions containing them and other small-molecule substances, such as sugars and salts.

The mixture is placed in a semi-permeable membrane, (cellophane or Visking bag) in a tank of water. In time the small molecule substances in the mixture *diffuse* into the water and large macromolecule substances remain behind in the bag.

2.8 FOOD OXIDATION AND REDUCTION

Oxygen, O_2, and *hydrogen*, H_2, are both important chemical elements, and between them they form the important chemical compound, water, H_2O.

Oxygen forms 21% by volume of the gas mixture air, which includes 78% *nitrogen* and 1% other rare gases.

Photosynthesis (see Section 3.8) in green plants is the *source* of oxygen.

Almost all *elements* combine with oxygen to form *oxides* by means of a chemical reaction called *oxidation*.

$$\text{Element} + \text{oxygen} \xrightarrow{(oxidation)} \text{Element oxide}$$

In addition many chemical *compounds* can be *oxidised* in oxidation processes (see Section 5.3).

Important oxidation processes

1. *Aerobic respiration* (see Section 5.5) is a process of oxidation of glucose in body cells; the carbon and hydrogen composing the glucose are oxidised to form carbon dioxide and water:

$$\underset{\text{(glucose)}}{C_6H_{12}O_6} + 6O_2 \qquad 6CO_2 + 6H_2O + \textit{energy}$$

2. *Chemical combustion* is a process of oxidation of foods and other substances in air by burning. The elements C, H, S and N in foods form *gaseous*, volatile oxides which enter the air, whilst the other elements form non-volatile *solid* oxides which remain in the food *ash* (see figure 2.3).

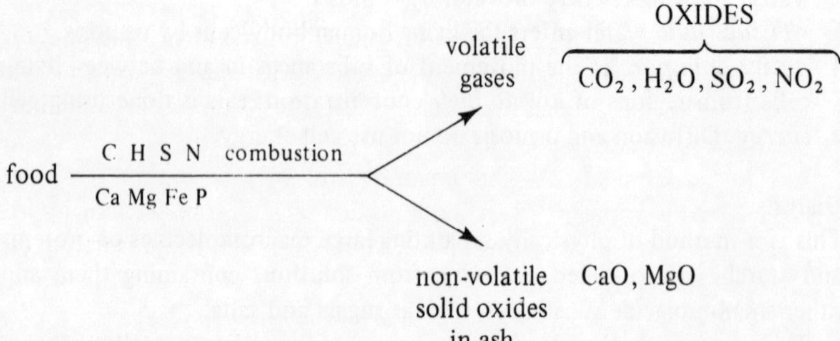

Important by-products of combustion are *heat* energy and *light* energy. The solid, liquid and gaseous *fuels* undergo combustion in the same way as food.

Fig 2.3 *chemical combustion of sugar in air or oxygen*

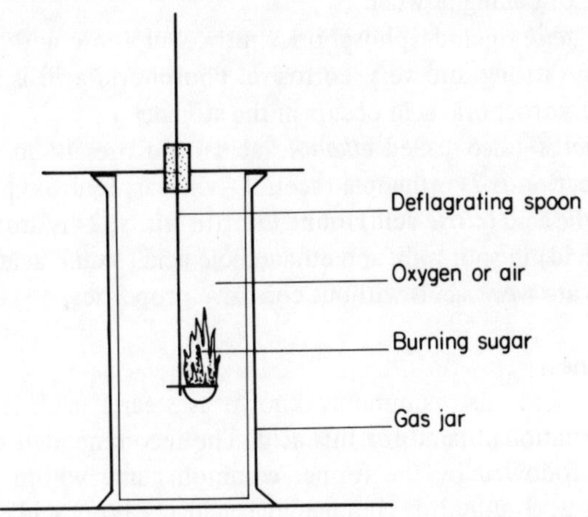

In Experiment 2.1 carbon and hydrogen in the food are *oxidised* by oxygen from the copper (II) oxide, to form carbon dioxide and water. *Hydrogen* exists as a colourless gas:

(a) Its most important chemical reaction is its oxidation to form *water*, a rapid process giving out considerable energy.

$$2H_2 + O_2 \longrightarrow 2H_2O + \textit{energy}$$

The reverse chemical reaction occurs in photosynthesis (see Section 3.8) when sunlight energy is used to *split* up water into oxygen gas and hydrogen atoms:

$$2H_2O \longrightarrow 2H_2 + O_2$$

(b) *Reduction* is a chemical process which is the *reverse* of oxidation, and involve the loss of oxygen by hydrogen removing oxygen from substances, or adding itself onto substances – a process sometimes called *hydrogenation*.

In Experiment 2.1 the nitrogen and sulphur in the foods are *reduced* by means of hydrogen provided by soda lime forming hydrogen compounds of nitrogen (or ammonia, NH_3) and sulphur (or hydrogen sulphide, H_2S).

2.9 FOOD ACIDS, BASES AND SALTS

Acids are those substances which may have a sour taste, and turn the colour of an *indicator* such as litmus, red. All acids contain hydrogen and most will release carbon dioxide from sodium hydrogen carbonate - a component of baking powder.

Inorganic acids include phosphoric, nitric, sulphuric and hydrochloric acids, all very strong and very corrosive. Phosphoric acid is a food component, and hydrochoric acid occurs in the stomach.

Organic acids (also called *alkanoic* acids) are present in a variety of foods (see Section 6.7); ethanoic (acetic) - vinegar; hydroxypropane 1, 2, 3-tricarboxylic acid (*citric* acid) found in citrus fruits; 2-hydroxypropanoic acid (*lactic* acid) in sour milk and ethanedioic acid (*oxalic* acid) in rhubarb leaves. These are *weak* acids without corrosive properties.

Chemical names

Octadecanoic acid, also commonly known as stearic acid, is the *recommended* international name for this acid. The recommended name will be written first followed by the former common name within brackets, as for example, 2, 3-dihydroxybutanedioic acid (tartaric acid). The choice of the chemical name is left to the reader.

Bases which are soluble in water are called alkalis; they are compounds which react chemically with acids to form salts and water by a chemical change called *neutralisation*.

$$\textit{base or alkali} + \textit{acid} \xrightarrow{(\textit{neutralisation})} \textit{salt} + \textit{water}$$

Ammonium, sodium, calcium and potassium hydroxides are examples. Most alkalis turn the colour of indicators - red litmus turns blue.

The organic bases containing nitrogen which occur in foods are called *amines* and *amino*-compounds. Amongst the most important organic bases found in foods and cells are the bases *adenine*, *guanine*, *cytosine*, *uracil*, and *thymine*; these are important components of nucleic acids or polynucleotides (see Section 3.4 and 4.10).

Salts are the compounds formed from an acid and alkali. Most are *neutral* to indicators, for examples, sodium nitrate and sodium chloride; others are *alkaline*, for example, sodium hydrogen carbonate; and others are *acid*, for example, ammonium chloride. The inorganic constituents or minerals in foods are usually in the form of different salts called *mineral salts*.

2.10 NUTRIENT IONS

Most *inorganic* acids, bases and salts and a few organic substances will conduct a current of electricity when the substances are dissolved in water. These are called *electrolytes* and are composed of positively and negatively charged atoms or groups of atoms called *ions*.

Common or table salt (sodium chloride NaCl) consists of *sodium* and *chloride* ions. The sodium ion is positive, Na^+, and chloride negative, Cl^-. *Salt substitute* is called potassium chloride (KCl).

Non-electrolytes do not form ions and their solutions in water do not conduct electricity. This group includes *glucose* and many other organic substances.

Tissue fluid and other body fluids, blood plasma, saliva, mucus and certain foods in solution will contain mineral nutrients as *ions* on Na^+, K^+, Ca^{++}, Mg^{++}, Cl^-, $HCO_3{}^-$, $SO_4{}^{--}$, the non-electrolyte components will be glucose and certain lipid substances.

2.11 FOOD pH

Water ionises into *equal* amounts of hydrogen and hydroxyl ions and the liquid is neutral.

$$H_2O \xrightarrow{\textit{Ionisation}} H^+ + OH^-$$

The concentration of the hydrogen ions can be measured. Solutions with a *high* hydrogen ion concentration are *acid*, whilst a *low* concentration indicates *alkalinity*. A scale called the *pH scale* shows pH 7 as the neutral point, and values above pH 7 to pH 14 indicate *increasing* alkalinity, whilst pH 7 to pH 0 are of increasing acidity. Ginger ale, wines, vinegar, fruit juices are *acidic* with a pH range of 2.8–4.0; tomato juice and beers have a pH of 4.3, whilst milk is of almost neutral pH 6.5–7.0. Coffee and tea infusions have a pH 5–pH 7.

Universal indicator papers are used to find the pH of a solution by dipping the paper into the solution and matching the colour change with a pH colour chart.

Tissue fluid has a pH 7.4, being almost neutral with very slight alkalinity. *Proteins* are important for keeping pH in and around body cells constant; they mop up any acidity or alkalinity which may develop to upset homeostasis. They are called pH *buffers* because of this property.

2.12 CHEMICAL REACTIONS

When two or more substances interact chemically, they are called *reactants*; they will produce one or more new substances or *products* by means of a *chemical reaction*. During chemical reactions *bonds* are made or broken between atoms.

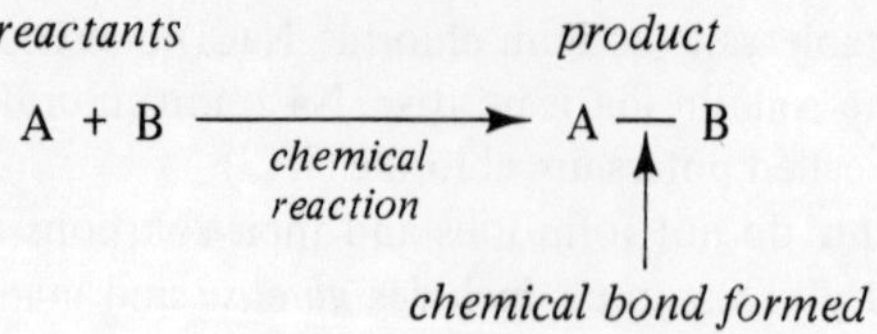

A *chemical equation* summarises the chemical reaction using words or chemical formulae for reactants and products.
Word equation:–

Carbon dioxide + water → glucose + oxygen

Chemical formula equation:–

$$6CO_2 + 6H_2O \rightarrow C_6H_{12}O_6 + 6O_2$$

Rates of chemical reactions

The *rate* is a measure of how fast or how slowly a chemical reaction takes place. The rates of food metabolism in human body cells are affected by the same conditions which affect chemical reactions in laboratory test-tubes.

(i) *Concentration of reactants* The more concentrated the reactants are in a solution, the greater will be the rate of reaction. Reactions are more rapid between ions than between molecules.

(ii) *Temperature* An *increase* in temperature of 10°C *doubles* the rate of reaction. At low temperatures the rate is very slow. This is only partly true for organic chemical reactions whose rate generally increases to a maximum or optimum temperature then declines quickly thereafter. The human body cell uses an *optimum*, or most favourable temperature of 37°C. This is kept constant by homeostasis and is disturbed only during body fever. Homeostasis ensures that metabolism proceeds at a steady rate.

(iii) *Catalysts* These are substances called *enzymes* in living cells, which alter the rate of reaction – usually by *increasing* the rate. The catalyst remains unchanged at the end of the reaction and can be used again in some cases. Enzymes control almost all the processes of metabolism.

Experiment 2.3 *to show effects of catalysts*

Procedure

(i) Prepare a dilute solution of hydrogen peroxide and place a portion in each test-tube.

(ii) Add a pinch of powdered manganese dioxide *catalyst* to one test-tube and observe its *catalytic action* in releasing a foam of oxygen gas.
(iii) Add a piece of fresh meat or apple to another test-tube and note how its *biological catalyst* or enzymes release oxygen.
(iv) Add a piece of *boiled* and cooked meat or apple and note how the gas is not released, since heat *destroys* the enzyme. Similarly *blanching* destroys fruit and vegetable enzymes by treatment with steam or boiling water.

Types of chemical reactions
The various chemical reactions which occur in food metabolism are given names as follows, and will be referred to by name in future chapters:

1. *Neutralisation*, a reaction between an acid and base to form a salt and water

$$\text{acid} + \text{base} \longrightarrow \text{salt} + H_2O$$

2. *Hydrolysis*, a *breakdown* of a compound by means of *water*

$$\text{AB} + \text{water} \xrightarrow{\textit{(hydrolysis)}} \text{A} + \text{B}$$

3. *Condensation* is the *elimination* of water when two substances react

$$\text{A} + \text{B} \xrightarrow{\textit{(condensation)}} \text{AB} + H_2O$$

4. *Oxidation* is the addition of oxygen as described in Section 2.8.
5. *Reduction* is the addition of hydrogen as described in Section 2.8.
6. *Deamination* is the removal of amino- groups from amino-acid compounds (see Section 8.17).

2.13 QUESTIONS

1. Construct a pie diagram showing the chemical composition of the human body using the figures listed in Table 2.3.
2. What are ions? Which substances are used by the human body in the form of ions? Explain the term hydrogen ion concentration, or pH.
3. Explain the difference between heat and temperature. Explain the following physical terms: condensation, specific heat capacity, and heat convection.

4. Explain each of the following terms:
   (a) concentration (b) diffusion
   (c) dispersion (d) distillation.
5. What are acids, bases and salts?
   What factors affect the *rate* of a chemical reaction?

CHAPTER 3

FOOD BIOLOGY

3.1 VARIETY OF FOODS

Biology is the study of *living organisms* and *life* in plants and animals.

A wide range of different plants and animals exist; each group of similar plants or animals which are able to breed amongst themselves is called a *species*. There are about one million different species of animals, and about half a million different species of plants. Consequently, human beings can select food items originating from about $1\frac{1}{2}$ million different sources, since the *omnivorous* diet of human beings permits selection from a wide range of foods of different plant or animal origin.

Human nutrition is concerned with eating selected parts or products, or the whole body, of foods of plant or animal origin.

Plant origin foods form 75% of the world's food supply and include vegetables, fruits, cereals, nuts, non-alcoholic and alcoholic beverages, herbs and spices. The majority of *fresh* unprocessed foods of plant origin, seeds, roots, stems etc. are *living* and remain so until processed or cooked. These living fresh foods continue the life process of respiration, and in many cases are the means to continue plant life in seeds, bulbs and tubers.

Animal origin foods form 25% of the *world's food supply* and include meat from different mammals, birds and fish, together with their *products*. This includes milk and eggs.

By contrast, food of animal origin is *dead* or non-living and shows no characteristics of respiration or means to continue life. *Fresh* eggs are living foods providing suitable incubation conditions are utilised. Similarly *fresh* oysters are eaten alive.

3.2 CLASSIFICATION

The $1\frac{1}{2}$ million different species of living organisms are classified as follows; the groups which contribute to or affect human nutrition are indicated.

A. Plant classification

Bacteria are one-celled organisms important in food-processing, fermentation and vitamin manufacture in the human gut. They are also responsible for certain human diseases, food poisoning and food decay (see Sections 11.3, 11.10).

Algae are green, red and brown, unicellular or multicellular. The multicellular *seaweeds* yield food products; carrageen, laver and dulse are edible seaweeds.

Fungi are colourless, unicellular yeasts and multicellular mushrooms; the latter include the edible field mushroom and highly poisonous Deathcap mushroom. Yeasts are important in food-processing as raising agents and fermentation agents in alcoholic beverage production (see Sections 7.11 and 6.12), and as a source of nutrients in yeast extracts.

Liverworts, mosses and ferns are green multicellular plants which are not sources of food in human nutrition.

Conifers are the cone-bearing plants and have a resin content which makes them unsuitable as a food source; an exception is in the use of pine *seeds.*

Flowering plants include 0.3 million different species of plants which produce *flowers* and later form *seeds* contained within a *fruit*. This great class of plants is the main source of food of plant origin in human nutrition. All fruits, seeds, nuts, cereals, sugars, vegetables and vegetable oils, together with herbs and spices, are derived from different species of flowering plants (angiosperms).

B. Animal classification

The one million different species of animals are classified as follows, those contributing to human nutrition being indicated in greater detail.

Animals without backbones invertebrates

Protozoa are unicellular animals and some inhabit the human gut without harm, others cause disease (see Section 10.6).

Sponges and jellyfish are multicellular animals of no value in human nutrition.

Flatworms and roundworms are multicellular inhabitants of many other animals including fish, poultry, cattle and human beings; they are mainly *harmful*, and of no value in human nutrition (see Section 10.6).

Segmented worms include multicellular worms related to the earthworm.

Arthropods include animals with jointed legs attached to segmented bodies. These include:

(i) *crustaceans*, the crabs, lobsters, crayfish, prawns, and shrimps.

(ii) *insects*, such as locusts, grasshoppers, crickets, termites, and certain grubs and caterpillars, are useful protein sources in certain developing countries.

Molluscs, the multicellular animals with a soft body protected by a hard shell, one shell in *univalves*, two shells in *bivalves*. Edible molluscs include cockles, mussels, oysters, scallops or queens, whelks, winkles, abalone or UK ormer and NZ paua, snails, octopus and squid, and the sea slug, *bêche-de-mer.*
Echinoderms, spiny-skinned animals, include the sea urchin whose brightly-coloured reproductive organs are used as a tasty uncooked food.

Animals with backbones - vertebrates
The vertebrates are the major source of food of animal origin in the human diet and include 6000 different species.
Fish are either *bony* - herring and trout, or *cartilaginous* - shark and ray. Freshwater and sea fish of different species form an important part of the diet of people throughout the world.
Amphibia include frogs.
Reptiles are the scaly-skinned crocodiles, alligators, snakes and turtles.
Birds are the warm-blooded animals covered in feathers and include *poultry* (hens, ducks, geese, turkey, guinea-fowl) and *game* birds such as pheasants, quails and pigeons. A range of eggs is also an important food source.
Mammals are the warm-blooded animals covered in hair or fur. This group includes a wide range of mammals used as food: *cattle*, cows, pigs, sheep, goats, horses; *game*, deer, rabbits, hares, bush animals, monkeys and elephants, and, in certain areas, dogs, seals and whales.

3.3 CELLULAR NATURE OF FOOD

Multicellular living organisms and most of the foods derived from them consist of millions of cells; a human body can contain about *one hundred million million*! These cells are grouped together as *tissues* which perform a similar function; but all cells share the ability to *live* or metabolise, *grow*, *reproduce* or *divide. Non-cellular* foods include milk, butter, lard, cooking oils, refined sugar and starches.

Microscopes
These are instruments of two kinds: *light* microscopes which by combined eye and objective *lenses* provide magnifications of from 50 to 1000 *times* as shown in figure 3.1. *Electron* microscopes can produce magnifications up to 500 000 times.

Photographs taken through a light microscope are called *photomicrographs*, whilst *electron micrographs* are obtained by means of electron microscopes (see Plate 3.1).

The light microscope shows the *cellular* structure of living organisms and foods, and the following general information is known concerning plant and animal cells.

fig 3.1 *parts of a light or optical microscope*

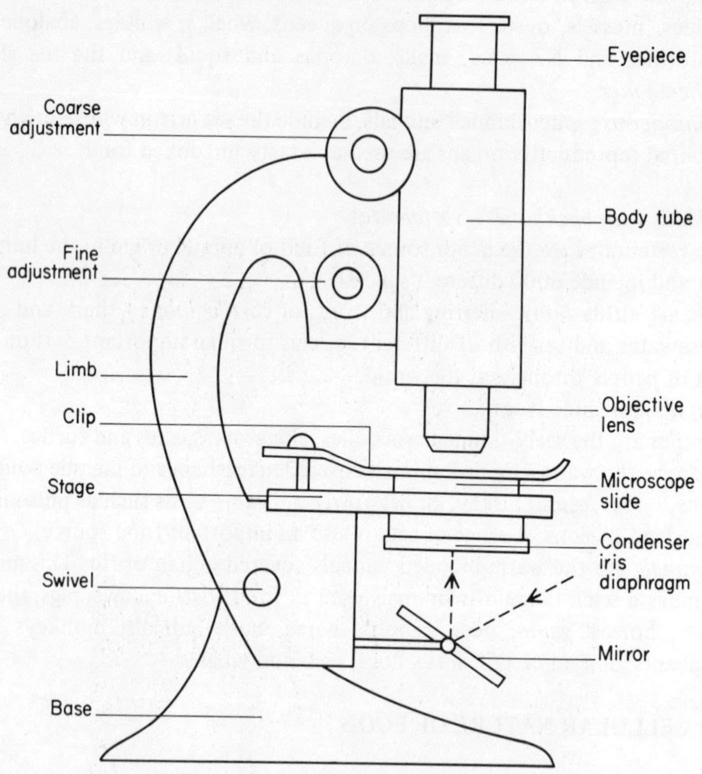

Cell structure

Chemical composition

The *living substance* composing a cell is called *protoplasm* and this is composed of water, mineral ions, proteins, carbohydrates, lipids and other substances, for example, vitamins.

Physical structure

The cell protoplasm consists of three main parts:

(a) the *cell membrane* or plasma membrane; this is the important living semi-permeable membrane for diffusion and osmosis (see Section 2.7).

(b) *Cytoplasm* or cell substance which is mainly in a sol condition (see Section 2.6) and contains important organelles (see Figure 3.2).

Plate 3.1 *the electron microscope produces magnifications of over 500 000 times (Sandoz, Ltd)*

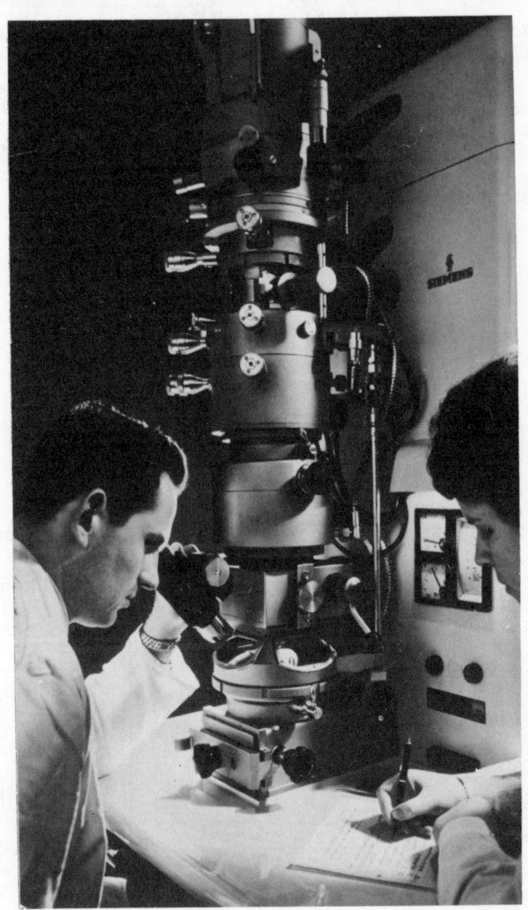

fig 3.2 *generalised structure of (a) an animal cell and (b) a green plant cell showing organelles*

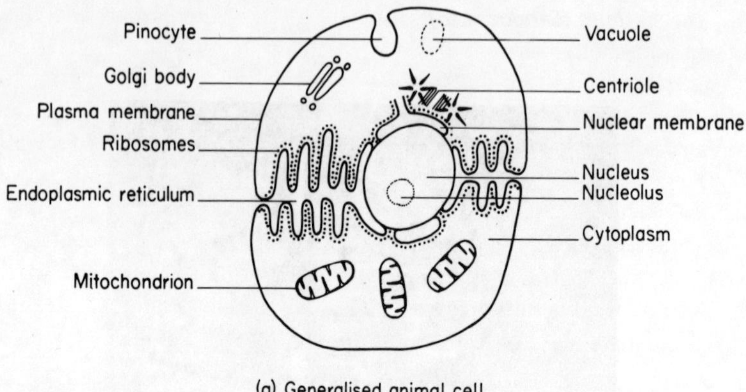

(a) Generalised animal cell

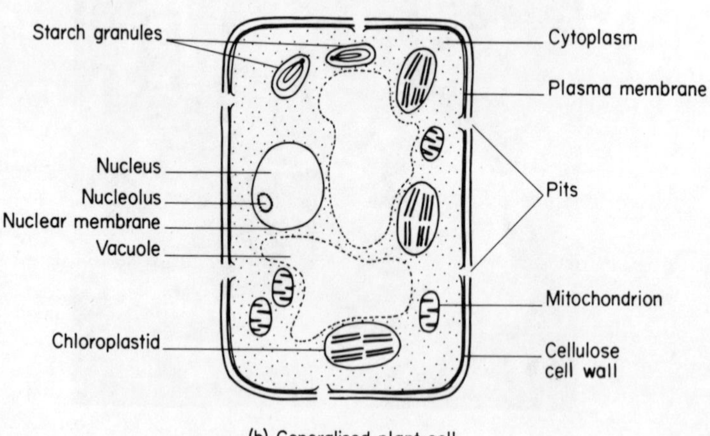

(b) Generalised plant cell

(c) *Nucleus* of a spherical shape surrounded by a porous nuclear membrane and may contain a nucleolus. Bacteria cells are without a definite nucleus, whilst human red blood cells are without a nucleus of any kind (see also Section 3.4).

Cell wall

Only the cells of *bacteria* and *plants* have a cell wall enclosing and close to the plasma membrane.

The cell wall of green plants is *permeable* and is composed of *cellulose* sometimes strengthened with a woody material, *lignin*. Plant cells are cemented together by an intercellular substance consisting of *protopectins*.

Plant cell vacuoles

These are seen only in plant cells as clear fluid-filled spaces containing *soluble* chemical substances and occupying almost 80% of plant cell space. This vacuole fluid is important in osmosis and in maintaining the turgidity providing support for the plant and fresh vegetable foodstuffs.

Organelles

These are the important *functional units* within the cytoplasm where different catabolic and anabolic processes of metabolism occur.

(i) *Mitochondria* are organelles concerned with the catabolic process of *energy-release* from energy-providing nutrients, and formation of the *energy-rich* substance called ATP, *adenosine triphosphate* (see section 5.4).
(ii) *Endoplasmic reticulum* is an infolding of the cell membrane covered with granular *ribosomes.* Their function is to *secrete* proteins (see Section 3.4).
(iii) *Chloroplasts* are large organelles (found *only* in green plant cells) whose function is the anabolic synthesis of carbohydrates.
(iv) *Lysosomes* are spheres surrounded by membranes present mainly in animal cells. (In plant cells the *vacuoles* may function as lysosomes). These organelles can *engulf* foreign particles and then digest them; they act as scavengers within the cell cytoplasm.

In extreme cases the lysosome membrane breaks down releasing enzymes which cause *cell* and *tissue destruction* through *self-digestion*; this happens in dead animal foodstuffs through post-mortem changes called *autolysis.* It is an important process in tenderising meat and game by 'hanging' (see Section 6.16). It also occurs in foods of plant origin and is partly prevented by 'blanching' (see Section 10.2), otherwise it is the process *preceding decay* of plant and animal origin foods.

Experiment 3.1 *look at cells*

A. *Animal cells* (see figure 1.1)

(i) Gently scrape inside the cheek of the mouth with the blunt end of a previously cleansed spoon handle.

(ii) Transfer the cloudy substance which collects from the spoon handle end onto a clean microscope slide and allow it to *dry*.

(iii) Add two drops of a *microscope stain*, methylene blue, to the dry smear, leave for two minutes and rinse gently with clean water.

(iv) Add one drop of propanetriol (glycerine) to the stained specimen and cover with a glass cover slip.

View the preparation through a light microscope and observe the structure of a human cheek epithelium cell.

B. *Plant cells* (see figure 1.2)

(i) Strip off the translucent tissue from the inner surface of a fleshy onion scale.

(ii) Spread a small portion out on a microscope slide, and add two drops of iodine solution to stain the specimen for two minutes. Cover with a glass cover slip and view these leaf scale cells through a microscope. Note the *intercellular* spaces which contain the cellular cement called *protopectin.*

3.4 CELL NUCLEUS

A cell nucleus is composed of a definite number of threadlike *chromosomes*; the number is constant for a species, human beings having 46, cows 60, maize 20 and common wheat 42 chromosomes. Plate 3.2 shows chromosomes in a human cell nucleus.

Genes are arranged along the length of each chromosome and it is these genes which *control* cell metabolism, protein synthesis, and cell reproduction. The genes are composed of *polynucleotides* or nucleic acids (see Section 4.10).

Cell function control

Each nucleus will have thousands of different genes, each of which controls *protein formation* within the cells ribosomes. Thousands of different types of proteins are formed, each having a function in building the different *cell structures* or making different *cell enzymes*.

The nucleic acid in the genes called *deoxyribose nucleic acid* or DNA controls another nucleic acid, called *ribonucleic acid*, RNA (see Sections

Plate 3.2 *photomicrograph of 46 chromosomes seen in a human cell nucleus (World Health Organisation (WHO))*

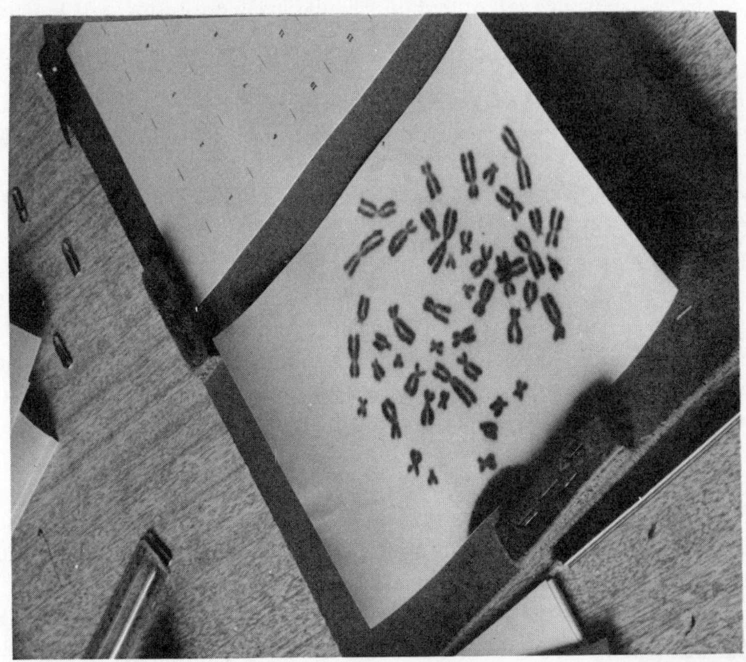

4.10 and 3.7), which passes into the cell from the nucleus to control cell functions.

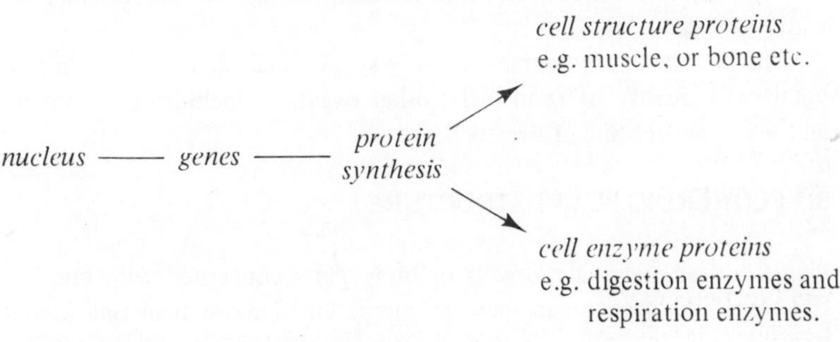

Cell growth and repair

(i) *Growth* by *increase in size* of *cells* is due to formation of new cell structure proteins, and certain carbohydrates cellulose in plants. *Repair* of damaged cells occurs by the same process.

(ii) *Growth* can also occur by controlled cell *division* or *reproduction*. This occurs by a process in which the nucleus divides into two and is followed by the cell splitting into two new cells. This process is called *mitosis* and is responsible for growth in *size* and *old cell* replacement in human beings and other multicellular living organisms.

Cancer or neoplasm

This is the *uncontrolled* growth and division of certain cells in a tissue to form tumours; cancer cells or *neoplasms* deprive healthy cells of their nutrient supply.

Gene abnormalities

The type of gene in the human body is inherited from parents. Some genes may become changed or abnormal by *mutation*. These mutant genes cause disorders of metabolism by not being able to produce certain enzymes. A number of disorders of metabolism are inborn and due to faulty genes which affect carbohydrate and protein metabolism. For example, PKU or *phenylketonuria* is treated partly through a special *diet*.

Food genetics

The study of genes and inheritance, *genetics*, is important in agriculture and food production. *Wheat* is an important food for most of the world, and there are many different *species* of wheat.

Early Neolithic-age man (see Section 11.1) had a small-grained wild wheat of chromosome number 14 which accidentally crossed with a wild grass to give a better-sized wheat grain, in the Iron Age, with a chromosome number of 28. Today wheat growers have produced a larger-grained wheat by *selection* and careful breeding, with a chromosome number of 42, that is, three times the chromosome number of the original wild wheat (see Plate 3.3).

This is but one example of the way in which genetics can improve yields and quality of foodstuffs; other examples include rice, tomatoes and selective breeding of livestock.

3.5 FLOWERING PLANT STRUCTURE

Plants and animals have *organs* or body parts concerned with one main function, and each organ may be composed of more than one kind of tissue.

Flowering plant organs include the flower, leaf, bud, stem and root. The flower is a *reproductive* organ, whilst the leaf, bud, stem and root are *vegetative* organs concerned with food manufacture, storage or transport.

Some vegetative organs can become modified; *bulbs*, *tubers* and *swollen roots* are some examples of modified stems and roots respectively.

Plate 3.3 *an improved variety of wheat grown in Ethiopia: over half of the world's population eat wheat (Food and Agriculture Organisation of the United Nations (FAO, UN))*

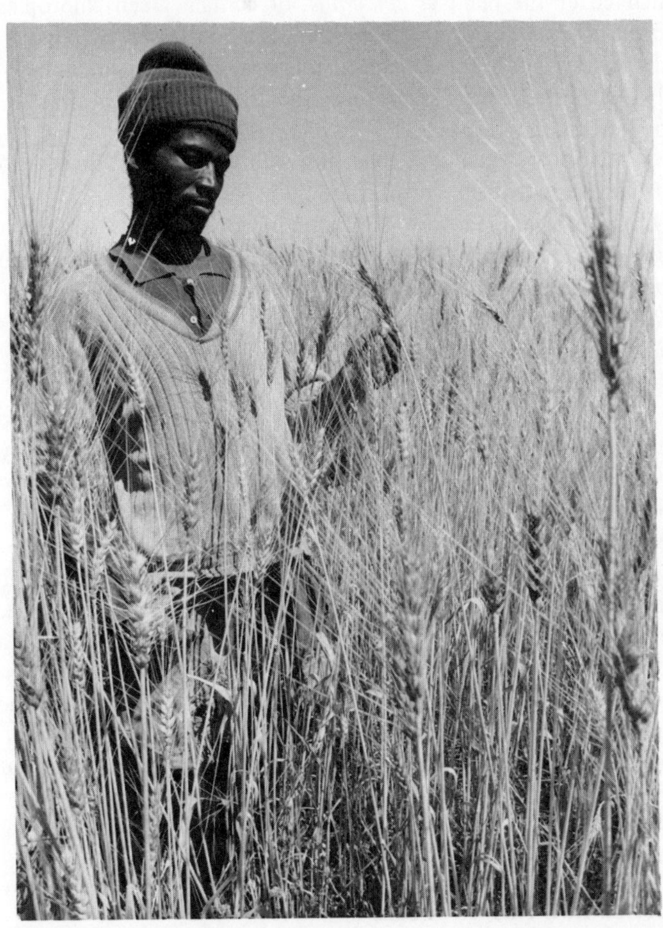

(a) *Stem* vegetables are recognised by having *buds* closely associated with a *leaf* or leaf scar as in the potato and Jerusalem artichokes.
(b) *Leafy* vegetables are composed of a broad or narrow leaf *blade*, together with a stalk or *petiole*, as in cabbage, lettuce and parsley.
(c) *Buds* are closely telescoped forms of stems with attached leaves, evident in Brussels sprouts.
(d) *Root* vegetables are without leaves or buds and are mainly swollen *taproots* as in carrots and horseradish.

Flowering plant tissues

The following tissues are involved in the structure of vegetative organs:

1. *SOFT cellulose wall tissues* form the majority of flowering plant tissues which cover the plant as *epidermis*, or contain green chloroplasts in *photosynthetic* tissue, or fill the stem and root as *packing* tissue. Cell walls of seaweeds become *mucilaginous* as in carrageen and dulse.
2. *HARD lignified wall tissues* form the tubular *vascular* tissue within roots, stems and leaves. The cells are thickened with woody *lignin.* They transport water and ions throughout the plant, in addition to providing support to the plant.

   Elongated lignified *fibres* are found in woody carrots, stringy runner beans, and asparagus spears. Gritty lignified *stone cells* are found in certain pears and nuts.

   Herbaceous vegetables and fruits are mostly composed of soft tissues only, compared with woody trees and shrubs which are composed of mainly hard tissue.
3. *Fatty wall tissue* includes the surface epidermis cells with an outer waterproof layer of fatty *cutin* and cork cells with a coating of waxy *suberin.*

Storage organs

Food is manufactured but not stored in leaves. Food can be stored inside the packing cell-tissue of stems and roots, also within seeds and nuts, and in modified organs such as bulbs, tubers and swollen roots. Vegetables which are also food storage organs - for example, onions, potatoes and turnips - will have a higher nutrient content than leafy vegetables such as cabbages and lettuce.

Sugar *sucrose* is stored in sugar cane *stems* or in the *swollen roots* of sugar beet.

3.6 HUMAN BODY STRUCTURE

The structure of the human body closely resembles the *basic* structure of the other vertebrate animals, being composed of *organs* with a particular function and composed of different tissues.

The following list summarises the tissues present in vertebrate animals:

1. *Covering and lining* tissue, called epithelial tissue, covers the outer skin and lines all internal cavities of the gut, lungs, glands and blood vessels.
2. *Supporting and binding* tissue called connective tissue forms the structure of bones, ligaments and tendons.

3. *Muscle* tissue is a *contractile* tissue, present in heart, limbs and trunk, and also in the gut wall.
4. *Blood and lymph* tissue is important because it *circulates* between other tissues.
5. *Nerve tissue* in brain and sense organs.
6. *Reproductive* tissue in the male and female reproductive organs.

Human body systems

The human body can be subdivided into major functional *systems* also called *organ systems* as they can be composed of more than one organ.

1. *Skeleton and muscle system* consists of *bones* connected by *ligaments* to other bones across *joints. Skeletal muscle* is composed of millions of muscle fibres, and is connected to bones by muscle *tendons.* This system functions in support and movement, called locomotion.
2. *Nervous system* is composed of the *brain, spinal cord* and *peripheral nerves* to arms and legs. The *sensory* portion is concerned with taste, smell, sight, hearing and touch, and a *motor* portion controls muscles. The *autonomic nervous system* regulates the gut, glands, blood vessels and bladder muscles.
3. *Alimentary system* is composed of organs concerned with *nutrition*, ingestion, digestion, absorption of food and elimination of indigestable or unabsorbable food materials (see Sections 8.5 and figure 8.1).
4. *Circulatory system* consists of the blood, lymph and its circulation by the *heart*, blood and lymph *vessels.* This system functions in the *transport* of nutrients and other substances between other body organs and systems and formation of *tissue fluid.* (See figure 3.3).
5. *Homeostatic metabolic system* is concerned with maintaining homeostasis of the *tissue fluid* around cells, and includes the homeostatic organs skin, liver (figure 8.5), pancreas (figure 8.2) and kidneys (figure 8.6) which are also an excretory system. Homeostasis also depends on the function of other body systems: the circulatory system to supply and remove tissue fluid components, the nervous system to sense changes in tissue fluid concentration and the alimentary system to supply nutrients to the blood.
6. *Respiratory system* is concerned with the *exchange* of oxygen in air for carbon dioxide in blood by a system of air passages and blood vessels in the *lungs*, aided by the muscles of the chest wall and *diaphragm* dividing the chest cavity from the abdominal cavity.
   Oxygen functions in *energy release* in the cell *mitochondria* (see figure 3.4).
7. *Reproductive system* includes the male and female reproductive organs which serve to form male *sperm* (which is ejaculated in a *seminal fluid*

fig 3.3 *general arrangement of human blood circulatory system*

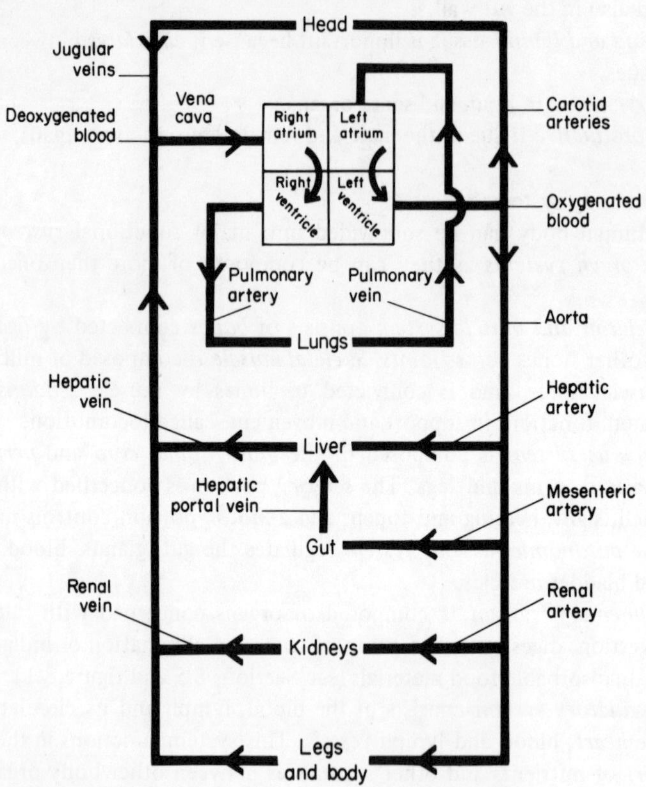

containing many nutrients to feed the active sperm) and female *ova* respectively.

The female develops breasts or *mammae* which consist of *mammary glands*, secreting *milk* during the breast-feeding stage called *lactation*. The glandular tissue consists of *lobules* which pass the milk by *ducts* into wide milk collecting spaces called *sinuses* which connect with the nipple.

Human foetus and pregnancy

The human *embryo* develops within the female *uterus*, and the time from its conception to birth is called gestation and is approximately nine months or up to forty-one weeks. After the first *trimester* or 4–17 weeks, the embryo is called a *foetus*. The *second trimester* of pregnancy occupies 17–26 weeks, and the *third trimester* 28–41 weeks.

Feeding of the foetus occurs by nutrients and oxygen passing from the mother's blood across a *placenta* into the foetal circulation, by diffusion,

fig 3.4 *human respiratory system*

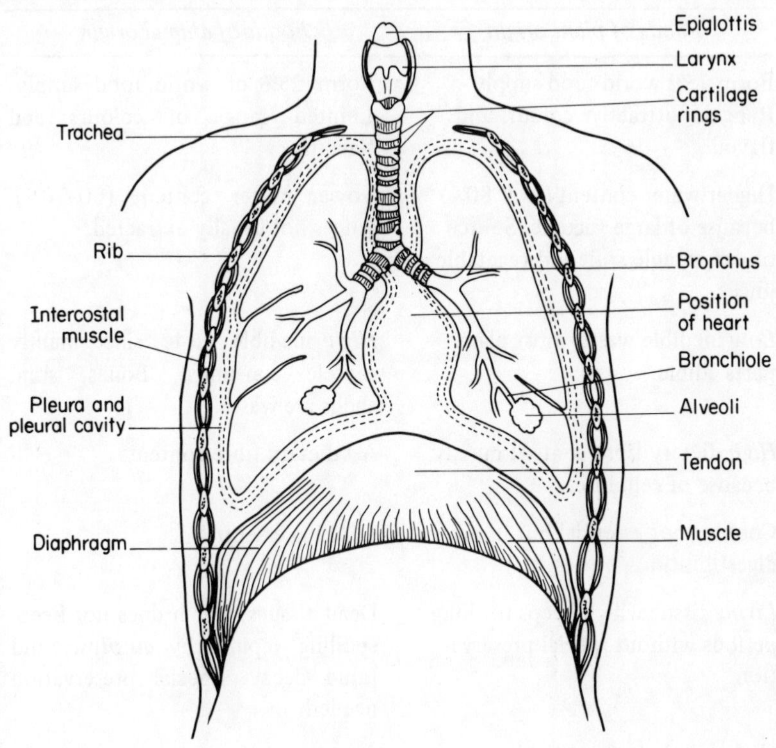

osmosis and active transport. Waste products pass back into the mother's blood via the placenta. During gestation the foetus composition changes from 90% water, 7% protein, 2% lipids, in the first trimester to 75% water, 11% protein, 13% lipids in the third trimester.

3.7 DIFFERENCES BETWEEN FOODS OF PLANT AND ANIMAL ORIGIN

Foods from plant and animal sources resemble each other in their *cellular* composition, and in having an almost similar chemical composition through similar metabolic life processes. The *main differences* between foods from plant and animal sources are summarised in Table 3.1. The differences refer mainly to *fresh* unprocessed foods.

Table 3.1 *a comparison of foods of plant and animal origin*

Foods of plant origin	*Foods of animal origin*
Form 75% world food supply. Range of attractive colours and flavours.	Form 25% of world food supply. Limited range of colours and flavours.
Higher water content (over 80%) because of large vacuole. Source of extractable fruit and vegetable juices.	Lower water content (60-70%). Juices not usually extracted.
Low inedible waste, most plant parts edible.	*High* inedible waste, since mainly muscle consumed. Bones, skin, shells are waste.
High dietary fibre content mainly because of cellulose.	*No* dietary fibre content.
Cooking *not* essential but improves digestibility.	Cooking essential.
Living tissue which keeps for long periods without special preservation.	Dead tissues, which does not keep, spoiling rapidly by *autolysis* and rapid decay. Special preservation needed.
Higher carbohydrate content mainly because of starches and cellulose.	*Lower carbohydrate* content mainly glycogen.
Low protein content, and deficient in certain essential amino-acids (see Section 4.9).	High protein content and more complete range of essential amino-acids.
Lipids mainly as unsaturated *liquid* oils (see Section 4.8).	Lipids mainly as saturated *solid* fats.
Sole source of vitamin K. [Vitamin A present as a *precursor form* – carotenes. Rich source vitamin C and folic acid.	Sole source of vitamins A retinol and D and B_{12}.
Most plant origin foods are produced within *one* year (annuals); some take *two* (biennials) years.	Most animal origin foods are reared over more than *two* years; exceptions are rabbits and broiler chickens.

Phytic acid content variable (see Section 4.4).	Nil.
Nil	Variable cholesterol content (see Section 4.3).

Note *Plant crops* yield *eight* times more edible *energy*, and between *four* and *six* times more *protein* per *hectare* than animals crops reared on a similar area of land, subject to land quality.

3.8 PHOTOSYNTHESIS

This is the main process of *nutrition* in all green plants. The following summarises the requirements and the products of *photosynthesis*:

light energy + *green chlorophyll* + *carbon dioxide* + *water* + *inorganic ions* ⟶ *organic compounds* + *oxygen*

organic compounds → *carbohydrates*, *amino acids*, *lipids*

(i) The sunlight energy is trapped in the cell chloroplasts by means of chlorophyll. Photosynthesis will only occur in chloroplasts containing cells found mainly in the *leaf* and sometimes the stem.

(ii) Carbon dioxide diffuses into the leaf cells, whilst water is already present in the cell; this reaches the leaves by absorption from the soil by a root system.

(iii) Mineral ions such as iron, calcium, magnesium, as well as nitrates, sulphates and phosphates are also needed for photosynthesis and for forming amino-acids. These enter the roots with water from the soil where they are present as fertilisers from artificial or organic soil manures.

Mechanism of photosynthesis

1. The *energy-rich* compound ATP, adenosine triphosphate, is formed by chlorophyll which traps sunlight energy.
2. Energy is then used to *split* water into *oxygen gas* and hydrogen *atoms.*
3. The ATP energy is used to combine hydrogen atoms with CO_2 (carbon dioxide) and *phosphate* ions to make the first product of photosynthesis, a simple sugar called *triose phosphate.*

$$\textit{hydrogen atoms} + \underset{\text{(carbon dioxide)}}{CO_2} + \textit{phosphate} \xrightarrow[\textit{energy}]{\text{ATP}} \textit{triose phosphate}$$

4. *Glucose* rapidly forms from triose phosphate; this can be changed and stored as starch in the leaf for a few hours. At night the *starch* is changed into *sucrose* sugar and transported for *permanent* storage in root and stem cells as *starch granules.* Alternatively it is used to provide *energy* or *cellulose* to build new cell walls.
5. *Amino-acids* are made in the cells at the tips of roots and stems using glucose and nitrate ions. Amino-acids are then used to make *proteins*, *enzymes* and *pigments* by means of the *genes'* RNA influence (see Section 3.4).
6. *Lipids* are synthesised by complex processes called *lipogenesis* from glucose.

3.9 INTERRELATIONS BETWEEN LIVING THINGS

The 1½ million different species of living things have a range of associations between one another; these associations range from beneficial to extremely harmful.

(a) *Symbiosis* is a *beneficial* relationship, for example human beings are the *hosts* to certain bacteria or *symbionts* which are present in great numbers in the large intestine of man. These symbiotic bacteria provide vitamins of the B group and vitamin H (biotin) in return for certain nutrients from our diet, and protection within our bodies. *Antibiotics* can destroy these beneficial bacteria. Herbivorous mammals digest cellulose by means of similar symbiotic bacteria.

(b) *Parasitism* is mainly a relationship in which the *parasite* benefits, whilst the host may or may not be harmed. Parasitic relationships in human beings include *plant* parasites causing skin ringworm, and *animal* parasites such as fleas and other blood-sucking insects. *Internal* parasites include tapeworms and roundworms in the human gut (see Section 11.6). Some of these internal parasites can be transmitted to man by *food*; these also include bacteria and viruses which cause *food poisoning* (see Section 11.10).

3.10 FOOD RELATIONSHIPS

All the living things which live together can be allocated a definite job in relationship to food and feeding. The three main jobs are as follows:

1. *Producers* are all green plants which trap energy and manufacture organic food.

2. *Consumers* are all those animals which obtain their energy *directly* from the producers and include the herbivores (sheep and other cattle) and those *indirect* consumers (the *carnivores*) which feed on herbivores. The *omnivore* feeds both directly and indirectly on producers or other consumers.

   Food can be consumed by *pests* as the food *grows*, or when the food is *stored* (see Section 10.2).
3. *Decomposers* are the non-green organisms such as *bacteria* and *fungi* moulds, which feed on surplus food, dead remains and wastes of producers and consumers. Decomposers are responsible for food spoilage and food decay (see Section 10.2).

Food chains

A food chain shows the *feeding relationship* and *energy transfer* between producers and consumers. For example, cereal grain crops are the world's largest single type of foodstuff for human beings. A *simple* food chain is shown as follows:

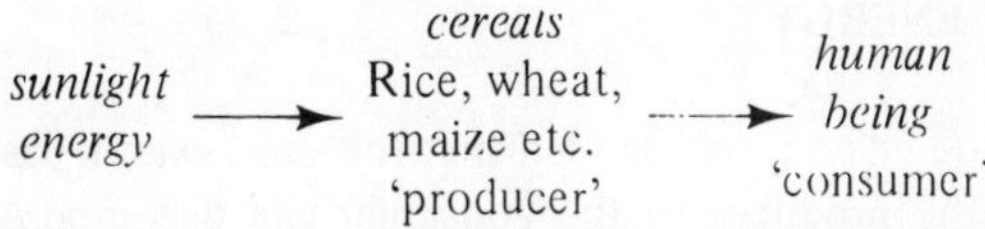

In this chain almost all the sunlight energy trapped in cereals become edible or food energy for humans.

Another food chain in which human beings consume beef is shown as follows:

sunlight energy ⟶ pasture grass ⟶ beef cattle ⟶ human being

'producer' 'secondary consumer' 'primary consumer'

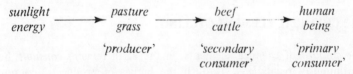

Only 10% of the energy in the grass or *feed* fed to cattle becomes edible or food energy for human beings. The feeding cattle *lose* 90% of energy from their bodies mainly as heat.

The following is a longer food chain:

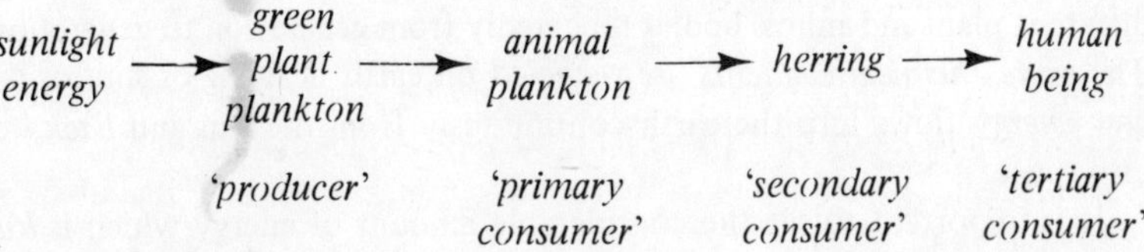

Food webs

The herring can feed on *many* different plant and animal organisms and the simple chain becomes a more complex *food web* before it reaches a human being. Similarly a human being is also part of a complex food web since we eat a vast *variety* of foodstuffs which are part of other food chains and webs.

Pyramids of weight and numbers

Food chains and webs only show the *species* of organism involved and do not indicate the number or weight of organisms.

A pyramid of weight will show the weight of food needed to feed a population of human beings. The present world population of over 4500m people is supported on top of a food pyramid of over 2600m tonnes, the amount produced in the world each year. This great food pyramid will have a tremendous base of plants to feed the human population *directly* and to feed all other living animals including those animals becoming food for a world human population.

3.11 FLOW OF ENERGY

Studying the food chain it will be seen that the sun's *energy* passes through or *flows* from the producer to the consumer and decomposer, and then radiates back into space. Meanwhile *heat* energy is lost at each feeding level; this also passes out into space. Of the total energy from the sun, only about 1% is trapped by the producers.

During its passage through different living organisms the energy is *changed* from one form into another, it is *not* destroyed in any way [see Section 7.2].

3.12 CHEMICAL ELEMENT CYCLING

The *amount* of chemical elements on the earth remains *constant*, being continuously *recirculated* through the bodies of producers, consumers and decomposers. There is no creation or destruction of new chemical matter, the chemical elements *recombine* to form different compounds in different organisms using *energy* to form new *bonds* between the atoms. The *same* carbon, hydrogen, oxygen, sulphur and phosphorus atoms remain today as when the earth was first formed, and circulate through different plant and animal bodies repeatedly from generation to generation. The *same chemical elements* are *recycled* on earth in living organisms but *new energy* flows into the earth continuously from the sun and *back* out into space.

It is important to see the considerable amount of energy which is *lost* to space, as it passes from one feeding level to another. Only 10 per cent of the producers' energy reaches the *consumers*, and in turn only 10 per cent of the consumers' energy reaches the *decomposers*.

3.13 FOOD AND AGRICULTURE

Modern agriculture in developed countries (see Section 12.3) aims at controlled production of one type of crop through *monocultures* or the growing of large areas of wheat, or a single vegetable on the same land each year; or *intensive* rearing of one kind of livestock – for example, poultry in batteries in the same area each year.

This single crop attracts equally large numbers of *pests* which in turn require extensive use of *pesticides* or *herbicides* to control them. Pesticides of the *organo-chlorine* type do not decompose but persist in the soil. They also have the property of *accumulating* in the fatty tissues of animals and consequently in foods causing *food contamination*. Since the same plant crop uses up chemical fertilisers, more *artificial* fertilisers must be applied to the soil, which in turn *leach* into rivers and lakes to *contaminate* drinking water.

The controlled feeding and rearing of one crop produces a foodstuff of uniform composition, compared with foods reared as *wild* stock such as sea-fish and game which tend to have variable composition. Organically-grown foods are those fruits and vegetables grown without the use of chemical artificial fertilisers and chemical pesticides, but employing natural organic composts and manures and biological control of pests. Such organically-grown foods would be free of harmful chemical pesticides. It is also preferable to re-use animal and vegetable wastes, instead of consuming irreplaceable chemicals and fossil fuels, to make artificial fertilisers.

Organically-grown foods, also known misleadingly as 'health' foods, are *whole* foods which are not *refined* or *processed* by canning or addition of chemical preservatives, hormones or antibiotics, or any form of *additive* (see Section 7.1).

3.14 QUESTIONS

1. Explain the term food chain. Trace the flow of energy through a food chain. What effect have organo-chlorine pesticides on a food chain?
2. If the main purpose of foods is to maintain health, why are 'health foods' misleadingly so-called? Suggest a more acceptable term describing these foods.
3. Compare the structure and composition of foods from animal with foods from plant sources.

4. Describe the structure of a plant and animal cell. Name four different kinds of cells composing a cabbage and a lamb chop.
5. What functions are performed by the following cell components:
(a) nucleus (b) mitochondrion (c) lysosome (d) chloroplast (e) ribosome.
6. Name foodstuffs for human beings which originate from:
(a) producers (b) primary consumers (c) secondary consumers; and (d) decomposers.

CHAPTER 4

FOOD COMPONENTS

4.1 INTRODUCTION

Almost every food component, except a few mineral components such as sodium chloride, is composed of *carbon* together with other elements in a range of *organic compounds.*

Carbon atoms are able to join with other carbon atoms through strong chemical bonds called *covalent links*, to form single and branched *chains* or *rings* or nets in macromolecules.

4.2 HYDROCARBONS

Hydrocarbons are organic compounds consisting of varying numbers of *hydrogen* (H) and *carbon* (C) atoms; the carbon atoms form the chain or ring, backbone of the molecule, and the hydrogen atoms are connected by covalent links to the carbon atoms. The three simplest hydrocarbons are shown as follows by *structural formulae*:

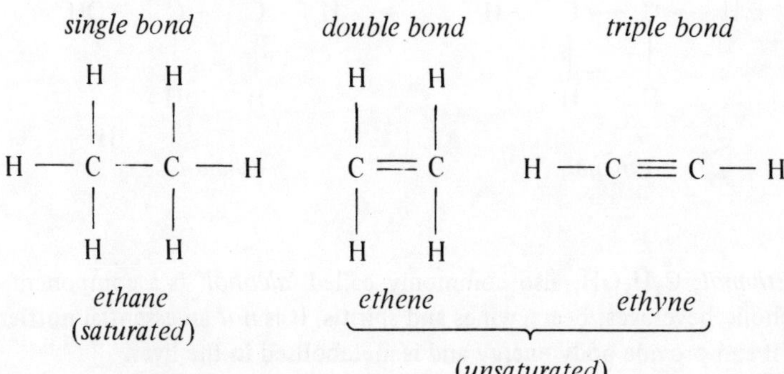

Hydrocarbons and other organic compounds like ethane which are composed of *single* bonds between carbon atoms are called *saturated compounds.*

Hydrocarbons like ethene and ethyne and other organic compounds composed of *double* or *triple* bonds are called *unsaturated compounds.*

Mineral oils are the different hydrocarbon components of crude petroleum composed of chain molecules with between *four* and *thirty* carbon atoms in the chain. *Propane*, C_3H_8, and *butane*, C_4H_{10}, are important gaseous fuels. *Liquid paraffin, soft* (petroleum jelly) and *hard* paraffin wax, none of which have a nutritive value, are used on a restricted basis for processing foods. Liquid paraffin (0.5%) as a *lubricant* prevents dried fruit clumping together, and is used to *glaze* certain sweets; paraffin *waxes* are coatings for certain cheeses for example, Edam, and can also be components of chewing gums. *Medicinal* liquid paraffin is a laxative and faecal lubricant, which acts as a vitamin A and D solvent withdrawing these vitamins from lipid foods in the intestine.

Essential oils or essences of fruit oils - for example, orange essence - contain the hydrocarbons called *terpenes*; *limonene* with ten carbon atoms in its macromolecule is a terpene responsible for the characteristic *flavour* of many citrus fruits.

4.3 **ALCOHOLS**

Alcohols are organic compounds of *carbon*, *hydrogen* and *oxygen*. They form a *series* of different alcohols with names ending in -ol - methanol, ethanol, butanol, etc. All alcohols possess a typical functional group called *hydroxyl*, (–OH) connected to one carbon atom by *replacing* a hydrogen atom in a hydrocarbon skeleton molecule.

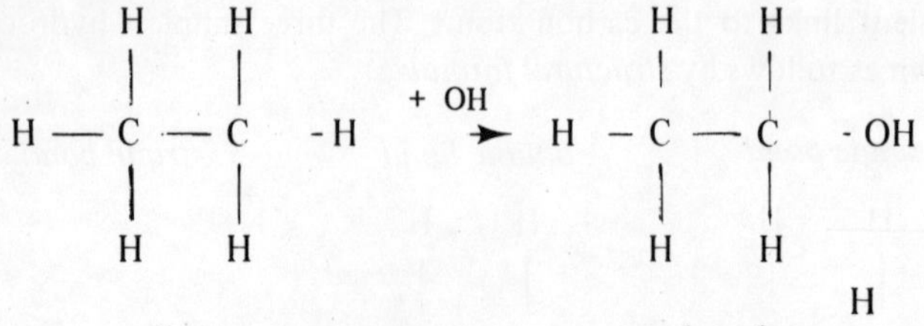

```
     H   H                     H   H
     |   |                     |   |
                + OH
H — C — C   - H      ➤    H – C — C   · OH
     |   |                     |   |
     H   H                     H   H

                                        H
    ethane                    ethanol
```

Ethanol, C_2H_5OH, also commonly called *'alcohol'* is a component of alcoholic beverages, beers, wines and spiritis. It is *not* an essential nutrient, but it can provide body energy and is metabolised in the liver.

Propane-1,2,3-triol (glycerol), $C_3H_8O_3$, is a component of many plant and animal *lipids.* It is a sweet syrupy liquid and is metabolised in the body. Formula of propane-1,2,3-triol (glycerol):

$$\begin{array}{c} CH_2 - OH \\ | \\ CH - OH \\ | \\ CH_2 - OH \end{array}$$

Sorbitol found in certain fruits, human semen fluid and used as a diabetic sugar substitute, is metabolised in the body. *Dulcitol* and *xylitol* are also sweet-tasting metabolised alcohols.

Inositol is a sweet-tasting alcohol found in muscle, heart and liver, formerly called meat sugar, present in plants. It is an essential nutrient for *certain* animals, but it is *not* known if it is essential for human beings.

Sterols are complex, non-essential alcohols which include *cholesterol*, a waxy solid, found only in foods of *animal* origin - meat, offal and egg yolk have large amounts (see also Table 4.1 showing approximate cholesterol content of foods). Plant origin foods contain only *phytosterols*. *Ergosterol* in yeast is used to make vitamin D_2.

Vitamin E is a mixture of complex alcohols called *tocopherols* (see Section 4.12).

Vitamin A, called *retinol*, is a hydrocarbon molecule with an alcohol hydroxyl group.

4.4 ORGANIC ACIDS

These are compounds of carbon, hydrogen and oxygen, which form a series of different acids with names ending in *-enoic acid* - ethanoic, hexadecanoic acid, etc. All organic acids have the functional group called *carboxylic*, –COOH, connected to a carbon atom of a hydrocarbon skeleton molecule:

$$\begin{array}{c} H \\ | \\ H - C - COOH \\ | \\ H \end{array}$$

ethanoic acid
(acetic acid)

Organic carboxylic acids range in physical condition from liquids in ethanoic (acetic) acid to solids: ethanedioic acid (oxalic acid) and waxy solids, octadecanoic acid (stearic acid).

Table 4.1 *approximate cholesterol content of some foods*

Food item	*Cholesterol range in g per 100g*
Vegetable cooking oils and margarine	ZERO
ALL foods of plant origin	
Milk, ice cream	0.01–0.02
Fish, sausage, meat pies, meat stews, meat puddings	0.05
Cheese, bacon, lard, dripping	0.085
Cooked meats, poultry, game	
Lobster, crab, shrimps, prawns	0.15
Butter, mayonnaise, sweetbreads, fish roes, liver	0.3
Kidneys	0.4
Whole eggs, chicken, goose liver and cod liver oil	0.5
Raw egg yolk	1.60
Brains	2.36

[NOTE:- The WHO recommended daily intake of cholesterol is less than 0.3g daily]

Ethanoic acid (acetic acid) component of vinegar (5%) is used to flavour and preserve foods and is metabolised in the body.

Ethanedioic acid (oxalic acid) present in rhubarb, beetroot, parsley and spinach, is poisonous in large amounts. It is not metabolised.

Alkanoic acids formerly called *fatty acids*, are important components of plant and animal lipids; they have a long hydrocarbon chain of between 4 and 24 carbon atoms. Some are *saturated* without double bonds: butanoic (butyric), dodecanoic (lauric), hexadecanoic (palmitic) and octadecanoic (stearic) acids.

Others have one double bond or are *mono-unsaturated*: 9-octadecanoic (oleic), and docosenoic (erucic) acids. The following have two or more double bonds and are *poly-unsaturated* alkanoic (fatty) acids (sometimes abbreviated to PUFA): octadecadienoic (linoleic), eiccosatetraenoic (arachidonic) and octadecatrienoic (linolenic) acids. All the alkanoic (fatty) acids are metabolised in the body.

Hyroxy carboxylic acids

These include a range of acids which possess a *hydroxyl*, –OH, in addition to a carboxylic, –COOH, group (see Section 6.8).

2-hydroxypropanoic (lactic) acid is an important acid metabolised in body cells when oxygen is in short supply. It is the acid component of sour milk yoghurts, and many prepared foods, such as *sauerkraut.*

2-hydroxypropane 1,2,3-tricarboxylic (citric) acid is the acid component of citrus and other fruits and some vegetables and is used as a food flavour. It is metabolised in body cells.

2-hydroxybutanedioic (malic) acid is present in most fruits, particularly apples and tomatoes. It is metabolised in body cells.

2,3-dihydroxybutanedioic (tartaric) acid is a component of wines and some fruits, is added to food as flavour and is a component of baking powder. It is *not* metabolised in the body.

Uronic acids are components of *pectins, chondroitin* cartilage, and plant gums.

Ascorbic acid of vitamin C, the component of fruits and vegetables, controls metabolic processes (see Section 4.6).

Phytic acid, present in large amounts in wheat bran, flour, cereals, peas, beans and nuts, is the phosphoric acid compound of inositol (see Section 4.3). This acid combines to form ***insoluble salts*** with calcium, zinc and iron *ions.*

Ethanedioic (oxalic) acid also forms insoluble salts with calcium and magnesium. Phytic and oxalic acids impair the absorption of calcium, magnesium, zinc and iron (see Section 8.11).

4.5 ESTERS

Esters are formed by the reaction between alcohols and organic carboxylic acids.

$$\textit{alcohol} + \begin{matrix}\textit{organic}\\ \textit{acid}\end{matrix} \longrightarrow \textit{ester} + \textit{water}$$

Esters are of two main kinds in foods:

(a) The *lipids* are mainly esters of propanetriol (glycerine) and different alkanoic (fatty) acids (see Section 4.8).

(b) The *flavour* esters are the components of *essences* of the different fruits, herbs or spices. These flavour essence esters can be either synthetically manufactured or natural *extracts.* Natural flavour extracts may have between 20 to 50 components drawn from different esters, terpenes, alcohols and alkanoic (fatty) acids.

The ester components of natural and synthetic flavours are *not* metabolised in the body.

4.6 POLYMERS

Polymers are formed by the linking together of *small* molecules called *monomers*, to form a large macromolecule called a *polymer*, by a process of *polymerisation.*

Plastic materials used in food packaging are examples of *addition polymers* made by joining together monomer units of unsaturated hydrocarbons containing double bonds. *Polyethene* is the polymer of unsaturated *ethene*, used for plastic bags. *Polypropylene* is a polymer of *propylene*. Polyvinyl chloride and polyester are further examples of plastic polymers used in packaging material. *Condensation polymers* are formed by monomer units joining together and eliminating a molecule of water. *Nylons* are condensation polymers, as well as the *food polymers* - proteins, polysaccharides, carbohydrate starches and polynucleotides or nucleic acids.

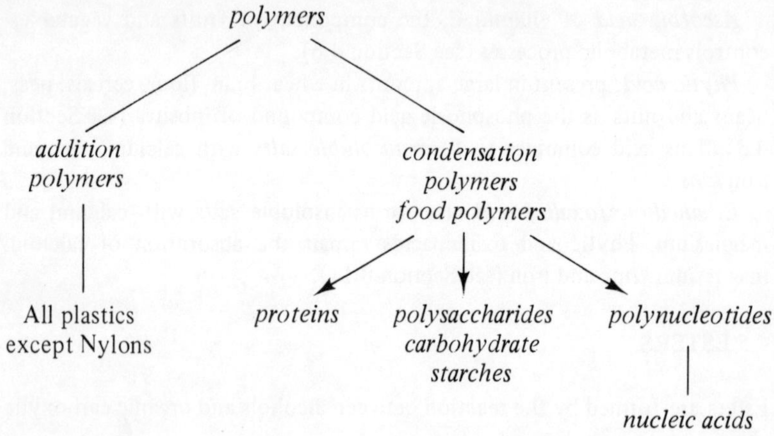

4.7 CARBOHYDRATES

Carbohydrates contain varying amounts of the elements *carbon, hydrogen* and *oxygen*, and include a wide range of different substances which are sugars, starches and fibres; this wide variety is classified into three groups: *monosaccharides, oligosaccharides* and *polysaccharides.*

Monosaccharides

This group includes the simplest water soluble sugars that cannot be split up into other sugars by *hydrolysis* (see Section 2.12). Since many have a sweet taste they are called sugars. The molecule is made up of between 3 and 7 carbon atoms linked together, and they contain as many hydroxyl (–OH) groups, making them resemble the polyhydric alcohols.

The following are the more important monosaccharides in human nutrition, all of which are metabolised in the body:

Deoxyribose, $C_5H_{10}O_4$, is the important component of DNA, *deoxyribonucleic acid*, the cell *nucleus* nucleic acid of all plants and animals.

Ribose, $C_5H_{10}O_5$, is the component of RNA, *ribonucleic acid*, the nucleic acid present in plant and animal cytoplasm.

Fructose or fruit sugar, $C_6H_{12}O_6$, is the sweetest of sugars present in many ripe fruits and honey; also present in human sperm fluid.

Glucose or blood sugar, $C_6H_{12}O_6$, is an important component of blood and tissue fluid, being the main *cell energy source* and found widely in plants. It differs from fructose in having a different arrangement of hydrogen and oxygen atoms on one carbon atom. It therefore shares a *simple* formula $C_6H_{12}O_6$ with fructose.

Galactose or brain sugar, $C_6H_{12}O_6$, is a component of substances in nerve tissue, and of milk sugar.

Oligosaccharides

This group includes sweet-tasting water-soluble sugars composed of 2 or up to 10 monosaccharide molecules.

Disaccharides consist of *two* similar or different monosaccharide units. They have a similar, simple or *empirical* formula - $C_{12}H_{22}O_{11}$, but a different *structural* formula. These sugars are split up into the component units by *hydrolysis* and metabolised in the body.

Lactose or milk sugar, $C_{12}H_{22}O_{11}$, is the slightly sweet carbohydrate component of cows' and human milk, composed of different monosaccharides, *glucose* and *galactose*.

$$\textit{lactos} \xrightarrow{\textit{hydrolysis}} \textit{glucose} + \textit{galactose}$$

Maltose or malt sugar, $C_{12}H_{22}O_{11}$ is formed when starch or glycogen is digested or hydrolysed. It forms in germinating or sprouting barley grain which can be used to provide *malt extract.* Maltose is composed of two similar monosaccharide units, viz. *glucose*.

$$\textit{maltose} \xrightarrow{\textit{hydrolysis}} \textit{glucose} + \textit{glucose}$$

Sucrose, cane or beet sugar, $C_{12}H_{22}O_{11}$, is present in all green plants and is commercially extracted from the sugar cane and sugar beet plants. Sucrose is composed of two different monosaccharides, glucose and fructose.

$$\textit{sucrose} \xrightarrow{\textit{hydrolysis}} \underbrace{\textit{glucose} + \textit{fructose}}_{\textit{invert sugar mixture}}$$

Honey made from flower *nectar* which is sucrose, is changed by bees' digestive enzymes into invert sugar.

Sweetness of the sugars is rated as follows: fructose, 170 per cent; sucrose, 100 per cent; glucose, 70 per cent; maltose, 33 per cent; lactose, 20 per cent. This indicates that fructose is 8.5 times sweeter than lactose.

Polysaccharides

Polysaccharides are the carbohydrate *polymers*, composed of monosaccharide monomer units mainly *glucose*. A polysaccharide can be composed of up to several thousand units. Some polysaccharides are broken down by hydrolysis.

Ordinary starch is found in wheat, rice, tapioca and potato food storage cells as *granules*, which consists of two carbohydrates: *water insoluble* 80% *amylopectin*, consisting of several hundred glucose units in a *branched* chain, and 20% *water soluble amylose*, composed of a *straight* chain of glucose units.

Waxy starch is 100% *amylopectin* and is found only in waxy varieties of maize, rice and sorghum. These form clear, jelly-like sticky solutions or *mucilaginous* pastes useful for certain pie fillings or *instant* puddings (see also *dietary fibre*).

Dextrins are mixtures of *water-soluble* large-molecule carbohydrate substances produced when starches are partly cooked or partly hydrolysed.

Glycogen or animal starch, found in meat and liver, has a similar *branched*-chain-molecule structure of *glucose* units to amylopectin. It is readily changed in the body into 2-hydroxypropanoic (lactic) acid.

Chondroitins are complex polysaccharides which form most of bone and cartilage.

Inulin is a water-soluble polysaccharide composed of about 40 fructose units and is found in Jerusalem artichokes.

Dietary fibre

This ia a *mixture* composed of those mainly polysaccharide substances which are *not* digested in the human gut, and are important components of foods of *plant* origin. The following are the main components of *dietary fibre*:

(a) *Cellulose* is the main polysaccharide component of plant cell walls and consists of *fibres* with large molecules composed of thousands of *glucose* units. Cellulose cannot be hydrolysed or digested within the gut. *Purified* forms of cellulose are cotton wool and *methylcellulose* used in appetite-suppressing preparations giving a feeling of fullness or *satiety* because of its ability to swell up with water in the gut.

(b) *Hemicelluloses* are mixtures of fibre polysaccharides called pentosans and xylans, closely linked with cellulose in cell walls.
(c) *Gums and mucilages* are not fibres, and are not digested. The *gums* include plant secretions called gum acacia, tragacanth and Indian gum which are used as thickeners in sauces and confectionery. The *mucilages* include seaweed extracts of agar, alginate and carrageen or Irish moss which are used also as thickeners in creams and sauces.
(d) *Pectins* are the non-fibrous polysaccharides which are found *between* cells as *intercellular cements*. They are important as setting agents in jams and jellies. Main sources of pectin are fruits, in particular apple and seville oranges.
(e) *Lignin* is a component of woody fibres present in tough carrots or in wheat bran. It is *not* a carbohydrate, but is closely linked to cellulose in thickened cell walls.

Food composition tables can indicate the carbohydrate content of food in two ways.

1st Method Carbohydrate content shown in the table as
(a) *Available carbohydrate* meaning starches, free sugars and dextrins which are digested and absorbed in the human gut (Section 8.7). The *free sugar* content of some foods is shown in Table 4.2.

Table 4.2 *percentage of free sugars in some foods*

Food item	*Percentage free sugars*
Refined cane, beet sugar, pure glucose powder and brown sugar	90–100
Honey, boiled sweets	80–90
Caramel toffee	70–80
Syrup, treacle, molasses, jams and marmalade, dried fruits	60–70
Liquid glucose solution	40–50
Liqueurs	20–30
Sweet wines, most fruits: especially oranges, melons, peaches, plums	10–20
Soft drinks, human and goats' milk, some fruits – raspberries, currants, peas and onions	5–10
Cows' milk, beans, carrots, potatoes, tomatoes, leafy vegetables and eggs	2–5
Rhubarb, canned peas, lettuce, cucumber, broccoli	1–2

(b) *Dietary fibre*, the cellulose, hemicelluloses, gums, pectins and lignin which are not absorbed. The dietary fibre content of some foods is shown in Table 4.3.

Table 4.3 *approximate indigestible dietary fibre content of some foods*

Food	*Indigestible dietary fibre (g/100 g)*
Meat, fish, cooking oils and fats, milk and milk products, sweets	ZERO
Apples, bananas, peaches, oranges, pears, strawberries, fruit jams, pastries and rice	0.5–2
Plums, lettuce, tomatoes, cake, biscuits, popcorn, white bread, soya beans	3–4
Dried fruits, blackcurrants, blackberries, carrots, potatoes, rolled oats, peanuts	5–10
Peas, beans, onions, wholemeal bread	10–15
Bran cereals, curly kale	20–30
Wheat bran	Over 50

2nd Method The carbohydrate content is shown in the food composition table in the Appendix of this book as *total carbohydrate.*

$$\text{Total carbohydrate} = \begin{matrix}\text{Available}\\\text{carbohydrate}\end{matrix} + \begin{matrix}\text{Dietary}\\\text{fibre}\end{matrix}$$

Experiment 4.1 *qualitative tests for carbohydrate nutrients in foods*
A range of food samples can be tested as follows:

1. *Monosaccharides*

   Glucose is specifically tested for by *test reagent strips*: 'Albustix', 'Quantan CI', 'Tes-tape', 'Clinistix', 'Diastix' and 'BM–Test Glucose'. *Tablet* preparations are also available: 'Quantan RC' and 'Clinitest'. A specific colour change is produced which in some cases can be used to estimate *quantities* in a solution.
2. *Reducing sugars.* These are sugars with *reducing* properties – able to remove oxygen from certain compounds – and include glucose, fructose, lactose and maltose. The sugar is added to a solution of freshly-mixed equal volumes of Fehlings A and B solutions, or to Benedict's solution, which is gently warmed in a water bath. Orange- to red-coloured precipitates indicate reducing sugars (see Figure 4.1).

fig 4.1 *testing for presence of reducing sugars*

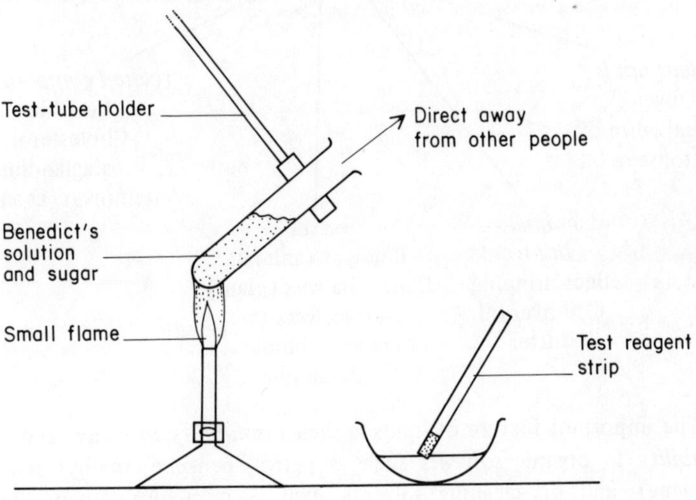

3. *Carbohydrate polysaccharides* produce different colours with iodine solution.
   Amylose in waxy starches - blue.
   amylopectin, dextrins and glycogen - red, brown, to black.
   Ordinary potato or cereal starch gives a blue purple black colour.
   Starch granules can be viewed using a light microscope by dispersing a few grains of starch powder from different sources in a drop of water on a microscope slide and covering with a glass coverslip.
4. *Chemical elements* present in carbohydrates can be tested for qualitatively by Experiment 2.1 - oxygen cannot be tested in this experiment.

4.8 LIPIDS

Lipids contain variable amounts of the chemical elements *carbon*, *hydrogen* and *oxygen*; there is a higher carbon content in lipids compared to carbohydrates. The term *lipid* covers edible oils, fats and waxes of plant or animal origin, and certain related compounds which include sterols and phospholipids. [Mineral *hydrocarbon* oils, greases and waxes are *not* edible or lipids.]

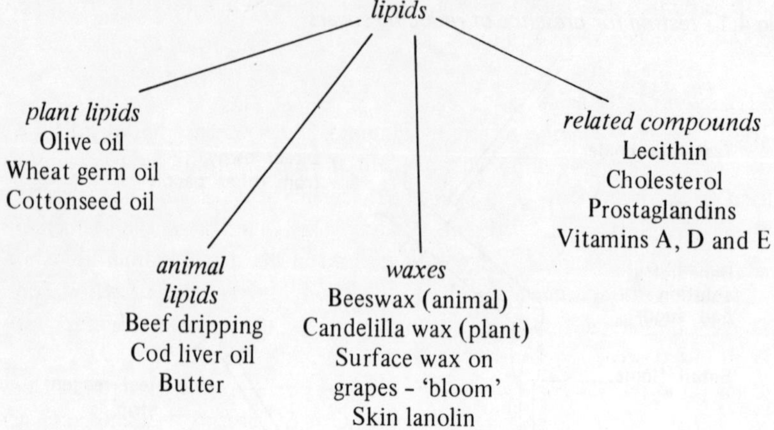

The important feature of lipids is their *insolubility in water*, and their *solubility* in organic *solvents* such as petrol, benzene, methyl benzene (toluene), and dry-cleaning solvents such as tetrachloro-ethane. These solvents are used to extract lipids from foods to determine the *total lipid content* as shown in the food composition tables in Appendix A.

The main *physical* difference between lipid oils and fats is that oils are *liquid* at room temperature, 20°C, and fats remain *solid* at this temperature. The exception is coconut oil which is normally a solid at room temperature.

Composition of lipid oils and fats

Lipid oils and fats are *esters* (see Section 4.5) of propanetriol (glycerol) and different alkanoic (fatty) acids. These esters are called *triesters* or *triglycerides.*

propane 1,2,3-triol (glycerol) + *alkanoic (fatty) acids* ⟶ *propane 1,2,3-triester (triglycerides) or lipid oils and fats*

Each propane 1,2,3-triol (glycerol) molecule combines with *three* (tri) molecules of alkanoic (fatty) acids to form *one* lipid *triester* or triglyceride molecule.

Adipose tissue or fatty tissue is the body lipid store of mammals and human beings. This tissue is found beneath the skin, around the kidneys, in muscle, around the heart and between the intestines, as *fat deposits.* The adipose tissue *cells* contain a large droplet of lipid surrounded by cytoplasm. In a human being the adipose tissue may form an average 14 per cent of the body by weight in males and 25 per cent in females.

Plant lipids are found as lipid *droplets* dispersed within the cell cytoplasm of certain seeds and nuts.

Alkanoic or fatty acids

There are over eighty different alkanoic (fatty) acids, about forty of which are found as components of plant and animal lipids and are *metabolised* in the living cell. Consequently there will be a vast range of triglycerides or triesters with *different* alkanoic (fatty) acids in their molecule structure. The alkanoic (fatty) acids found in plant and animal lipids are of three kinds: *saturated* (no double bonds), *mono-unsaturated* (one double bond), and *polyunsaturated* (two or more double bonds) (see Section 4.4). They are present in variable amounts.

(a) Lipids from *terrestrial animal* sources, beef, mutton and poultry are usually *solid* fats, having a high content of *saturated* alkanoic (fatty) acids mainly hexadecanoic (palmitic) acid, and octadecanoic (stearic) acid. The *mono-unsaturated* octadec-9-enoic (oleic) acid is also present in *high* concentration.

(b) Lipids from *marine* animal sources; fish, seal and whales, are usually *liquid* oils having a high content of the *polyunsaturated* alkanoic (fatty) acids: octadecadienoic (linoleic) and octadecatrienoic (linolenic) acids.

(c) *Plant* lipids with the exception of coconut oil and palm oil are all *liquid* oils and have a *high* content of *polyunsaturated* alkanoic (fatty) acids. The proportion of the different alkanoic (fatty) acids is shown in Table 4.4, also indicating sources of lipids in different foods.

Essential alkanoic or fatty acid

This is the polyunsaturated alkanoic (fatty) acid octadecadienoic (linoleic) acid which is an *essential* component of a human diet, because it cannot be made in the body cells. It is required to form cell membranes and the hormone-like substances called *prostaglandins* which affect the human womb (uterus) muscle contraction. (See also Section 4.13.)

Docosenoic (erucic) acid

This mono-unsaturated alkanoic (fatty) acid component of rape and mustard seed oils is known to have a harmful effect on heart muscle when fed to animals in large quantities. The amount of these oils is restricted to between 2 and 5 per cent in margarine and cooking-oil manufacture.

Waxes and complex lipids

Waxes from plant or animal sources are not essential components of a human diet. Their main purpose is as waterproofing agents for the outer surfaces of plants, fruits, vegetables and animals as in human skin *sebum* wax.

Table 4.4 *proportion of different alkanoic (fatty) acids present in different food lipids*

Food item	*Percentage alkanoic (fatty) acid*		
	Saturated	*Mono-unsaturated*	*Poly-unsaturated "PUFA"*
Plant sources:			
Corn oil	14	29	57
Margarine	34-68	14-38	10-31
Palm oil	52	37	11
Peanut oil	20	50	30
Rapeseed oil	7	68	25
Animal sources:			
Milk, cows	60	33	7
Cod	26	17	57
Beef	45	50	5
Pork	43	48	9
Chicken	35	48	15

Phospholipids include the substance *lecithin* which is a mixture of substances including triesters, propanetriol, alkanoic (fatty) acids, phosphoric acid and an organic base, choline. It is an important component of egg yolk and milk and has *emulsifying* properties.

Cephalins are similar to lecithin, but are components of nerve tissue and brain.

Sterols of animal origin include *cholesterol* (Section 4.3) and the important *bile* salts secreted by the liver (Section 8.9). The plant sterols are called *phytosterols.*

Experiment 4.2 *qualitative tests for lipids*

Procedure

(i) *Lipid extraction*
Visible lipids are lard, butter, margarine and cooking oils and fat on bacon or around kidneys and are easily seen. *Invisible* lipids are those lipids which are part of other substances in nuts, seeds and egg yolk. The invisible fat is extracted by an *organic solvent* such as tetrachloroethane or dry-cleaning fluid, by shaking a food sample in a test tube

with the solvent. The clear extract is poured into a shallow watch-glass and allowed to evaporate leaving the *non-volatile* lipid.

(ii) *Grease spot test*

The visible fat or lipid extract is tested by pressing a piece of writing paper on it and observing the translucent grease spot formed by lipids.

4.9 AMINO-ACIDS

Amino-acids are water soluble compounds composed of *carbon*, *hydrogen*, *oxygen* and *nitrogen*. Three amino-acids (cysteine, cystine and methionine) also contain *sulphur* whilst the amino-acids present in the thyroid gland also contain *iodine* in addition to C, H, O and N. These chemical elements, excepting iodine, can be tested for by the procedure in Experiment 2.1.

Essential amino-acids

There are over twenty-eight different amino-acids but of these only eighteen are important as components of the body tissue fluid, cell cytoplasm and blood. Ten amino-acids, called *essential amino-acids* are needed in the diet of human beings, these ten cannot be made in the body-cells, whereas the remaining *non-essential* amino-acids can be made in the human body cells from other nitrogen-containing compounds, or amino-acids, in the diet (see Table 4.5 and Section 10.1). Most foods of plant origin have a lower

Table 4.5 *the main amino-acids in human tissue and as food components*

Essential amino-acids (must be present in human diet)	*Non-essential amino-acids*
Isoleucine	Alanine
Leucine	Aspartic acid
Lysine	Cysteine
Methionine	Glutamic acid (used as a flavouring agent – SOY sauce)
Phenylalanine	Glycine
Threonine	Hydroxyproline
Tryptophan	Proline
Valine	Serine
Infants also require:	
Histidine, and possibly	
Arginine	

NOTE Cystine and tyrosine, although non-essential, have a sparing effect in the needs of methionine and phenylalanine

content of *methionine*, *tryptophan* and *cystine* than foods of animal origin. Certain cereals have a low content of *lysine* and *threonine* (see Table 10.3).

Functional groups

All amino-acids contain *two* functional groups, the *carboxylic*, –COOH, group present in organic acids (see Section 4.4) and an *amino*, $-NH_2$; this has *basic* properties similar to other organic bases or amines.

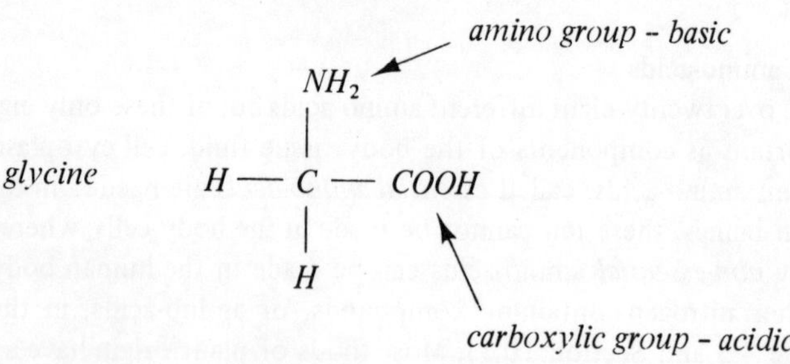

The formula of the amino-acid *glycine* (2-aminoethanoic acid) shows the presence of the two different functional groups.

All amino-acids are soluble in water the main component of cell cytoplasm.

Meat and yeast extracts have a high content of water-soluble *free* amino-acids, which are also present to a lesser extent in certain fruits, vegetables and fish. Soups and gravies may also contain *free* amino-acids. The sweetener *aspartame* is derived from aspartic acid and phenylalanine.

4.10 NUCLEIC ACIDS OR POLYNUCLEOTIDES

There are two main kinds of nucleic acids or polynucleotides in living cells: (a) the human body cells *nucleus* contains about 6 picogrammes of DNA (deoxyribonucleic acid) and (b) the *cytoplasm* contains RNA, ribonucleic acid (see Section 3.4).

Nucleic acids are very large macromolecules composed of three units, ribose or deoxyribose *sugar*, *phosphates* and organic *bases* called purines or pyrimidines. (See also Section 8.9.)

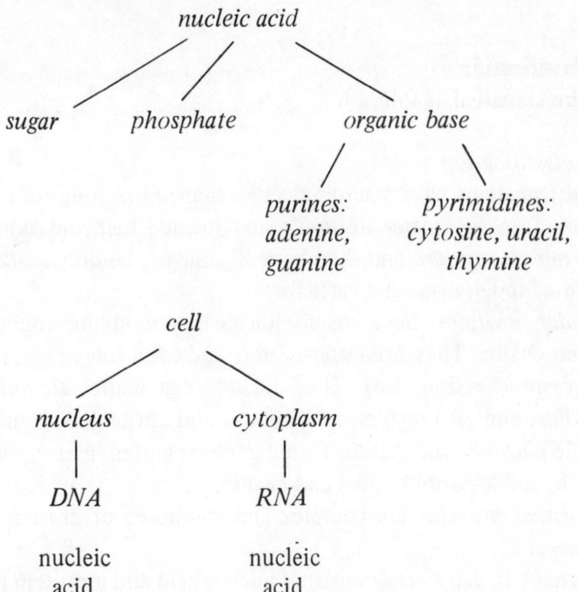

4.11 PROTEINS

The synthesis of proteins occurs in living cells using the twenty or more different amino-acids which are present in the cell cytoplasm and provided by the tissue fluid (Sections 1.4 and 4.9). The nucleus DNA nucleic acid *decides* which amino-acids are to be used to make a *specific* protein, it then *transmits* a *pattern*-coded message by the cytoplasm RNA nucleic acid which makes certain the correct type of protein is made on the *ribosomes* of the cell endoplasmic reticulum (Section 3.3).

Different amino-acids will be selected to make different proteins, for example human milk protein is made from a different selection of amino-acids from those used to make cows' milk protein.

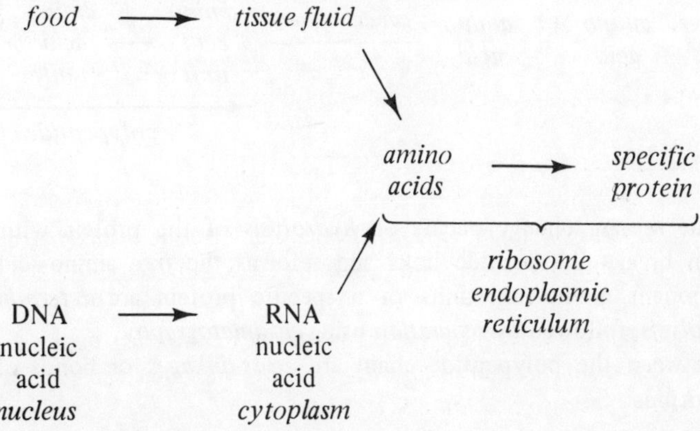

Protein classification
Proteins are classified as follows:

Chemical classification
(a) *Fibrous* proteins have macromolecules shaped like long coils or folded chains. They are *water insoluble* and include hair and skin *keratin*, meat muscle *myosin*, and skin, bone, ligaments, tendons, *collagen*, and *elastin* of tough meat and cartilage.
(b) *Globular proteins* have macromolecules resembling round shaped tangled chains. They are *water soluble* and form sols or gels in the cell cytoplasm (Section 2.6). They include egg white, *albumin*, blood *globulins*, and also enzymes, hormones and antibodies. Plant proteins include *glutenin* and *gliadin* forming wheat gluten, maize *zein*, potato *tuberin*, and *legumin* in peas and beans.
(c) *Conjugated proteins* are complex and composed of protein and non-protein units.

Nucleoproteins in cell nuclei consist of nucleic acid and a protein (histone).
Glycoproteins are uronic acids and proteins in lubricant fluids, mucous and bone joint fluid, and blood plasma.
Lipoproteins in cell membranes and blood are composed of lipid and protein units.
Phosphoprotein, for example, milk *casein* contains phosphate and protein.

Protein structure
Proteins are *polymers* formed by *condensation* of monomer units, the amino-acids (see Section 4.6). The amino-acid units join together by means of a *peptide link* to form a long *polypeptide chain.*

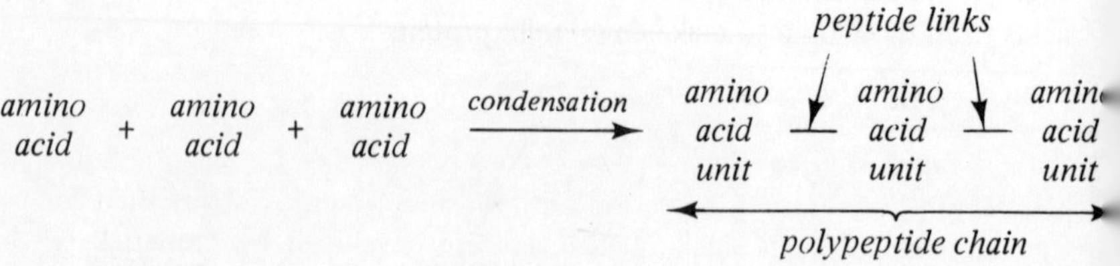

The *reverse* change occurs on *hydrolysis* of the protein with water which breaks the peptide links and reforms the *free* amino-acids. The component amino-acid units of a specific protein are *determined* by *hydrolysis*, followed by *separation* using *chromatography*.

Between the polypeptide chain are *cross-linkages* or bonds of three main kinds:

(i) *ionic* or salt bonds between electric charges of opposite chains,
(ii) *hydrogen* bonds by sharing a hydrogen atom between opposite chains;
(iii) *disulphide* bonds formed from two sulphur atoms from cysteine amino acid in opposite chains. These are very strong bonds compared with the weaker ionic and hydrogen bonds.

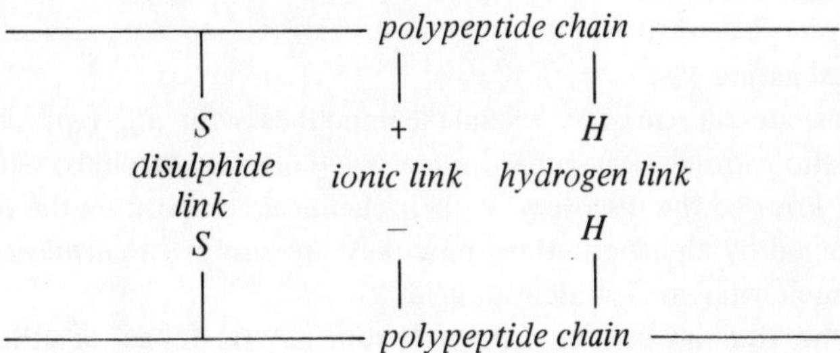

Food protein content

Food composition tables (see Appendix A) show the protein content as grammes per 100 gramme of the food item. This is determined *indirectly* by measuring the *nitrogen* content by complex chemical methods.

Experiment 4.3 *qualitative tests for proteins*

(i) *Biuret test* Add a few drops of sodium hydroxide solution to the sample, then add 3 drops of 1 per cent copper II sulphate solution. Leave to stand and observe a violet to pink colour which forms with most proteins.
(ii) *Protein test papers* 'Quantan DT', 'Albustix' and Boehringer 'Albym' test reagent strips are pressed against fresh moist samples. A colour change of yellow to green, or green to blue, indicates the presence of certain proteins.

4.12 **VITAMINS**

Vitamins are *organic substances* present in *minute* amounts, measured in *milligrammes* (mg) and *microgrammes* (μg) per 100g of natural food. For this reason they escaped detection until sensitive and accurate methods of measurement of such small quantities were developed by Frederick G. Hopkins (1861-1947) and later researchers. Prior to this it was believed that a diet of water, proteins, carbohydrates, lipids and certain *macro-minerals* was sufficient for a healthy human body.

It is now known that vitamins are essential for *controlling metabolic processes*, and when *absent* from the diet cause *deficiency* disorders seen as growth and metabolism defects, and other detectable clinical signs and symptoms, seen in scurvy, rickets and other vitamin deficiency diseases (see Section 9.3 and Table 9.4).

Vitamin-deficient diets prepared from pure 100 per cent lipids, sugars and proteins, together with pure calcium and iron minerals were fed to laboratory rats which later developed various deficiency disorders because of lack of essential vitamins. When a supplement of *fresh milk* was added to the diet the rats overcame the deficiencies by the vitamins present in small quantities in the milk.

Chemical nature

Vitamins are all complex organic compounds with *different* chemical composition from each other; some are complex alcohols, acids and amines. Prior to the discovery of their chemical composition the vitamins were named by alphabet letters, now they are also given *chemical names*, for example vitamin C *or* ascorbic acid.

All the vitamins can be *extracted* from natural foods, or other plant and animal sources. Many vitamins are now *synthesised* or manufactured chemically; a few are synthesised in the human body tissues, and by gut symbiotic bacteria.

Solubility

Vitamins are either *water-soluble* - for example vitamin C and vitamins of the B group and folic acid, or *lipid-soluble* - vitamins A, D, E and K.

Vegetable cooking water, clear soups, fruit juices and vegetable extracts will contain most of the water-soluble vitamins namely ascorbic acid vitamin C and members of the B group of vitamins. Meat dripping, gravies and thick soups will contain most of the lipid-soluble vitamins A, D, E and K. Similarly natural vegetable oils, butter and cream are the other sources. Table 4.6 summarises the main vitamins, their sources, and functions in the body. The food composition tables in the Appendix show the main vitamin content of foods.

Other water-soluble vitamins

Vitamin B_6 (*pyridoxine*) *pantothenic acid* and *biotin* are essential for human health and occur in sufficient quantities in a range of foods or are made in the gut by intestinal bacteria. Disorders caused by a shortage of these vitamins are uncommon.

Vitamin B_{12} (*cyanocobalamin*) is a bright red crystalline substance which contains an atom of *cobalt* in the complex molecule. It is found only in food from animal sources - liver, kidney, meat, milk, eggs, fish, cheese. Some cyanocabalamin is synthesised by symbiotic bacteria in the human intestine (Section 10.5). It is measured in *microgrammes* (μg). Strict vegetarians - vegans - are likely to suffer a deficiency of this vitamin and may develop *pernicious anaemia* (Section 9.3). It functions with folic acid in cell division and the formation of new red blood cells.

Other lipid-soluble vitamins
Vitamin E (tocopherols) and vitamin K, called the anti-haemorrhagic vitamin, are both essential for human health, and occur in sufficient quantities in a large range of foods. Disorders caused by shortage of these vitamins are uncommon in the UK diet. Vitamin K is formed by synthesis from symbiotic bacteria in the human intestine - the vitamin is involved in the blood-clotting mechanism in wound-healing. Table 4.7 shows the main lipid-soluble vitamins.

Experiment 4.4 *qualitative testing for vitamin C (ascorbic acid)*
A blue coloured solution of 2:6 dichlorophenol indophenol, DCPIP, is prepared by dissolving one tablet in 50cm^3 of distilled water. This blue solution is decolorised by *reducing agents* which include vitamin C ascorbic acid.

Fresh fruit juices or water extracts are treated with 5 per cent ethanoic (acetic) acid to inactivate enzymes that destroy vitamin C. Various food samples are then tested using the DCPIP reagent solution.

Preserved fruit juices may contain sulphur dioxide, (a reducing agent and preservative), this would decolorise the reagent.

4.13 **VITAMINOIDS**

These are substances with a *vitamin-like* action which are essential components of the human diet. Shortage of these substances in the diet may cause deficiency disorders with various symptoms.

Essential alkanoic or fatty acid (see Section 4.8) called octadecadienoic (linoleic) acid; a shortage in the diet of babies causes skin and hair disorders. Human milk contains almost *five* times more octadecadienoic (linoleic) acid than cows' milk whilst artificial milk feeds contain 10 to 8 times more (Section 10.9). Essential fatty acid deficiency is a rare condition in the UK. Sources of essential alkanoic or fatty acids include sunflower, maize, soya bean, and peanut *oils* (Section 4.8).

The following substances *may* be essential in human nutrition, but no *specific* deficiency disorders are known arising from their absence in the human diet:

(i) *Inositol* (Section 4.3), component of heart, brain and muscle.
(ii) *Choline*, a component of lecithin (Section 4.8), deficiency causes liver and kidney damage.

Table 4.6 *the main water soluble vitamins*

Letter, chemical name and diet measurement unit	*Main sources (In decreasing order of abundance)*	*Function in human body and storage*
B_1 *Thiamin*, mg. White crystalline solid, a complex amine.	Brewers' yeast, rice and wheat bran, yeast extract. Breakfast cereals, wholemeal flour, soya bean flour, pork, ham, bacon and pork fat, meat offal (heart, liver, kidney). Nuts, potatoes and green vegetables. Milk, eggs and cheese. *Added* to white flour and breakfast cereals in UK. *Small* amounts made by intestinal symbiotic bacteria. Levels can be affected by antibiotic drugs.	Catalyst in energy release from *carbohydrates* in cells of brain, nerves, heart, kidneys and muscles. No storage, excess excreted in urine.
B_2 *Riboflavin*, mg. Orange yellow fluorescent crystalline solid. Ribose sugar and coloured flavin compound.	Brewers' yeast, yeast extract, meat extract, liver, kidney, meat and fish. Milk, cheese, eggs, green leafy vegetables. Dried fruits, nuts, wholemeal flour. Beer. *Large* amounts made by intestinal symbiotic bacteria, and can therefore be affected by antibiotic drugs.	Catalyst in energy release and usage in cell respiration. Some storage in liver, heart and kidneys.
Nicotinic acid (formerly *niacin*), mg. White crystalline solid. Carboxylic acid compound. (Sometimes called vitamin PP)	Meat extract, yeast extract, wheat and rice bran, liver, kidney, meat, chicken and fish. Added to breakfast cereals. Human body makes nicotinic acid from the essential amino-acid *tryptophan*. SIXTY Tryptophan parts by weight —(Other B vitamins as catalysts)→ ONE Nicotinic acid. parts by weight Some also synthesised by intestinal bacteria, and therefore affected by antibiotic drugs.	Energy release catalyst in cell respiration. Stored in the liver, and found in all tissues.

Free *folic acid (folate)* μg. Orange yellow solid. Complex substance partly linked to amino-acid glutamic acid. (Sometimes called vitamin M or vitamin B_C)	Spinach, broccoli, liver, kidney, fish, peas, beans, yeast, milk, cereals and orange. Synthesised by intestinal symbiotic bacteria, and therefore affected by antibiotic drugs. (*Free* folic acid forms 25 per cent of the *total* folic acid in a food the remaining 75 per cent is in a poorly absorbed form combined with glutamic acid. Appendix A shows *free* folic acid content)	For synthesis of *nucleic acids*, and essential for *cell division*. Found mainly in liver, red blood cells, and blood plasma (See anaemias, Section 9.3)
C *Ascorbic acid*, mg. White crystalline solid. A simple sugar-like compound formed from glucose.	Found in all *flowering plant* cells, blackcurrants, citrus fruits, broccoli, cabbage, spinach, watercress, parsley; also in liver, milk, eggs, meat. Most animals *except* certain mammals and human beings can synthesise their own vitamin C in the *liver*. Aspirin and certain birth control 'pills' can affect the body's vitamin C level.	1. Essential for iron absorption in small intestine 2. Connective tissue metabolism – especially scar tissue, bones and teeth. 3. Anti-stress and protection against cold, chills and damp. Prevents muscle fatigue. 4. Anti-scorbutic, the prevention and cure of scurvy. 5. Important in breakdown of cholesterol. 6. Reduces formation of carcinogenic nitrosamines.

Table 4.7 *the main lipid soluble vitamins*

Letter, chemical name and diet measurement unit	*Main sources (In decreasing order of abundance)*	*Function in human body and storage*
A. *Retinol*, mg. Yellow solid. A complex hydrocarbon with an *alcohol* group in molecule. *Carotenes* are hydrocarbons, yellow to red pigments in fruits and vegetables; they are vitamin A *precursors*.	(i) Retinol or preformed vitamin A found in fish livers, halibut, cod, shark, and sheep or ox liver. Butter, margarine, eggs, cheese and milk. (ii) *Carotenes* are *changed into retinol* in the intestine lining. Found in palm oil, carrots, green leafy vegetables, sweet potatoes, apricots and tomatoes, as well as in milk, butter, cream and egg yolk, giving *creamy* colour. [Six parts by weight of β-carotene is equal to ONE part by weight of retinol. β CAROTENE six parts by weight $\longrightarrow$ Retinol ONE part by weight	1. Essential for night vision. 2. Healthy epithelial surfaces and mucous membranes. Storage in liver sufficient for many months without dietary intake. *Harmful* in large doses causing skin, hair, bone and liver disorders. Overdosage with certain vitamins is called *hypervitaminosis* (Section 9.4.)
and		
	Chief source – action of sunlight (ultra-violet ray) on skin	
D. *Calciferols* D_3 *Cholecalciferol* μg. A complex sterol.	Found only in animals. Tunny fish, halibut and cod liver oils. Herrings, salmon, margarine, eggs, milk, butter, liver, cheese.	1. Concerned with *calcium* and *phosphate* metabolism. 2. Necessary for bone and teeth development.
D_2 – *Ergocalciferol* An irradiated sterol.	This form of vitamin D is made by exposing yeasts to ultra-violet rays. It is added to margarine and processed milks and used in preparing vitamin *supplements*.	3. Anti-rachitic, prevents rickets or bending of bones through vitamin D deficiency.
Pro-vitamin D_3.	This substance is in the oily secretion of *human skin* as 7-dehydrocholesterol. It is changed into vitamin D_3 cholecalciferol by means of SUNLIGHT or ultra-violet rays.	Most stored in *fat depot* beneath skin, some in liver. *Hypervitaminosis* (Section 9.4.) *Very harmful* in large doses causing loss of appetite, vomiting, wasting, diarrhoea and kidney damage.

4.14 MINERAL SUBSTANCES

About twenty different mineral substances or ions are essential for life in most animals including human beings, the daily dietary unit of measurement being in milligrammes for the major elements Ca, Mg, P, Na, K, Cl and in microgrammes for the trace elements. Many mineral elements become *poisonous* to the body when taken in large amounts as in *accidental poisoning* by iron, iodine, fluorine; whilst lead, mercury, arsenic and cadmium are *cumulative body poisons* collecting in body tissues.

Table 4.8 lists the more important mineral substances essential to the human diet together with their sources and functions. Appendix A shows the *iron* and *calcium* content of foods.

Distribution in cell fluids

The mineral ions or electrolytes are found in the *tissue fluid* around the cells and also inside the cells in the *intracellular fluid*. The tissue fluid contains most of the *sodium*, *calcium* and *chloride* ions, whilst the intracellular fluid contains most of the *potassium*, *magnesium* and *phosphate* ions. The tissue fluid contains 14 times more *sodium chloride* salt than does the intracellular fluid, thus providing cells with an external environment somewhat similar to warm seawater, the environment of the first living organisms on earth.

Other mineral substances

The mineral substances listed in Table 4.9 are essential for human health, a shortage of these substances in the diet is rare since they occur in sufficient quantities in a range of foods. In addition to the subtances listed in the table the following are also essential for human health: chromium, cobalt, manganese, molybdenum, selenium, zinc.

Experiment 4.5 *qualitative testing for certain mineral substances*

(i) *Ash content of food*

Carefully place a 5g sample of a *dried* food in a porcelain or silica crucible. Heat gently at first over a bunsen burner flame and then more strongly as the protein, lipid, carbohydrate and vitamin content burn away. The remaining ash is the *mineral* substance content of the food.

(ii) *Flame testing food ash*

Carefully moisten the ash with a little concentrated hydrochloric acid (CAUTION – POISONOUS AND CORROSIVE). Hold a clean platinum wire in the bunsen burner flame and note how it glows *white* when hot. Dip the platinum wire in the acid-moistened ash and return it to

Table 4.8 *major mineral substances, sources and function*

Mineral substance and total in human body	*Sources (In decreasing order of abundance)*	*Function*
Ca *Calcium* 1 kg. Mostly in bones and teeth. Calcium ion content of tissue fluid is *twice* that of intracellular fluid.	*Calcium carbonate* (chalk) added to white wheat flour. *Hard* water. Cheeses; dried milk; skimmed, condensed and fresh milk; salmon; whitebait and sardines, eggs and meat. Nuts; vegetables; oatmeal; wholemeal flour; white wheat flour; bread, and baking powder.	1. Teeth and bone formation. 2. Blood clotting. 3. Muscle contraction.
PO_4 *Phosphate* 780 g. 88% in bones and teeth. PO_4 in intracellular fluid is 60 times the concentration in tissue fluid.	*Found in all foodstuffs* in adequate amounts. Meat; fish; cheese; eggs, milk and green vegetables. Yeast extract.	1. Teeth and bone formation as calcium phosphate. 2. Nucleic acid component DNA and RNA. 3. Energy-rich compound ATP adenosine triphosphate in muscles. *One phosphate bond breakage = 30 kJ energy.* 4. Nervous system component.

Fe *Iron* 5 g. 70 per cent in blood as compound *haem*. 15% in muscle as compound *myoglobin.* 15% in liver as iron store compound *ferritin.*	*Animal origin food*: Black pudding; liver; beef; mutton; eggs; fish, cockles, snails. Iron mainly as *organic* compound and is better absorbed in gut. *Plant origin food*: Black treacle; cocoa; curry powder; parsley; dried fruits; pulses; oatmeal, wholemeal and white flour. Red wines. Iron mainly as *inorganic* compound less easily absorbed. Ferric iron salts added to white flour. Ferrous iron salts used in medicines.	1. Blood *haemoglobin* formation in red blood cells and oxygen 2. Muscle *myoglobin* formation. *Harmful* in large doses in the inorganic form causing *siderosis* because of excess iron in body cells, resulting in liver disorders (Section 9.4).

Table 4.9 *mineral substances essential for human health*

mineral substance: amount in human body	*Main sources*	*Function*
Na^+ *Sodium* 100 g tissue fluid content 14 times that of intracellular fluid (*inside* the cell)	Table salt, cheese, bacon, kippers, butter, sausages and canned vegetables	These three substances have similar and closely related functions: 1. blood plasma and tissue fluid composition.
Cl^- *Chloride* 95 g tissue fluid content 25 times that of intracellular fluid	Table salt, cheese, bacon, kippers, butter, sausages and canned vegetables	2. nerve message transmission. 3. muscle contraction. 4. pH control in tissues. 5. water and ion control in body (see Section 8.19). Chloride also important in formation of gastric juice (hydrochloride acid)
K^- *Potassium* 140 g intracellular fluid content 30 times that of tissue fluid	Fruit, vegetables, milk, meats and potatoes	As above except for gastric juices
Mg^{++} *Magnesium* 19 g intracellular fluid 10 times that of tissue fluid	Green vegetables and cereals	1. Component of bones and teeth 2. ATP energy metabolism in muscles
Cu^{++} *Copper* 0.07 g	Liver, green vegetables, oysters	1. Blood haemoglobin formation 2. Skin and hair pigment formation
I^- *Iodine* 0.01 g	Fish, table salt and drinking water	Thyroid gland function
F^- *Fluoride* 2.6 g	Fish, drinking water and tea; toothpaste	Bone and teeth formation; prevents tooth decay (*dental caries*)

the burner flame. Observe if any of the following colours are seen in the burner flame: bright yellow - sodium.

The following are best confirmed by viewing through a cobalt blue glass:
brick red - calcium
lilac - potassium
blue-green - copper.

4.15 QUESTIONS

1. Explain the differences between a hydrocarbon, a carbohydrate and a lipid. To which group of these substances can the term unsaturated apply?
2. Give a brief outline classification of the carbohydrates, discuss their occurrence in foods of plant and animal origin. What is dietary fibre composed of?
3. Write short explanatory notes with reference to food and nutrition on: (a) essential oils; (b) essential amino-acids; (c) essential alkanoic or fatty acid.
4. Which vitamins and mineral substances are mainly concerned with energy release from food? Which minerals and vitamins are mainly concerned with the body structure and maintenance?
5. Construct a table showing food components which are water-*soluble* and those which are *insoluble* in water.
6. The main chemical elements composing the human body are carbon, hydrogen, oxygen, nitrogen, phosphorus, sulphur, iron and calcium. Which *nutrients* provide these chemical elements, and which *foodstuffs* are good sources for these nutrients.

CHAPTER 5

FOOD ENERGY

5.1 ENERGY

Compounents of living cells are able to *release energy* stored in certain food nutrients. This energy is able to do *work* for various kinds of cell activities; muscle contraction, protein synthesis or the production of heat.

Energy exists in different *forms*; those of importance in nutrition are:

1. *Light or solar energy*, also called electromagnetic radiation, X-rays and ultra-violet rays (see Figure 7.2). This is the *main* source of energy on Earth for photosynthesis (Section 3.8) and vitamin D synthesis in the skin.
2. *Chemical energy* provided by certain food nutrients in the form of the *energy-rich* compound, adenosine triphosphate (ATP) (Section 5.4).
3. *Mechanical energy* seen as the movement of muscles or muslce *contraction*.
4. *Electrical energy* is essential to the functioning of nerves and the brain; this is detectable by electroencephalograph (EEG) for brain activity, and electrocardiography (ECG) for heart muscle activity.
5. *Heat energy* (detectable by thermometers) provides the essential warmth for cell homeostasis (Sections 1.3 and 3.6).

Living cells are able to *change* energy from one form into another:

light energy —— *cell chloroplasts* ——→ *chemical energy*

chemical energy —— *muscle cells* ——→ *mechanical energy*

chemical energy —— *nerve cells* ——→ *electrical energy*

The release of *heat* energy accompanies most energy conversion processes; it is also the form into which other forms are finally changed in living cells. This *heat* then radiates from the body into outer space (see Section 3.11, flow of energy).

5.2 ENERGY MEASUREMENT

Since the various forms of energy can be *converted* into *heat*, energy is measured in one unit called the joule (J) kilojoule (kJ) or megajoule (MJ).

One kilojoule (kJ) = 1 000 J

One megajoule (MJ) = 1 000 00 J = 1 000 kJ

(See Section 2.4.)

Prior to 1970 the *calorie* was used, one calorie being approximately equal to 4.2 joules:

One calorie = 4.2J

A *calorie* is equal to the amount of *heat* needed to raise the temperature of *one gramme of water* through one degree Celsius; this temperature rise is achieved also by 4.2 Joules.

Calorimeters

Calorimeters are the instruments used to measure heat energy, the heat produced being gathered in a known weight of water and the temperature rise recorded.

The *bomb calorimeter* (as shown in Plate 5.1) is used to measure the *energy value* of foods and also certain fuels.

5.3 CHEMICAL COMBUSTION OF FOODSTUFFS

Glucose, $C_6H_{12}O_6$ is available as a white, sweet-tasting solid which can undergo *chemical combustion* or burning; the chemical change is shown in the following equation:

$$C_6H_{12}O_6 + 6O_2 \longrightarrow 6CO_2 + 6H_2O + \text{heat energy}$$

180g *glucose*	*oxygen from air*	*carbon dioxide gas*	*water vapour*	2.8 MJ

Plate 5.1 *a ballistic bomb calorimeter used to measure energy values of foods (Gallenkamp)*

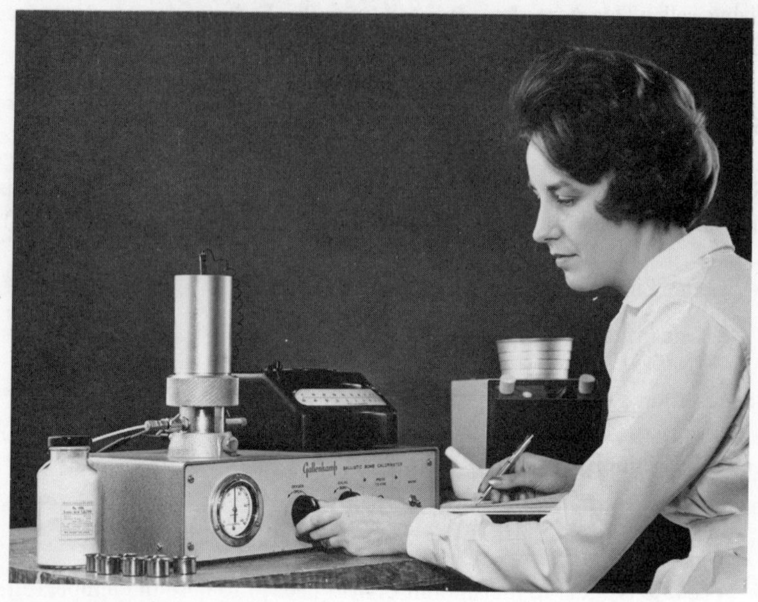

The heat produced by the complete combustion of one mole (or molecule weight in grammes) or 180g glucose is measured in a bomb calorimeter and found to be 2.8MJ or 2 800kJ; this is called the *heat of combustion* of glucose (see Section 2.8 and Figure 2.4).

Features of chemical combustion of glucose

1. *Occurrence* Takes place outside living cells as a laboratory reaction.
2. *State* The glucose is in a *solid* state surrounded by gaseous oxygen or air.
3. *Mechanism* The reaction mechanism is chemical and occurs rapidly, and is controlled by increasing or decreasing the oxygen supply.
4. *Energy* All the energy is released in *one* form as *heat* at a high temperature.
5. *Products* Both the carbon dioxide and water are in gaseous forms.

The *heat of combustion*, measured in a bomb calorimeter in kilojoules per gramme, for different pure food substances, is shown in Table 5.1.

Table 5.1 *heats of combustion for pure food substances*

	Food substance	*Heat of combustion* kJ/g
Carbohydrates	Glucose	16.1
	Starch	17.2
Lipids	Peanut oil (100% lipid)	37.0
	Butter (80% lipid)	30.2
Protein	Meat protein	22.4
	Egg protein	23.4
Alcohol	Ethanol	29.8
Salts	Sodium chloride	NIL
	Water	NIL

Experiment 5.1 *to estimate the heat of combustion of a cooking oil*

Procedure

(i) Place a *known weight* of cooking oil in a glass burner lamp.

(ii) Place exactly 200cm^3 of water in the large test tube supported as shown in figure 5.1, and insert a narrow range thermometer and stirrer into the water.

(iii) Record the initial temperature of the water.

(iv) Light the cooking oil at the burner wick and allow the flame to impinge on the test tube to heat the water. Stir the water gently.

(v) Allow the water temperature to rise by exactly 20°C, then extinguish the flame.

(vi) Carefully weigh the burner to determine its *decrease* in weight due to combustion of oil.

Calculation

(a) Let weight of oil burnt equal A grammes.

(b) Heat produced by combustion of A grammes of cooking oil in joules = Weight of water × Temperature rise × 4.2.

(c) Heat of combustion of cooking oil in joules per gramme

$$= \frac{\text{Weight of water} \times \text{Temperature rise} \times 4.2}{\text{Weight of oil burnt}}$$

5.4 CELL ENERGY RELEASE

Living cells release energy from the *energy-rich* compound *adenosine triphosphate* (ATP) which is mainly formed from *glucose* present in the

Fig 5.1 *simple apparatus to determine approximate energy value of a cooking oil*

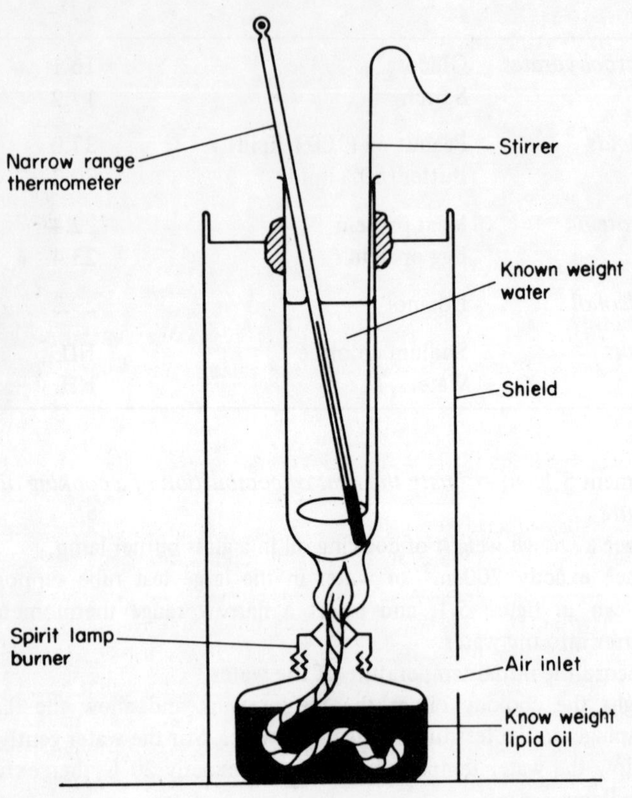

cell fluid. This *biological* process of energy release is called *respiration*, and is very different from the chemical process of combustion.

Respiration occurs by two methods in the human body. The main method of respiration is *aerobic* respiration using air oxygen, and a secondary method called *anaerobic* respiration – without air oxygen.

In *both* processes of respiration ATP is formed. Aerobic respiration forms *twenty* times the amount of ATP that is formed by anaerobic respiration.

Energy release from ATP

When energy is needed for a cell activity it is drawn from the cell store of ATP. One mole (molecule weight in grammes) of ATP will provide 33kJ of energy, and at the same time the compound adenosine *di*phosphate

(ADP) is formed; this can be *recycled* to reform more ATP by joining with more phosphate ions. Karl Lohmann (born 1898) a biochemist, was the first to discover ATP.

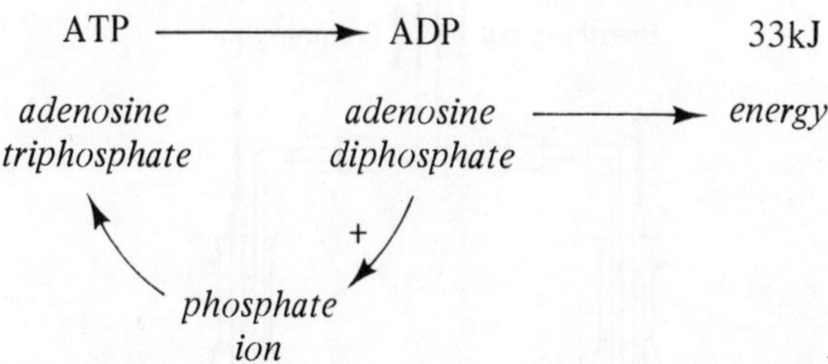

It is seen from these chemical changes how important *phosphate* ions are as mineral components of a diet, in bringing about energy transfer and release.

5.5 CELL RESPIRATION WITH OXYGEN

Oxygen is drawn into the *lungs* (Fig. 3.4) where it *diffuses* through the thin moist cell walls of the *alveoli* into the blood and is combined with the iron-containing *haemoglobin* of the red blood cells to form *oxyhaemoglobin*. The heart circulates the blood cells and fluid plasma to supply living cells with the *tissue fluid* (see Table 1.1, Section 8.14 and Fig 8.6). Oxygen then passes by diffusion into the living cell, whilst glucose enters by active transport using cell energy for this purpose.

Both oxygen and glucose reach the cell *mitochondria* where the actual process of energy release occurs. The mechanism of energy release is complex and passes through many intermediate stages, all of which are catalysed by *enzymes* and *coenzymes* of vitamins of the *B group*. Sir Hans Krebs (1900–81) a biochemist, discovered the chemical mechanism which takes place in cell mitochondria.

Products of aerobic respiration

One mole (molecular weight in grammes) or 180 grammes of glucose provides the following important products by aerobic respiration:

1. *Carbon dioxide* which is returned to the lungs dissolved in the blood for expulsion into the air (see Figure 5.2).
2. *Metabolic water* which becomes an important component of the body fluid.
3. *ATP* is formed, 38 molecules of this energy-rich substance is produced either for immediate use or for temporary cell storage. It has an energy value of about 1.1MJ.

Fig 5.2 *apparatus to demonstrate that carbon dioxide is present in exhaled human breath*

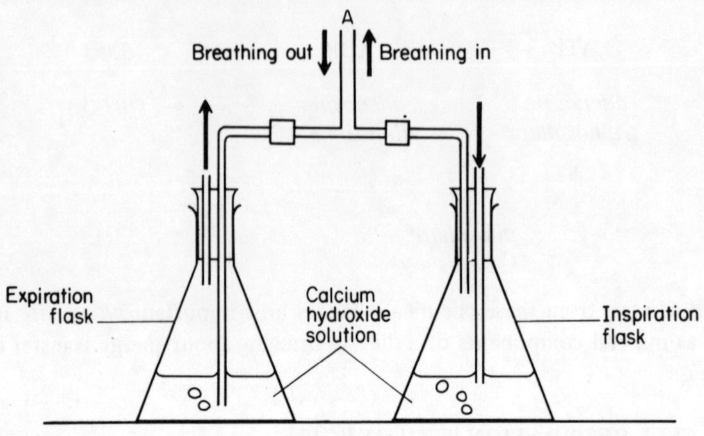

4. *Heat energy* amounting to about 1.7MJ is produced providing the body cells with warmth which is then radiated or lost from the body as heat.

Aerobic respiration of one mole (180g) of glucose can be summarised as follows:

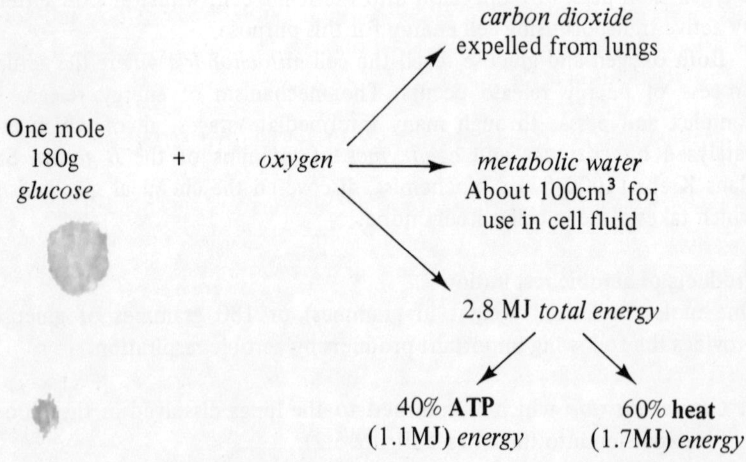

5.6 CELL RESPIRATION WITHOUT OXYGEN

When the human body undertakes very strenuous exercise *insufficient* oxygen may reach the cells. In these circumstances the cell obtains energy from its ATP stores, and also by anaerobic respiration of glucose. The glucose present in *skeletal muscle* cells is changed by cell enzymes into *lactic acid* (2-hydroxypropanoic acid) and *two* molecules of ATP produced together with *heat* energy.

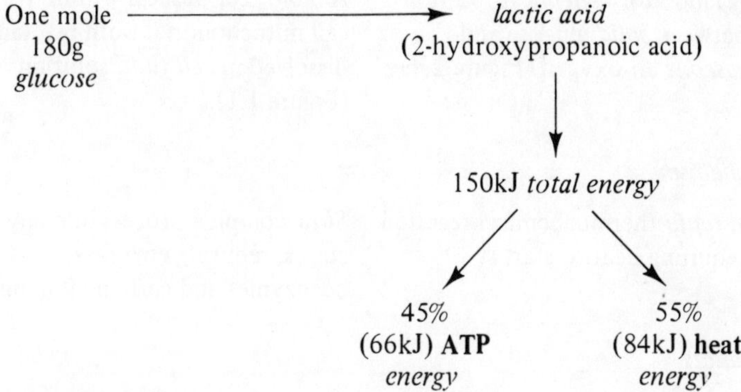

This process can only occur for a *short time*, otherwise lactic (2-hydroxypropanoic) acid accumulates in the muscle cells causing poisoning experienced as cramp, pain and fatigue. The lactic (2-hydroxypropanoic) acid is rapidly changed back into glucose on *resting*. At the same time breathing is very rapid and deep after strenuous exercise to repay the *oxygen debt* needed to restore homeostasis in the cells.

By contrast, anaerobic respiration can occur in green plants, and certain fungal yeasts, to produce ethanol, carbon dioxide, ATP and heat energy (see Section 6.12).

5.7 COMPARISON OF RESPIRATION AND COMBUSTION

Chemical combustion (see Section 2.8 and Figure 2.4) and cell aerobic respiration of glucose are processes which resemble one another by being represented by the *same chemical equation* and in the *total energy* produced:

$$C_6H_{12}O_6 \quad + \quad 6O_2 \longrightarrow 6H_2O \quad + \quad 6CO_2 \quad + \quad \text{ENERGY}$$

$C_6H_{12}O_6$	$6O_2$	$6H_2O$	$6CO_2$	ENERGY
One mole 180g *glucose*	*oxygen*	*water*	*carbon dioxide*	2.8MJ

Otherwise the two processes are very different from each other as shown in Table 5.2.

Table 5.2 *comparison of chemical combustion and respiration*

	Chemical combustion	*Aerobic respiration*
Occurrence		
	A laboratory *chemical* reaction between *solid* glucose and *gaseous* air oxygen (Figure 2.4)	A *biological* process within living cell mitochondria. Both reactants dissolved in *cell fluid* solution (Figure 1.1)
Mechanism		
	A *rapid* thermochemical reaction requiring heat to start it	*Slow* complex process in many stages, requring enzymes, coenzymes and certain vitamins
Products		
	Both gases, CO_2 and H_2O H_2O vapour	One a gas, CO_2, and liquid *metabolic water*
Energy forms		
	100% heat	55% heat 45% ATP

When ATP is *used* in cell activities a *further* quantity of heat is produced as in muscle contraction, thus explaining how the human body heats up during muscular exercise.

5.8 ENERGY VALUE OF FOOD NUTRIENTS

The main source of ATP in the human body cells is *glucose* provided by various carbohydrates, together with *fatty (alkanoic) acids* from different *lipids*. Other *secondary* sources can include *amino-acids* and glucose made from *proteins*, together with propanetriol (glycerine) from *lipids*.

Mineral ions, water and vitamins have *no energy value* to the body, whilst dietary fibre which is not digested in the human gut is also of no energy value. Consequently the energy content of a foodstuff is located in the carbohydrate, lipid, protein and ethanol content of a food. This is measured by *analysis* and recorded as a *percentage* (or grammes per 100 grammes) in *food composition tables*.

Metabolisable or available energy
The energy provided to *living cells* by energy-providing nutrients, can *differ* from the heat of combustion of the same nutrients listed in Table 5.1. This is caused by losses arising from incomplete digestion when some nutrient is lost in the faeces. This loss may amount to about 1 per cent in carbohydrates and 5 per cent in lipids, and is *nil* in the case of ethanol

$$\text{Metabolisable or available energy} = \text{Heat of combustion} - \text{Digestive losses}$$

In the case of proteins the losses due to digestion and in the formation of carbamide (urea) excreted in the urine, can be between 25 and 29 per cent.

The metabolisable or *available energy* of different nutrients is compared with their heats of combustion in Table 5.3.

Table 5.3 *available energy values of different nutrients,*

Nutrient	*Digestion loss (%)*	*Heat of combustion of (kJ/g)*	*Metabolisable or available energy to cells (kJ/g)*
Carbohydrate	1	17.2	17.0
Lipid	5	39.4	37.0
Ethanol	nil	29.0	29.0
Protein	29	24.0	17.0

5.9 CALCULATION OF FOOD ENERGY VALUE

The available energy values become important factors, in calculating the energy value of a foodstuff; the factors are carbohydrate *and* protein 17, lipid 37, ethanol 29.

In order to calculate the energy value of a foodstuff it is necessary to know the *composition* of the food either by carrying out an *analysis* to measure the amount of carbohydrate, lipid, protein or ethanol in a 100g portion, or more conveniently referring to *food composition tables* which are published in many countries throughout the world.

Method
To determine the energy value of fried potato chips, *first* find the composition from tables; *second, multiply* the amount of each energy-providing

nutrient by its available energy factor. Then total each energy value for all nutrients.

Table 5.4 *determination of energy value of fried potato chips*

Nutrient	*Amount per 100g*	×	*Conversion factor*	*Energy (kJ/100g)*
Protein	5.3		17	90
Lipid	39.8		37	1472
Carbohydrate	50.0		17	850

Total energy value of 100g potato chips = 2412kJ

Food composition tables

The available energy value shown in Appendix A (food composition tables) is calculated from the lipid, carbohydrate, protein and ethanol content of the food, using the factors as shown in Tables 5.3 and 5.4. The energy value is not measured directly by the bomb calorimeter which would provide heat of combustion values.

Factors affecting food energy values

1. *Fatty foods* rich in lipids will have a *higher* energy value than most other foods since the available energy from gramme weights of pure 100 per cent lipid, carbohydrate and protein is 37kJ for lipids and only 17kJ for carbohydrate and protein; the lipids have *twice* the energy value of the others.
2. *Watery foods*, soups, salad and other vegetables and fruits, with a *high* water content of no energy value to the body. The water content *dilutes* or lowers the food energy content. *Dried* fruit will have a higher energy value than fresh fruit. For example: fresh grapes have an energy value of 290kJ/100g, whilst dried raisins have an energy value of 1200kJ/100g, that is four times that of fresh fruit.
3. *Dietary fibre content* represents carbohydrate *not available* to living cells since it cannot be digested in the human gut (Section 4.7). The higher the fibre content the lower the energy value as shown as follows:

Wheat bran	44 per cent fibre	850kJ/100g
Wholemeal flour	10 per cent fibre	1300kJ/100g
White wheat flour	3 per cent fibre	1500kJ/100g

5.10 DIETARY ENERGY SOURCES

Most foodstuffs are *mixtures* of varying composition made up of carbohydrates, fats and proteins, and water. The average range of energy value for different foods is summarised in Table 5.5, from which it is seen that the *high energy foods* are cereals, legumes, nuts, seeds, dried fruits, together with edible oil and fats, sugar and confectionery.

Table 5.5 *energy values of the main groups of foodstuffs*

Foodstuff	*Energy value range (MJ/100g)*
Cereals	1.1 -1.6
Sugar and confectionery	1.1 -2.3
Starchy vegetables	0.2 -0.5
Other vegetables	0.05-0.2
Legumes, nuts and seeds	1.3 -2.5
Fruits, fresh	0.08-0.3
dried	1.0 -1.3
Meat, poultry, fish	0.4 -1.2
Fats and oils	2.8 -3.7
Dairy products: cheeses	0.4 -1.7
milk fresh/dried	0.25-2.0
Alcoholic beverages	0.2 -1.20
Non-alcoholic beverages	0.09-0.2

5.11 CELL USES OF ENERGY

The ATP provides energy for the following cell processes:

1. *Muscle* contraction resulting in mechanical work in *skeletal* muscles to move and support the body, in *heart* muscle to circulate the blood and in other *involuntary* muscles of the chest and lung walls and the gut wall, to move air and food in the body.
2. *Membrane transport* which involves the continual use of energy to allow mineral ions and nutrients to move into and out of the cells across the cell membrane by *active transport* (see Section 2.7).
3. *Synthesis* of cell protein used in growth and repair, carried out by cell DNA and RNA nucleic acids, and for making enzymes, hormones and other functional proteins (Section 3.4).

4. *Thermic or thermogenic effect of feeding* (formerly called specific dynamic action). This is the use of energy *following* the intake of nutrients either by mouth, or intravenously by drip feed directly into the blood, or the extra heat produced after feeding. This thermic or thermogenic effect uses energy to *metabolise* food, particularly the proteins. Sugars are changed into *glycogen* or fats, and amino acids are broken down into other substances informing *carbamide (urea)* (Section 8.17). The amount of total energy intake used in the way after feeding amounts to 15% for protein, 5% for carbohydrate, and 2% of lipid.

Experiment 5.2 *ATP and skeletal muscle contraction*

(i) Lay a strand of fresh lean meat on a clean microscope slide placed over squared graph paper as shown in Figure 5.3. Note the length of the meat strand.

Fig 5.3 *to demonstrate action of ATP on muscle tissue or meat*

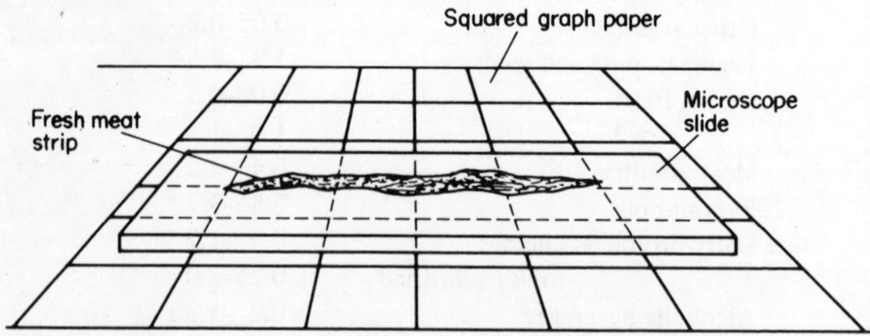

(ii) Add a few drops of 1 per cent glucose solution to the meat by means of a dropper and note any change in length of the meat strand.

(iii) Add a few drops of a prepared ATP solution from an ampoule and again note any change in length of the meat strand.

Glucose solution alone is unable to cause contraction, but ATP provides energy to the muscle cells resulting in a shortening of the muscle strand. Glucose must enter the aerobic respiration cycle to form ATP.

5.12 THE BODY ENERGY STORES

Primitive human beings seldom had a regular food supply nor ate meals at regular mealtimes; in the circumstances they depended partly on stores of food energy in their body tissues. In times of food shortage or famine or enforced starvation, the cells are able to draw on a considerable energy store (see Section 9.3). Provided the body is kept *warm* and has a supply of *water*, a *healthy* person can do without food for up to two weeks, and if he or she has a good reserve of *fat* can survive for up to one or two months without food.

Exposure to severe *cold* can kill a person in two to three *hours*, whilst being kept without *water* causes death in two to three *days*.

The *brain* and *nerve* cells must have a *continuous* supply of glucose, usually present in tissue fluid at a concentration of 0.1 per cent approximately. If the brain and nerve cells are *deprived* of glucose as in extreme fasting or starvation, the nerve cells are damaged and the body suffers *convulsions*, enters a *coma*, and the eye nerves are damaged with resultant *blindness*.

The main reserves of energy are found as *glucose* or *glycogen* (animal starch) stored mainly in the liver and muscles, together with glucose (blood sugar) in the blood. The lipid reserves are found in the skin, and kidney fat reserves, whilst the protein of muscles and skin is a store and supply of amino-acids.

The available body stores of energy in an adult human being (70kg) are summarised in Table 5.6, together with their amounts and estimated time of duration as a reserve supply.

Table 5.6 *energy reserves in a 70kg adult*

Reserve	*Tissue*	*Amount (g and kg)*	*Energy value, (MJ)*	*Approximate duration of supply*
Glucose	Blood and tissue fluid	15g.	0.25	½–1 hr.
Glucose and mainly glycogen	Muscle	300g	7.0	1 day
	Liver	100g		
Proteins	Muscle	4kg	72.5	10 days
	Skin	250g		
Lipid	Skin and kidney reserves	12kg	470.0	up to 2 months
	Muscle	600g		

The *total* energy reserves in a 70kg adult man equals about 550MJ which could last between forty and eighty days in a fasting man, depending on whether he was active or resting during the fast.

5.13 BASAL OR RESTING METABOLISM

The energy needed for a healthy human being lying down at *complete physical and mental rest* in a comfortably *warm* room, 20°C, some twelve hours *after* a meal, is called the energy of *basal metabolism*. In this state of basal metabolism energy is being used for the *minimum* energy needs of the body to maintain breathing, blood circulation, muscle tone, digestive system activity, cell metabolism and body temperature. It *excludes* energy used for all physical activity and any form of skeletal muscle movement, and also the thermic or thermogenic effect (Section 5.11).

Measurement

The *rate* of basal metabolism or BMR basal metabolic rate can be measured *directly* using a human calorimeter, or by the *indirect* human calorimeter. The indirect human calorimeter is most frequently used and measures the amount of *oxygen* used by the body in a certain time.

Careful measurements show that 1000cm^3 of oxygen releases 20.25kJ of energy from food in the body.

The average BMR for a healthy adult man of 70kg is about 290kJ/hr or 7MJ per day and is about 10–12 per cent or 6.3MJ per day for a 70 kg woman.

Calculation of BMR

The energy needs of a human body for basal metabolism are related mainly to body *size*, weight and height, or to *body surface area*. Large-frame or well built people need relatively more energy than people of small frame or build. An adult male requires 168kJ for every *square metre* (m^2) of body surface per hour, whilst an adult female requires 155kJ/m^2/h.

Body surface area can be measured from a formula as in Section 1.10 (Experiment 1.1) and BMR is then determined from the following relationship:

BMR adult male per hour = surface area (m^2) × 168 (kJ)

BMR adult female per hour = surface area (m^2) × 155 (kJ)

Example: If a man has a surface area of $1.67m^2$, his *daily* BMR will be calculated as follows:

BMR hour rate = 1.67 x 168

BMR daily rate = 1.67 x 168 x 24

= 6733 kJ/day

Daily BMR = 6.73 MJ per day.

Body weight measurement can be used to calculate BMR from the following relationships:

BMR daily rate adult MALE = 4.36 x body weight x 24

BMR daily rate adult FEMALE = 4.17 x body weight x 24

Example: A 56kg woman requires a daily BMR calculated as follows:

BMR daily rate = 4.17 x 56 x 24

= 5604 (kJ per day)

= 5.6 MJ per day.

The Nomogram is a graphical table showing relationship between body surface area, height and weight (or mass).

An adult with a height of 175cm and weight 105kg will have a body surface area of $2.2m^2$ as shown by drawing a connecting line between the height and weight values shown in the nomogram in Figure 5.4. Similarly, an adult of height 125cm and weight 50kg has a body surface area of $1.25m^2$.

5.14 FACTORS AFFECTING THE BASAL METABOLIC RATE

The *rate* of energy release in body cells also affects the BMR. The following list shows the more important factors affecting the BMR. It is important to realise that there is a *variation* in BMR for different individual people although they may be of identical body size and sex. There is also a variation in the BMR of different body *organs*; the liver and brain have the *highest* rates, followed by heart and kidneys.

1. *Thyroid gland disorder* This gland activity is related to the amount of iodine in the diet; and *excessive* secretion of its hormone *thyroxine* speeds up the rate of energy release and *increases* the BMR, a *decrease*

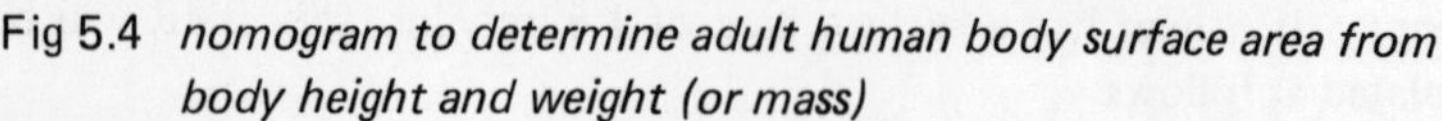

Fig 5.4 *nomogram to determine adult human body surface area from body height and weight (or mass)*

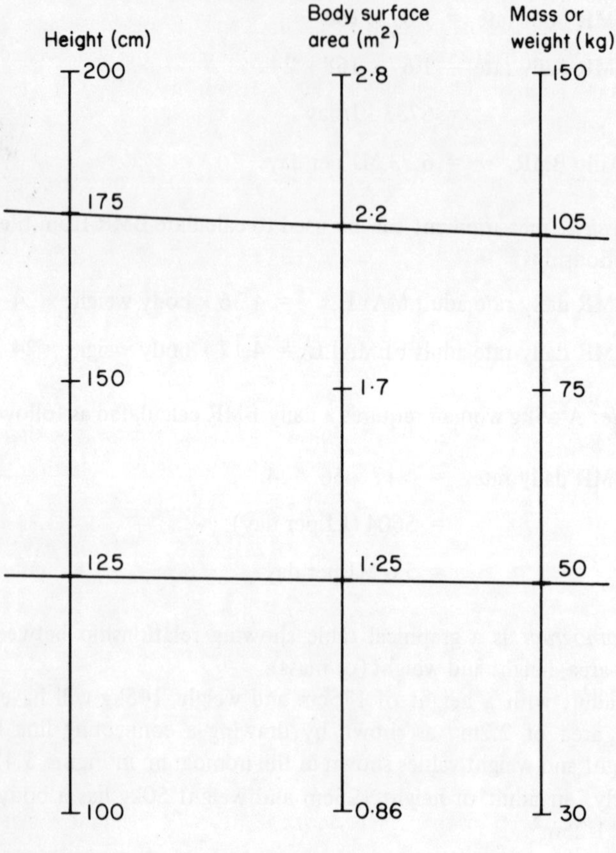

in its secretion *decreases* the BMR. These effects are only evident in people suffering from thyroid gland disorders (see also Table 9.6 and Plate 9.5).

2. *Adrenal glands and nervous stimulants* The secretion of the adrenal glands (close to the kidneys) (see Figure 8.7) and secretion of certain nerves, or anti-obesity drugs which stimulate these nerves can *increase* the BMR. It is essential that a person must be free from fear, tension, anxiety or other nervous stress conditions when BMR is being measured.
3. *Climate* Tropical climate temperatures tend to lower the BMR in most human beings who respond by being less active and lowering their heat output. In cold climates the BMR is raised automatically by *shivering*.

4. *Time of day* The BMR fluctuates through a twenty-four hour day, being at its *lowest* value at 4 a.m. or 04.00 hrs.
5. *Age and sex* The BMR is *highest* in newborn babies and *decreases* steadily with age after *20* to reach its lowest levels in old age. Females have a lower BMR than males, and women show a 10–12 per cent decrease compared with men. The variation in BMR with age and sex is shown in Figure 5.5.

Fig 5.5 *graph comparing basal metabolic rate in males and females*

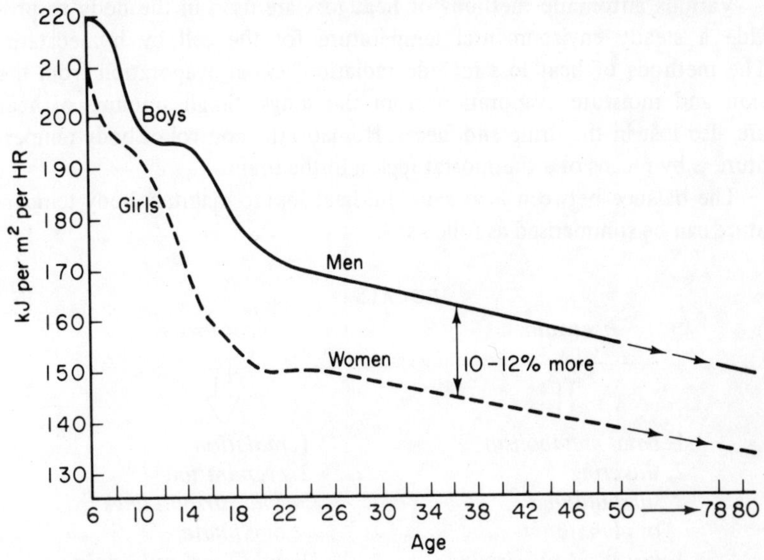

6. *Motherhood* During pregnancy the BMR of expectant mothers *rises* as extra energy is needed for growth of the baby, birth organs and breasts. Similarly mothers who are *lactating* or breast-feeding also show increased BMR since energy is needed for milk-production when the body is in a state of basal metabolism.
7. *Exercise or physical activity* Since the measurement of BMR precludes all exercise and physical activity, the energy requirements for different activities will be considered in Section 9.9.
8. *Smoking* seems to increase the BMR thus causing people to eat more on giving up the habit.

5.15 BODY TEMPERATURE

The human body temperature is approximately constant at 36.9°C (98.4°F); it can rise to 37.8°C (100°F) with strenuous exercise or after a hot bath and can fall to 36.0°C (96.5°F) in the early morning when a person is asleep.

Body temperature is the product of *basal metabolism*, and involuntary muscle activity or shivering. In addition the body may gain heat energy from its surroundings and from hot food.

All food energy is ultimately changed into heat energy; if the body had no means of losing this heat, its body temperature would rise by 1°C for every hour, finally resulting in death from heat stroke with the cells burning themselves out.

Various automatic methods of heat loss are used in the body to provide a steady environmental temperature for the cell by homeostasis. The methods of heat loss include radiation, sweat evaporation from the skin and moisture evaporation from the lungs. Small amounts of heat are also lost in the urine and faeces. Homeostatic control of body temperature is by means of a thermostat region in the brain.

The balance between heat gain and heat loss to maintain body temperature can be summarised as follows:

EQUALS

heat gain	*heat loss*
	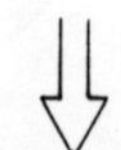
1. *basal metabolism*	1. *radiation*
2. *shivering*	2. *evaporation*
3. *surroundings* or *climate*	3. *cold surroundings* or *climate*
4. *hot food and drinks*	4. *cold food and drinks*

5.16 QUESTIONS

1. Explain the terms *heat of combustion* and *available energy* of an energy-providing nutrient. What units are used to measure food energy values?
2. Calculate the energy value of the following food item from the chemical composition provided: protein 10 per cent, lipids 18 per cent, carbohydrates 6 per cent. The conversion factors are carbohydrate and protein 17kJ/g and lipids 37kJ/g. The heat of combustion of this food was measured and found to equal 1010kJ/100g. Explain the differences between the heat of combustion and *calculated* energy value.
3. Explain the term basal metabolism and how it is measured. What conditions affect the basal metabolic rate in an adult woman? Why do men require more energy than women?

4. Which pure food nutrients provide energy? In what form is it available in the cell? List those food commodities with a *high* energy content and those with a *low* energy content.
5. Refer to the food composition tables in Appendix A, and determine the energy content of the following food snack: cornflakes 25g, fresh milk 50g, sugar 10g, bacon 33g, egg 50g.
6. For what purposes is food energy used in the body cells?

CHAPTER 6

FOOD

6.1 FOOD COMPOSITION

Whole foods, are usually fresh, raw, unrefined, and unprocessed *foodstuffs*, food *commodities* or food *materials* and mainly *mixtures* of the *nutrients* described in Chapter 4. An essential feature of a *mixture* is that it has a *variable composition* (see Section 2.5); this contrasts with the *fixed composition* of *chemical* compounds such as the different nutrients which compose foods.

Chemical analysis indicates the composition of a food, showing the amounts of each nutrient present in a known weight of food, usually a 100g portion. The chemical analysis of nutrients present in foods is recorded in *food composition tables*: these are produced by governments of different countries and also by the international Food and Agriculture Organisation (FAO) of the United Nations. Food composition values for a range of foods is listed in the table in Appendix A.

6.2 VARIABLE COMPOSITION OF FOOD

Foods from similar *groups*, for example, cereals, nuts. legumes, fish, meat and eggs have a similar *general composition*, and will show differences in composition *within* a group, for example, the cereals wheat and rice differ from each other and so do fish such as herring and whiting since they are also different biological *species.*

Differences in composition can occur within the *same species*; the individual herring fish can show varying amounts of lipids for several reasons, for example the female contains more than the male and starving fish have less lipids than feeding fish. Similarly different *varieties* of apples have varying sugar composition in cooking and eating apples; cooking apples have 9 per cent free sugars, and eating apples may have over 12 per cent free sugars.

Variation in composition also occurs in *different parts* of an individual, for example there is more lipid near the head region of a salmon than in the tail, and more of certain vitamins in the outer coating of cereal grains (Section 7.5) and potato tubers.

Different methods of *feeding* and *rearing* also affect food composition; the vitamin A, B_{12} and folic acid content varies for eggs from battery-reared and free-range hens, whilst wheat grown in different climates shows different protein composition - English wheat has less protein than Canadian wheat.

Home-processing of food including preparation, cooking, storage and preservation will affect food composition to different extents (Section 7.6), whilst individual *recipes* for a cooked food item can show a wide variation in composition. Consequently the tables of food composition are intended for *reference* and as a guide indicating the *average* composition of specific samples.

6.3 DISTRIBUTION OF NUTRIENTS IN FOODS

The food composition tables are of value in showing the *distribution* of nutrients in different foods. The nutrients are unequally divided between foods from plant and animal sources, for example, foods from plants have a generally higher content of carbohydrates, vitamins C, folic acid and dietary fibre, whilst foods from animals have a generally higher protein, lipid and vitamin D and B group content (see Table 3.1).

Different foods will therefore be deficient in certain nutrients, and consequently a *mixture of different foods* should be consumed in a *meal*, with each food making up the deficiencies present in the other, to provide a *balance* of nutrients in the meal or diet.

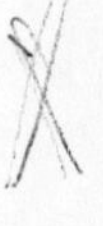

In the following sections the *general composition* of foods in the food group will be given; this is an overall average for the main members of the group. Details of the composition of *individual* food items are available from the food composition tables in Appendix A.

A FOOD FROM PLANT SOURCES

This forms about 75 per cent of the world's food supply (see Plate 6.1).

6.4 VEGETABLES

Vegetables form about 24 per cent of the world food supply and are foods of plant origin derived mainly from the *flowering* plants or angiosperms (Section 3.2). They can be conveniently grouped on the basis of their structure (Section 3.5) and composition into *leafy*, *root*, *starchy* and *other* vegetables. The *legumes* or *pulses* are grouped separately.

Plate 6.1 *an FAO home economist displaying a selection of foods from plant sources which form a major part of the diet in many developing countries worldwide (FAO, UN)*

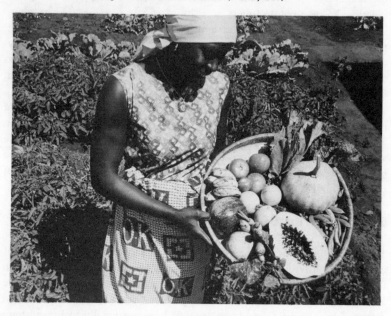

Leafy vegetables

This group includes the green cabbage, Brussels sprouts, spinach, spring greens, broccoli, waterleaf lettuce and watercress.

General composition

In sections which follow, and in Tables 6.1-6.17 the starred (*) items are those particular nutrients which are present in moderate to good amounts.

Leafy vegetables are useful sources of the vitamins B_2, C, and carotenes vitamin A, together with folic acid named from the Latin word *folium* meaning leaf. Because of the absence of phytic acid they are also useful sources of the minerals calcium and iron.

The low energy value and protein content, together with the high dietary fibre, 20 per cent in cabbage, 30 per cent in curly kale, make green leafy vegetables and salads attractive components of weight-reducing diets.

Quality

The higher water content affects leafy vegetable quality. Fresh produce will be firm and crisp, with attractive fresh green colour. Stale produce is limp, floppy and with brownish yellow discolouration.

Table 6.1 *general composition of raw leafy vegetables per 100g portion*

Water	92g	*Vitamins*:		
Energy	75kJ	A	Carotene*	1800μg
Carbohydrate	2g	B_1	Thiamin	0.08mg
Protein	2.5g	B_2	Riboflavin*	0.14mg
Lipid	trace	Nicotinic acid		0.54mg
Dietary fibre*	3g	C	Ascorbic acid*	53mg
Phytic acid	NIL		(cabbage, sprouts 100g)	
		Folic acid*		110μg
		Minerals:		
	Calcium 80mg		Iron 1.35mg	

Root vegetables

This group includes carrots, parsnips, turnips, swedes, beetroots and radishes. Table 6.2 shows the general composition of raw root vegetables.

Root vegetables are useful sources of dietary fibre (carrots contain 10 per cent) and being of a *low* energy value feature in weight-reducing diets. They are a moderate source of vitamin C (ascorbic acid) whilst carrots are a good source of carotenes vitamin A.

Table 6.2 *general composition of raw root vegetables per 100g portion*

Water	90g	*Vitamins*:		
Energy	110kJ	A	Carotene	trace
Carbohydrate	5.6g		(carrots*	12 000μg)
Protein	1.1g	B_1	Thiamin	0.05mg
Lipid	trace	B_2	Riboflavin	0.05mg
Dietary fibre*	2.75g	Nicotinic acid		0.60mg
Phytic acid	low	C	Ascorbic acid*	17mg
		Folic acid		40μg
		Minerals:		
	Calcium 50mg		Iron 0.6mg	

Quality
Fresh root vegetables are *firm* and snap crisply and are free of soil and mud. Stale root vegetables are limp and soft.

Other vegetables
This group includes leeks, onions, cauliflower, marrow, peppers, tomatoes and okra – a cucumber-like vegetable. These vegetables are forms of stems, bulbs, fruits or flowers. Table 6.3 shows the general composition of various raw vegetables other than leafy root or starchy vegetables.

Table 6.3 *general composition of various other raw vegetables (per 100g portion*

Water	92g	*Vitamins*:	
Energy	75kJ	Carotenes, vitamin A	130mg
Carbohydrate	3.5g	[tomatoes* 600μg]	
Protein	1.5g	B_1 Thiamin	0.045mg
Lipid	trace	B_2 Riboflavin	0.03mg
Dietary fibre*	3g	Nicotinic acid	0.40mg
Phytic acid	Nil	C *Ascorbic acid	27mg
		Folic acid	25μg
		Minerals:	
	Calcium 35mg	Iron 0.6mg	

These are low energy value foods with useful amounts of vitamin C (ascorbic acid) and vitamin A (carotenes) together with dietary fibre as high as 10 per cent.

Quality
Fresh produce is firm with bright-coloured skin. The green-coloured parts have a fresh green appearance without roughness or blemishes.

Starchy vegetables
This group includes those vegetables with a high starch (carbohydrate) content; they are modified roots or stems botanically called tubers and corms and in some cases are fruits. Potatoes, sweet potatoes, yams and cassava are underground tubers, whilst taro (cocoyams) are underground corms. Plantains are banana-like fruits. Breadfruit is a starchy fruit, staple seasonal food in the Caribbean countries. Table 6.4 shows general composition of raw starchy vegetables.

Table 6.4 *general composition of raw starchy vegetables (per 100g portion)*

Water	70g	*Vitamins*:	
Energy*	450kJ	Carotene, vitamin A	15μg
Carbohydrate* (starch)	25g	[yellow sweet potatoes*	4000μg]
Protein	1.5g	B_1 Thiamin	0.08mg
(cassava 0.9g)		B_2 Riboflavin	0.04mg
Lipid	0.25g	Nicotinic acid	0.70mg
Dietary fibre	3.5g	C Ascorbic acid*	18mg
Phytic acid	moderate	Folic acid	10μg
	Minerals:		
Calcium	20mg	Iron	0.6mg

Starchy roots, tubers and plantains are *staple* foods in thirteen *less developed* countries of the world including African countries, whilst cassava is an important food in Latin America, particularly Brazil, and in South India, Indonesia and the Philippines. Like the potato, these starchy vegetables are easy to grow and can be left in the ground until required.

Starchy vegetables have a high energy content with useful amounts of vitamin C (ascorbic acid) with vitamin B_1 (thiamin) and nicotinic acid in moderate amounts.

Potatoes contribute useful quantities of protein and iron and have a 10 per cent dietary fibre content since this starchy vegetable is consumed in larger amounts than other vegetables in the Western diet. Cassava is a very poor source of dietary protein.

Quality

Fresh underground produce is undamaged and firm. Stale product is soft, sprouting, stained or dark green in colour.

6.5 LEGUMES AND PULSES

Legumes are the seeds and pods of the pea and bean family and include peas, beans, lentils, cow-peas, mung beans and soya beans. *Pulses* are the *dried* seeds of legumes, various peas, beans or lentils, in contrast to the *fresh* green pods and seeds of other *leguminous* plants such as runner beans and garden peas. Table 6.5 shows their general composition. Many pulses are staple foods in the less developed countries of the world.[Peanuts are botanically legumes as the seed forms within pods – see Section 6.6].

Table 6.5 *general composition of dried raw legume seeds or pulses per 100g portion*

Water	12g	*Vitamins*:	
Energy*	1200kJ	Carotenes, vitamin A	80μg
Carbohydrate*	50g	B_1 Thiamin*	0.50mg
Protein*	21g	B_2 Riboflavin*	0.18mg
[soya 35g]			
Lipid	1.5g	Nicotinic acid*	1.25mg
[soya* 17g]		C Ascorbic acid	trace
Phytic acid	high	Folic acid*	80μg
Dietary fibre*	15g		
	Minerals:		
Calcium	80mg	Iron*	6.0mg

Dried legume seeds or pulses have a high energy and dietary fibre content and valuable protein content. The seeds contain all the food needs for the early growth of a plant and are good sources of vitamins of the B group, B_1, B_2 and nicotinic acid, and of folic acid. Fresh and soaked legume seeds will have a *lower* nutrient content, about a quarter that of the *dried* legume seed. Their high phytic acid content affects the calcium and iron availability.

Although the seeds do not contain vitamin C (ascorbic acid) the vitamin forms in useful amounts in *sprouted* bean seeds, such as sprouted mung beans in Asian and African diets.

Soya bean is a valuable pulse with a high protein content (40 per cent) and high lipid oil content (20 per cent) which finds application in the preparation of cooking oil, *textured vegetable protein* (Section 7.10) cereal products and as an important famine relief food in various forms such as soya milk, soya chutney, de-fatted soya flour, alone or blended with wheat flour.

Quality
Fresh legume products have a fresh green appearance with well-filled pods, and firm but *not* hard seeds inside. Runner beans or snap beans break crisply. Stale legumes have discoloured slimy pods.

6.6 NUTS

Nut *kernels* are mainly the *seeds* found within the hard-shelled fruits of hazel, brazil, almond and cashew nuts. The FAO includes peanuts or groundnuts in this group because of the high lipid content. (See Table 6.6).

Table 6.6 *general composition of dry nuts (per 100g portion)*

Water	10g	*Vitamins*:	
Energy*	2.5MJ	Carotene, vitamin A	trace
Carbohydrate	5g	B_1 Thiamin*	0.5mg
Protein*	15g	B_2 Riboflavin*	0.2mg
Lipid*	60g	Nicotinic acid	1.5mg
Dietary fibre*	10g	[peanut* 16mg]	
Phytic acid	high	C Ascorbic acid	trace
		Folic acid	low
		[peanut* 110μg]	
	Minerals		
Calcium	100mg	Iron*	4.0mg

Nuts are somewhat similar to pulses in their composition and nutritive value, they have a *high* energy content because of a high concentration of protein and lipid. They are good sources of the vitamins B_1 and B_2 and of folic acid. The iron and calcium content is high, together with the phytic acid content which may reduce the availability of these minerals.

6.7 FRUIT

Fruits form about 4 per cent of the world's food supply. Botanically fruits are seed-containing organs formed from the ripened ovary of a flower. The majority of fruits are fleshy or *juicy*, whilst the botanically *dry* fruits include cereal grains, nuts and legume pods. Table 6.7 shows the composition of ripe fleshy fruits.

Table 6.7 *general composition of fresh raw ripe fleshy fruit (per 100g portion)*

Water	85g	*Vitamins*:	
Energy	200kJ	Carotenes, vitamin A*	200μg
Carbohydrate	10g	[mango, apricot,	
Protein	0.9g	melon	1500μg]
Lipid	0.5g	B_1 Thiamin	0.04mg
[olive*	12mg	B_2 Riboflavin	0.04mg
[avocado pear*	20mg]	Nicotinic acid	0.40mg
Phytic acid	low	C Ascorbic acid	20mg
Dietary fibre*	3g	[blackcurrant 200mg]	
[berries		Folic acid	15μg
	6–8g		
currants		[avocado pear* 60μg]	
	Minerals:		
Calcium	20mg	Iron	0.5mg

The important features of fruit are their attractive colour and flavour. Ripe fruits have a *high* water and free sugar content in which almost all the nutritive components are soluble, to provide *fruit juices.*

The useful *dietary fibre* content consists mainly of *cellulose* and *pectin*. Carbohydrates present in ripe fruits are mainly *fructose* and *glucose* in amounts from 2 per cent in water melons to 22 per cent in bananas.

Lipids are found only in avocado pears (20 per cent) and olives (13 per cent) whilst proteins are found in negligible amounts in all fruits.

Fruits are important sources of vitamin C (ascorbic acid) present in a range of variable amounts, the highest concentration in blackcurrants and guava fruit (200mg/100g). The orange coloured mango, apricot, and melon fruits contain useful amounts of *carotenes*, the vitamin A precursor. *Six* parts by weight of carotenes are needed to make *one* part by weight of *retinol* vitamin A.

Since fruits and fruit juices are consumed in *large amounts* they also provide useful sources of the vitamins B_1 and B_2, nicotinic acid and minerals calcium and iron.

Dried fruits are partly *processed* foods and are a more *concentrated* source of most fresh fruit nutrients, with the exception of vitamin C (ascorbic acid) which is destroyed in the fruit-drying process. The general composition of dried fruit per 100g portion is summarised as follows: water, 22g; energy, 1.1MJ; carbohydrate, 70g; protein, 2.5g; fibre, 5-10g; iron, 2.0mg; calcium 100mg.

Fruit acids
Fruits contain variable amounts of organic acids which contribute to flavour and can provide limited amounts of *energy*; unripe fruits contain the highest concentrations.

1. *Citric acid* (2-hydroxypropane-1,2,3-tricarboxylic acid) is present in citrus fruits, lemons, limes, oranges and pineapples.
2. *Malic acid* (2-hydroxybutanedioic acid) is found in apples, pears and plums.
3. *Oxalic acid* (ethanedioic acid) is present in rhubarb and strawberries.
4. *Tartaric acid* (2,3-dihydroxybutanedioic acid) is present in grapes.

Quality
Fresh fruits have *clean* unblemished skin, unbruised with generally firm but not hard flesh; the colour is well-formed and attractive.

6.8 SUCROSE PRODUCTS

These are *processed* or refined foods.

1. *Sucrose*, commonly called sugar, is the main component of juices or syrups extracted from the sugar cane, sugar beet plants and the North American maple tree. *Refined* cane and beet sugar consists of 100 per cent pure sucrose and contains no other nutrients; the by-products of sugar-refining include treacle, golden syrup and molasses as syrups.
2. *Syrups*, including maple syrup, are concentrated solutions of sucrose 60-70 per cent, and water 40-30 per cent, which in addition contain useful amounts of vitamin B_2 (riboflavin) a rich source of iron, 6mg/100g, and calcium, 200mg/100g. They have a high energy value of 1.0MJ per 100g portion.
3. *Honey* is an 80 per cent solution of mixed carbohydrates glucose and fructose or invert sugar, made by *digestion* of *sucrose* flower-nectar in the honey bee's stomach. It has a high energy value of 1.3MJ per 100g portion.
4. *Liquid glucose* is a syrup *manufactured* from maize starch and is called corn or starch syrup, consisting of 70 per cent glucose.
5. *Boiled sweets or confectionery*, caramel, candy and toffee consist of about 70 per cent sucrose, 10-15 per cent lipid, and have an energy

value of 1.8MJ/100g. They contain small amounts of calcium and iron. *Black* liquorice sweets made from treacle and gelatine have a high iron content of 8mg/100g.

6. *Chocolate* is a concentrated source of energy, 2.3MJ/100g, and consists of 50 per cent carbohydrate, 35 per cent lipid, 7 per cent protein, with a useful content of calcium (200mg) and iron 2.5mg/100g. With added cereal biscuit, or dried fruit and nuts, the food is a valuable component of survival packs.

6.9 CEREALS

Cereals form 45 per cent of the world's food supply. The *cereals* rice, wheat, maize, millet and sorghum are the main source of nutrients for most of the world's population living in the *less-developed* countries. *Less-developed* countries comprise those countries which *exclude* Europe, North America, Australia, New Zealand, USSR and Japan which are called *more-developed* countries (Section 12.3). Rice is the staple food of thirty-six countries in Asia, the Far East and parts of West Africa and Latin America. Plate 6.2 illustrates the development of new strains of rice. *Maize* is the staple food in twenty-one countries parts of Latin America and Africa, whilst *millet* and *sorghum* are staple foods in fifteen countries of West Africa, East Africa and Arabia. It is important to note that 33 per cent of the world's cereal grain supply is used as *feed* for livestock rearing.

Wheat forms an important part of the diet of thirty-five European, Asian and other countries throughout the world, in the form of bread, pasta and other food products made from wheat.

Botanically the whole cereal grain is a fruit called a *caryopsis* and strongly resembles a *berry*. The cereal grains are the fruits of a large family of flowering plants called the *gramineae* or grain producing plants (see figure 7.1). Table 6.8 shows their general composition.

Starch is the main carbohydrate present in cereals (70-7 per cent) whilst the main protein is *gluten* (a mixture of *glutenin* and *gliadin*) (Section 8.12); maize contains the protein *zein*, and being without gluten is not used in bread-making. Similarly the protein *avenin* in oats is non-gluten-forming.

The high lipid content is found in maize (4 per cent), and oats (8 per cent); the maize oil is an important cooking oil.

The *high* energy value 1.3-1.6MJ/100g indicates their concentrated source of energy.

Whole cereals are a good source of vitamins B_1, and B_2, nicotinic acid and folic acid; these are located close to the grain skin or *bran* and in the embryo or *germ*. *Bran*, and wheat *germ* are products of *milling* wheat (see Section 7.5). (*Threshing* is a process of removing the loose husk from

Plate 6.2 *rice, a major food of many countries, is the subject of development of new strains at the International Rice Research Station in the Philippines (FAO, UN)*

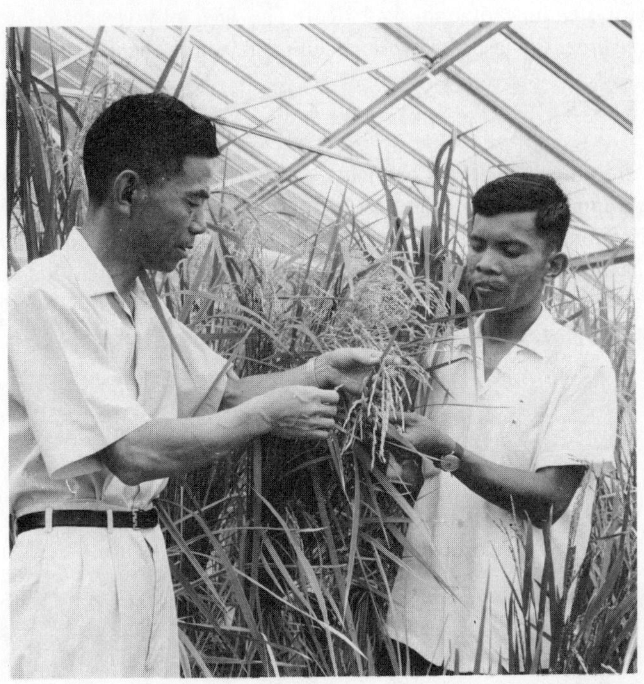

Table 6.8 *general composition of whole grain cereals (per 100g portion)*

Water	10g	*Vitamins*:	
Energy	1500kJ	Carotenes, vitamin A	trace
Carbohydrate*	74g	[yellow maize* 800μg]	
Protein*	10g	B_1 Thiamin*	0.4mg
Lipid	2.0g	B_2 Riboflavin*	0.12mg
(oats 8.0g)		Nicotinic acid*	3.5mg
Phytic acid	High	C Ascorbic acid	Nil
Dietary fibre*	4g	Folic acid*	40μg
	Minerals:		
Calcium	30mg	Iron	3.0mg

wheat grain. Rice husk is more difficult to remove from paddy rice and is done by *pounding* and *winnowing* to produce brown or dehusked rice. Paddy rice in the husk can also be dehusked by *parboiling* involving boiling or steaming of unhusked rice). The *high* phytic acid content of cereals *reduces* the availability of calcium and iron in the intestine.

6.10 YEASTS

Yeasts are unicellular fungi or plants without chlorophyll, and are of considerable importance in relationship to food nutrition and food production. Different varieties of yeasts are used in the production of *ethanol* or alcoholic beverages, in baking, and alone as medicinal and food supplements and sources of protein minerals and vitamins. Plate 6.3 shows yeast cells multiplying. Table 6.9 shows the composition of brewers' yeast.

Plate 6.3 *the unicellular structure of the fungus yeast is seen in this photomicrograph showing the yeast cells multiplying (Distillers Company Ltd)*

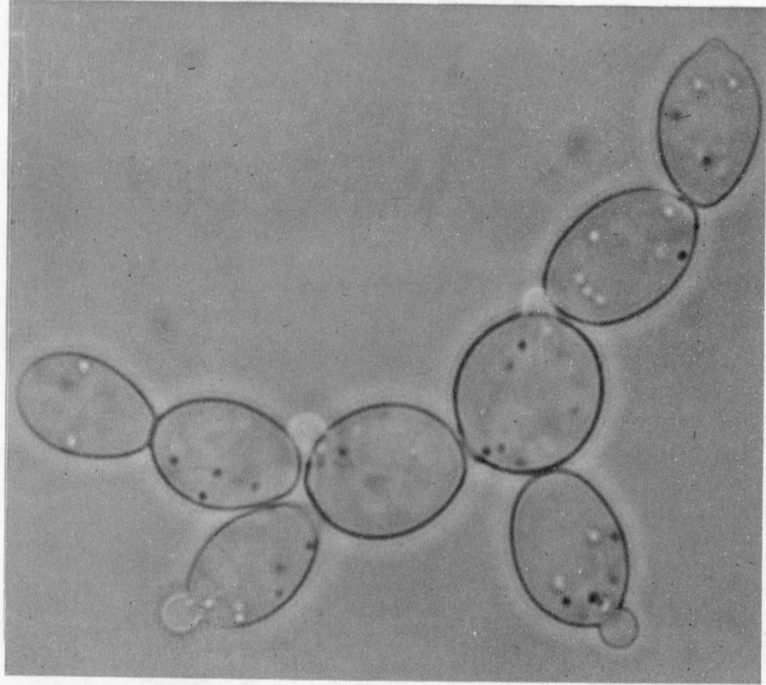

Table 6.9 *composition of dried brewers' yeast (per 100g portion)*

		Vitamins:	
Water	5g		
Energy	1200kJ	B_1 Thiamin*	15mg
Carbohydrate*	34g	B_2 Riboflavin*	4mg
Protein*	38g	Nicotinic acid*	40mg
Lipid	1g	C Ascorbic acid	trace
Dietary fibre	22g	Folic acid*	4000μg
	Minerals:		
Calcium	210mg	Iron*	17mg

The composition shows the importance of yeast in human nutrition as a *rich* source of vitamins of the B group, B_1 and B_2 and folic acid, and as an important source of *protein*.

6.11 **WATERS AND NON-ALCOHOLIC BEVERAGES**

Beverages are processed foods and include *extracts* or infusions in hot water of various plant organs; *leaf* extract - tea; *bean* extracts - coffee and cocoa; *root* extract - chicory (a coffee substitute), *meat* extract and *yeast* extract (see Section 6.10).

The *waters* include domestic drinking water, well-water and various *bottled* waters; Appollinaris, Evian, Malvern and Vichy. Waters can also be *carbonated* or treated with carbon dioxide as in soda-water and a range of sweetened carbonated mineral waters.

Fruit juices are processed or squeezed or expressed from the fruits and the fruit juice may have some water removed to form *concentrated* juice.

The nutritional content of unsweetened waters and beverages without added milk is summarised in Table 6.10.

6.12 **ALCOHOLIC BEVERAGES**

Alcohol present in alcoholic beverages is in the form of *ethanol*. Ethanol is formed as a product of *anaerobic respiration* or *fermentation* of glucose by different varieties of *yeasts* (Section 5.6). Carbon dioxide gas is also a product.

$$\textit{glucose} \xrightarrow[\textit{yeasts}]{} \textit{ethanol} \text{ (or 'alcohol')} + \textit{carbon dioxide} + \textit{energy}$$

Table 6.10 *nutritional content of unsweetened, non-milk beverages, fruit juices and waters (per 100g portion)*

Beverage	*Water content (%)*	*Nutritional value*
Drinking water	soft	Flat-tasting, with little natural *calcium* or *iron*.
	hard 99.9	Pleasant-tasting, with useful *calcium* and sometimes *iron* content. Both types may have natural *fluoride* or *added* fluoride content.
Bottled waters Vichy Appollinaris Saint-Yorre	99.6	Pleasant-tasting, with varying amount of *calcium*, *sodium*, *magnesium*, *chloride* and *fluoride*. Dissolved carbon dioxide gives a sparkling effect.
Tea-leaf extract	99.8	Bitter-tasting and coloured because of *tannin*, stimulating because of *caffeine*. Useful source of *fluoride*. Flavour given by essential oils.
Coffee-bean extract	99.1	Bitter-tasting and coloured because of *tannin*, stimulating because of *caffeine*. Some *nicotinic acid*. Flavour given by essential oils, and roasting products.
Cocoa-bean extract	Various over 98	Cocoa in suspension in a beverage is a source of *lipids*, *starches*, *calcium* and *iron*. Colour derived from pigments and tannin. Stimulant because of *theobromine*. Valuable in chocolate (see Section 6.8).
NATURAL Fruit juices	86	Pleasant-flavoured because of essential oils, *sugars* (10 per cent) fruit *acids*, and *vitamin C* (ascorbic acid) 50 mg. (see fruit composition, Section 6.7).
SYNTHETIC Fruit drinks and squashes	85	Variable composition, of *sucrose*, *vitamin C*, *saccharin*, mixtures of pure fruit juices, artificial flavours and colouring.

SYNTHETIC Carbonated mineral waters lemonade cola drinks	90–95	Sucrose 5–10 per cent, synthetic and natural plant extract flavours, colours, fruit acids, preservatives and dissolved carbon dioxide.

Glucose or other sugars are provided from a range of carbohydrate sources such as *fruit* (apples, grapes, etc. for wines and spirits) *cereal* grains (sorghum and barley) *vegetables* (potatoes) and *milk*. More than 9 per cent of the world's grain supply is used in beers and spirits.

Alcoholic beverages may be grouped according to their alcohol content (beers (2–6 per cent) wines (9–10 per cent) fortified wines, sherry and port (15 per cent) and spirits (31–40 per cent). For their general composition see Table 6.11.

B FOOD FROM ANIMAL SOURCES

This forms about 25 per cent of the world's food supply. *Foods from animal sources* - fish, meat, eggs, milk products and animal fats - can be regarded as the *staple diet* of mainly the wealthy, more developed countries. These foods feature in Sections 6.13–6.18.

About 25 per cent of the world's population in wealthy, industrialised more developed countries (Europe, North America, USSR, Australia, New Zealand and Japan) are able to afford these mainly luxury foods from animal sources, together with certain fruits and vegetables. Livestock-raising countries in South America have a high intake of food from animal sources.

It is only people with *high incomes* who can afford to eat these foods, high in lipid, protein and sugar content. By contrast staple foods rich in *starch* - cereals, roots and pulses which form the diet of the less wealthy developing countries.

6.13 SHELLFISH AND INSECTS

Shellfish include the *crustaceans*, shrimps, lobsters, Antarctic krill and crabs, together with the *molluscs*, mussels, cockles and snails. The insects consumed as food include grasshoppers, locusts, crickets and certain caterpillars or other insect larvae. The *shell* forms up to 75% of inedible waste in shellfish and the general composition of the *edible* matter is shown as follows.

This first group of foods from animals, like other foods from this source, is *deficient* in dietary fibre and phytic acid. In contrast to foods from plant sources, these foods now show the presence of cholesterol, Vitamin B_{12} (cyanocobalamin) and vitamin A (retinol) instead of carotenes.

Table 6.11 *general composition of alcoholic beverages (per 100g portion)*

Alcoholic beverage	*Water* (%)	*Energy* (kJ)	*Ethanol* (%)	*Carbohydrate* (%)	*Vitamins*	*Minerals*
Beers	94–98	110	2–6	1–6	Some vitamins B_1, B_2, and nicotinic acid	Calcium trace.
Wines	90	250	9–10	1% (Dry) 6% (Sweet)	Traces to NIL of B group	Calcium trace Iron 0.3 (red wines)
Fortified wines (Ethanol content increased by adding brandy) Sherry/Port	70–80	600	15	15	Traces to NIL of B group	Calcium trace Iron 0.3 (port)
Spirits Brandy, whisky etc.	60–70	1000	30–40	Trace	NIL	NIL
Liqueurs (Sugar-sweetened and flavoured spiritis)	50	1200	20	30	Trace	NIL

Table 6.12 *general composition of edible shellfish and insects (per 100g portions)*

Water	75g	*Vitamins*:	
Energy*	450kJ	A retinol	trace
Carbohydrate	4g	D cholecalciferol	trace
(glycogen)		B_1 thiamine	0.08mg
Protein*	15g	B_2 riboflavin	0.12mg
Lipid	3g	Nicotinic acid	1.00mg
Cholesterol	100mg	B_{12} cyanocobalamin	0.2μg
		Folic acid	15μg
		C Ascorbic acid	trace
	Minerals:		
Calcium	100mg	Iron 1.5mg]	
		[Insects, molluscs*	15mg]
Trace minerals	Iodine* and zinc* present		

Most shellfish and insects are sources of protein which can be collected freely to supplement the diet and previously formed a major part of the diet of primitive man in coastal regions, as seen in the evidence of shells in settlement waste heaps. *Luxury* foods in this class include lobster and oysters.

Molluscs have a high iron content in a form better absorbed than iron in foods from plants.

Quality

Fresh crustaceans should be purchased *alive* and moving. Fresh molluscs should be clean and free from sewage contamination.

6.14 FISH

Fish forms about 3 per cent of the world's food supply: about one third is used as animal feed. The world catch of fish comes from *freshwater* (10 per cent) or *seawater* (90 per cent) and is of two main kinds:

(i) *White fish* include cod, haddock, whiting, plaice and sole from Northern waters, and include snapper, groper, bonito, bluefish, croaker and stockfish or South African hake elsewhere.

(ii) *Oily fish* include herring, tuna, mackerel, salmon and smaller fish often eaten in their entirety such as sardines, sprats, anchovies and pilchards.

Most fish have considerable *waste* in heads, skin and bones amounting to about 40 per cent of the gutted body. Such fish is consumed as *fillets* of skeletal fish muscle, composed of *muscle blocks* (myotomes) connected together by a small amount of *connective tissue* (myocommata). When cooked the fish muscle separates into *flakes*. Figure 6.1 shows the flesh structure of a bony fish. Table 6.13 shows the general composition of fish flesh.

fig 6.1 *flesh structure of a bony fish*

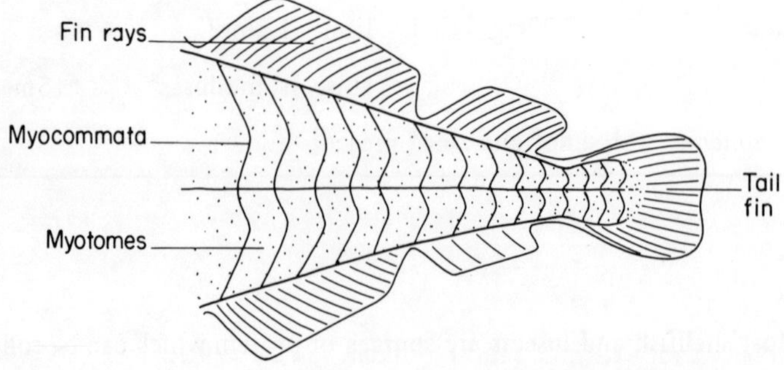

The proteins in fish are similar to meat, being mainly *myosin* and *actin.* Fish are important sources of protein, together with vitamin A (retinol) and vitamin D (cholecalciferol) from *oily* fish. The minerals calcium and iron are present in a useful form and amounts, more calcium being consumed in small whole fish such as sardines and whitebait.

Vitamin B_{12}, fluoride and iodine are present in oily sea fish. Fish *liver* oils are rich sources of vitamins A and D.

Quality

Fresh fish fillets have a pleasant white firm appearance and smell, stale fish fillets are soft and flabby, grey-coloured and smell unpleasant. Fresh whole fish have shiny smooth skin, bright raised eyes and bright red gills and smell fresh compared with stale whole fish with dry slimy skin, sunken eyes, grey gills and an unpleasant odour. Quality is also affected by the season of purchase.

Table 6.13 *general composition of fish flesh (per 100g portion)*

	White	*Oily*		*White*	*Oily*
Water	82g	70g	*Vitamins*		
Energy	300kJ*	800kJ*	A retinol	trace	45μg*
Carbohydrate	trace	trace	D cholecalciferol	trace	23μg*
Protein	17g*	17g*	B_1 thiamin	0.07mg	trace
Lipid	0.5g	13g*	B_2 riboflavin	0.07mg	0.2mg
Cholesterol	60mg	60mg	B_{12} cyano-cobalamin	1.5μg	10μg*
Minerals					
Calcium	17mg	32mg [600mg sardines, pilchards]	Nicotinic acid	5.0mg*	7.0mg*
			Folic acid	10μg	10μg
Iron	0.3mg	0.7mg*	C ascorbic acid	trace	trace
Trace minerals in seafish:	Iodine 0.15mg*	Fluorine*			

6.15 POULTRY AND EGGS

Poultry includes chicken, turkey, duck, goose, capon, and *game birds* - grouse, partridge, pheasant, guinea fowl, pigeon, quail and woodcock.

The *dressed carcase* consists mainly of *flesh* (lean meat, skeletal muscle and fat 63 per cent), *bones* (28 per cent) and *giblets* (9 per cent). Table 6.14 showing general composition refers to the *edible* flesh, minus bones and giblets.

Eggs form about 1 per cent of the world's food supply and are available from hens, ducks, geese and other birds, and Table 6.14 showing the general composition refers to a whole hen egg (*less* the shell) which has a similar composition to eggs from other birds.

Poultry meat is a useful source of protein, all the vitamins of the B group and of folic acid; it is deficient in vitamins A, D and C, and contains moderate amounts of calcium and iron.

Egg consists of 65 per cent white and 35 per cent yolk, which in contrast to *cellular* poultry lean meat muscle is a mainly *non-cellular* substance which provides a food supply for a developing chick embryo, as shown by Figure 6.2.

fig **6.2** *internal structure of a bird's fertilised egg*

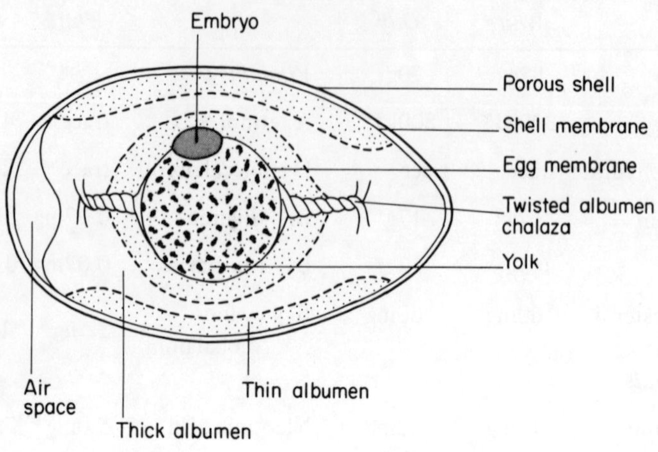

Table 6.14 *general composition of poultry flesh and whole hen egg (per 100g portion)*

	Poultry meat	*Egg*	*Vitamins*	*Poultry meat*	*Egg*
Water	76g	74.5g	A retinol	trace	354μg*
Energy	500kJ	680kJ	D cholecalciferol	trace	5μg*
Carbohydrate	trace	0.7	B_1 thiamin	0.15mg*	0.12mg*
Protein	20g*	12.8g*	B_2 riboflavin	0.3mg*	0.3mg*
Lipid	4g	11.5g*	Nicotinic acid	8.0mg*	0.1mg
Cholesterol	80mg	500mg*	B_{12} cyano-cobalamin	1.5μg*	2.0μg*
Minerals:			Folic acid	18μg*	25μg*
Calcium	10mg	54mg*	C ascorbic acid	trace	trace
Iron	1.0mg	2.3mg			
Trace minerals:					
Iodine present in eggs					

Note Proteins in poultry meat are *myosin* and *actin* (Section 6.16)

Egg yolk has an energy value *eight* times that of the egg white; the lipid content is mainly in the yolk. The egg *proteins* are distributed between the yolk and white, *lipoproteins*, namely lipovitellin, lipovitellenin and livetin in the yolk and *ovalbumins* called ovomucin, ovoglobulin and conalbumin, in the white. The vitamin content is in the yolk which provides a rich source of vitamin A (retinol) and vitamin D (cholecalciferol). Egg iron is in a form not easily available to the body in human nutrition. It is important to note that the cholesterol content of egg yolk is more than five times that of poultry meat.

Quality

(a) *Fresh* young birds have a pliable breastbone tip, with clean white, moist, fresh-looking skin, with bright pink legs.
Stale birds have flesh turning blue, and dry skin with unattractive off-colouring.
Certain *game-birds* are *hung* for three to seven days. When meat or poultry is stored or *hung*, the muscle fibres are separated by certain protein-splitting enzymes which attack connective tissues and separate the muscle fibres. The storage or hanging process gives the meat a flavour.

(b) *Fresh* whole eggs have a firm, raised domed yolk, with a large amount of thick white surrounded by an outer circlet of a small amount of thin white.
Stale eggs have weak yolks which break easily and have a large amount of thin, spreading white. Stale shelled eggs float in a 10 per cent solution of sodium chloride (table salt) in water; fresh shelled eggs sink in this solution. Stale eggs lose water through the porous shell and develop a large air space causing the egg to float.

6.16 MEAT AND OFFAL

Meat forms about 4.5 per cent of the world's food supply.

The *dressed carcase* of beef, lamb, pork, venison or goat consists of approximately 14 per cent bone, 25 per cent fat and 60 per cent lean meat or skeletal muscle.

Cuts of mainly lean meat are then purchased each with a varying composition of fat, muscle and bone. It is mainly the lean meat which is consumed, whilst some people consume the fat in addition to lean. Figure 6.3 shows the structure of the main meat tissue.

Lean meat is composed of muscle fibres (55 per cent), surrounding with connective tissue *perimysium* (12 per cent) enswathing and binding the muscle fibres. In addition there are minute blood vessels with streaks of

fig 6.3 *structure of striped voluntary muscle, the main component tissue of meat*

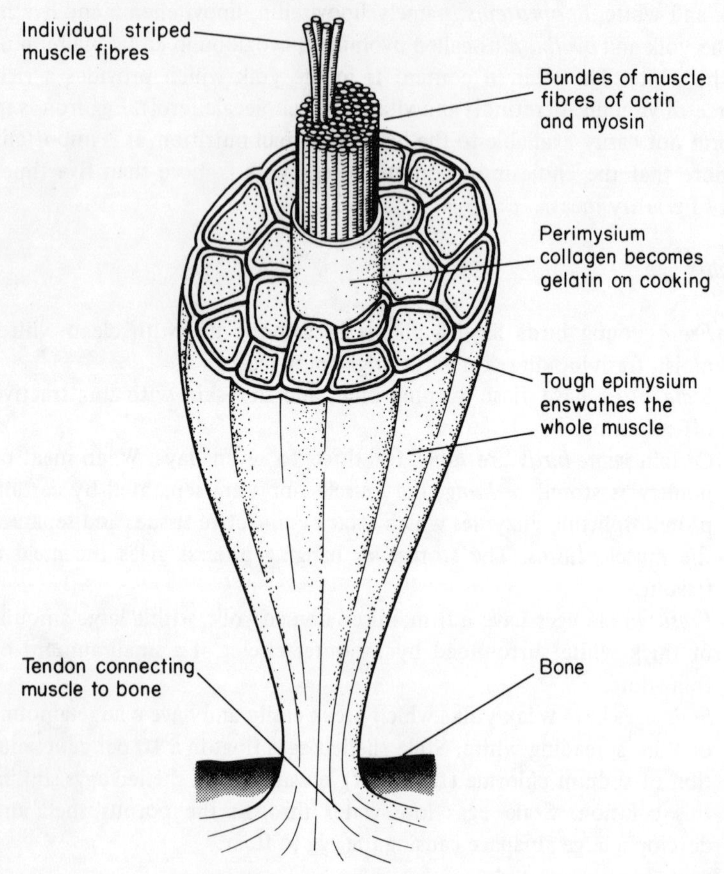

lipid fat close to them producing the 'marbling' of meat. This fat is therefore *within* the meat muscle. The whole muscle is surrounded by an outer *epimysium*.

The general composition of raw lean meat in Table 6.15 is based on an analysis of such meat from different species – beef, lamb, pork, etc. Considerable variation will exist in the composition of meat from the *same species*. This variation can be attributed to: (a) *breed* of animal (b) its *age* (c) its former *feeding* (d) the particular *muscle* from which the cut is obtained and (e) the changes brought about by *conditioning* after slaughter.

The main protein in meat muscle fibres is *myosin* (55 per cent) with *actin* (25 per cent) and other proteins called *troponins* and *tropomyosins* (25 per cent).

Table 6.15 *general composition of lean raw meats (per 100g portion)*

Water	74g	*Vitamins*	
Energy	550kJ	A retinol	trace
Carbohydrate	1g	D cholecalciferol	trace
(glycogen, (glucose)		B_1 thiamin*	0.25mg
		B_2 riboflavin*	0.18mg
Protein*	20g	Nicotinic acid*	7.5mg
Lipid	5g	B_{12} cyanocobalamin*	2.3μg
Cholesterol	70mg	Folic acid	7μg
Minerals		C ascorbic acid	trace
Calcium	7mg		
Iron*	2.5mg		

Meat is a source of good quality protein, absorbable iron, and vitamins of the B group, including folic acid. It is devoid of vitamins A, D and C, and is a poor source of calcium.

Quality

The edible quality of meat is very much a specialist area of knowledge of the butcher and meat scientist, and depends on many factors such as the breed and age of the animal and conditioning, chilling and cooking of the carcase which affect tenderness and flavour.

Offal

The liver, heart, kidneys and tongue are the meat offal of considerable nutritional value. These food items as purchased have little, if any, waste. Liver, kidneys and sweetbread (pancreas) have cells with large *nuclei*, and consequently have a high content of nucleic acids (DNA) and, in turn, a very high purine content (see Sections 8.9 and 4.10). Heart is composed of cardiac muscle, different in structure from skeletal muscle, being composed of *myoglobin* and other proteins, with glycogen carbohydrate. Table 6.16 lists its main nutrient components.

Liver is an outstanding source of all the vitamins of the B group, including folic acid, and vitamins A, C and D. It is the best source of iron, but is low in calcium. It is of similar composition to meat in protein and lipid content.

Table 6.16 *General composition of raw offal (per 100g portion)*

Water	74g	*Vitamins*	
Energy	500kJ	A retinol	100μg
Carbohydrate (glycogen)	2g	(Liver 1400μg)	
		D cholecalciferol	trace
Protein*	16g	(Liver 1μg)	
Lipid	7g	B_1 thiamin*	0.3mg
Cholesterol*	775mg	B_2 riboflavin*	2.5mg
Minerals		Nicotinic acid*	7.5mg
Calcium	10mg	B_{12} Cyanocobalamin (Liver 100μg)*	25μg
Iron*	15.0mg	Folic acid (Liver 240μg)*	12μg
		C ascorbic acid*	14mg

The very *high* cholesterol content exceeds that of egg yolk, whilst its purine content is high at 100mg per 100g (Section 8.9).

Meat extracts are produced by processing meat in hot water, and consist of vitamins of the B group, amino-acids, and certain minerals, potassium phosphates. They are also rich in purines.

6.17 MILK AND CHEESE

Milk and milk products form about 16 per cent of the world's food supply.

Milk is a non-cellular *almost complete* food with no waste and ready to be consumed. It is derived from the human breast, cows, sheep, goats, buffaloes and horses. Cheeses of various kinds and composition are prepared by *processing* different fresh or sour milks, which are *clotted* by means of *rennet* enzyme or acids in the milk or produced by bacteria. The cheese curd is then drained and ripened.

The major proteins in milk and cheese are *caseins, lactaglobulins* and *lactalbumins.* For general composition, see Table 6.17.

Cheeses are *concentrated* forms of milks with respect to most nutrients excepting carbohydrates, vitamin B_1 (thiamin), nicotinic acid and vitamin C (ascorbic acid), the nutrients and energy being concentrated *five* to *six* times in the cheeses.

Table 6.17 *general composition of milks and cheeses (per 100g portion)*

	Milks	Cheeses		Milks	Cheeses
Water	87g	45g	*Vitamins*:		
Energy	300kJ*	1500kJ*	A retinol	40μg*	300μg*
Carbohydrate (lactose)	5g*	2g	D cholecalciferol	0.1μg*	0.15μg*
			B_1 thiamin	0.04mg	0.04mg
Protein	3g*	22g*	B_2 riboflavin	0.15mg*	0.45mg*
Lipid	4.5g*	30g*	Nicotinic acid	0.20mg	0.10mg
Cholesterol	15mg	100mg	B_{12} cyanocobalamin	0.3μg*	1.3μg*
Minerals			Folic acid	5μg*	35μg*
Calcium	10mg*	115mg*	C ascorbic acid	4mg*	NIL
Iron	0.07mg	0.5mg			

The composition of milks *varies* considerably between the sources or *species* of animal making the milk. This difference in composition of milks is important when comparing cow's milk with human breast milk for feeding babies (see Section 10.8). Similarly the composition from a female mammal or human mother can vary as to the milk-producer's own nutrition and physical and mental health.

Both milk and cheese are valuable foods by virtue of their protein, lipid, vitamin and calcium contents. The cholesterol content is *less* than meat offal and egg yolk, but is present at a reasonably high level.

Quality

Milk and cheese are both examples of foods which are *processed* commercially in the UK and elsewhere. Consequently the processors need to maintain strict controls in the quality of their products – *freshness, hygiene*, and *uniform* composition etc. (see Section 7.12).

6.18 FATS AND OILS

Lipid fats or oils are extracted or separated from a wide range of foods of plant or animal origin which have a high lipid content, and include nuts, cereal germs, fruits, olives and soya beans (Section 7.5). Animal sources include oily fish (particularly their livers) and a range of mammals including cattle, pigs, sheep and buffalo.

Lipid oils and fats find important use:

(a) in *cooking* foods when they also increase the food's lipid content.
(b) when *added* to foods as spreads, dressings or creams as they increase the food's lipid and fat-soluble vitamin content.
(c) when *vitamins A and D* are extracted mainly from fish liver oils and are used as additives to enrich other food products such as margarine. The vitamin E (tocopherols) content of natural vegetable oils is useful as a *preservative* and *antioxidant*.

Plant sources include peanuts, olive, palm, sunflower, soya bean, coconut, maize, sesame and rape seeds and nuts. The oils from these sources have a *high* polyunsaturated fatty acid (PUFA) content. (Section 4.8 and Table 4.4).

Animal sources include lard (pork fat), dripping and suet (beef) tallow (mutton) ghee (buffalo milk) butter (cows milk) fish liver oils, for example cod and halibut, and fish oils, such as herring and pilchard.

1. *Energy* The nutritive value of lipid fats and oils is mainly as a *concentrated source* of energy, ranging from 1.5MJ/100g in thick cream and low energy spreads, to 2.5MJ/100g in peanut butter and salad dressings, to 3.8MJ in pure 100 per cent cooking fats and oils.
2. *Vitamins* The vitamins A (retinol) and D (cholecalciferol) are present mainly in animal origin lipids particularly fish liver oils, butter and cream. Palm oil has a high content of vitamin A as carotene.
3. *Essential fatty acid* Linoleic acid is found in large amounts in many vegetable oils, together with many other *unsaturated* fatty acids. Safflower oil contains 72 per cent, sunflower oil 63 per cent, soyabean oil 60 per cent, maize oil 56 per cent, peanut oil 30 per cent. Very small amounts of essential fatty acid are found in coconut oil 1.4 per cent, olive oil 8 per cent and palm oil 9 per cent.
4. *Cholesterol* is present in large amounts, 150–250mg per 100g in cream and butter, and to a lesser extent in lard, dripping and suet. Little, if any, is found in vegetable oils.

Margarine

This is *manufactured* or processed from either vegetable oils or a *mixture* of vegetable and animal lipids. The liquid lipid oil is treated with *hydrogen* gas which combines with *unsaturated* double bonds in the lipid molecule to form *saturated* single bonds by *hydrogenation*, forming a *solid* white fat. This may be used as *cooking* fat or *high ratio* cooking fat.

Otherwise the fat is treated with milk products to flavour it, and *additives* such as vitamin A and D and salt. *Colouring* matter is also added.

Low energy spreads are prepared in a similar way but with a higher *water* content to reduce the energy value. *Soft* margarines have a high PUFA content of up to 60 per cent of the total lipid, whilst *harder* margarines for cooking purposes have 10 per cent PUFA.

Quality

The majority of fats and oils and related food items are *processed* commercially in the UK and elsewhere; the *processors* therefore maintain uniform standards of freshness, hygiene and composition.

6.19 QUESTIONS

1. Summarise and compare the main nutrients and other components provided by foods from *plant* sources with foods from *animal* sources. Indicate those components which are absence or deficient in each.
2. Which foods are valued for their high energy content?
3. Which foods are valued for their high protein content?
4. Name and describe one group of foods from plant and one from animal sources which could be considered as almost complete in most nutrients.
5. Compare the contributions made by starchy vegetables, green leafy vegetables and fruits to the diet. Indicate which nutrients are deficient and which are present in useful quantities.
6. Write short notes on each of the following:
   (a) gluten; (b) myosin; (c) ovalbumin; (d) caseins, (e) zein.
7. Comment on the distribution of the following nutrients in foods:

   (a) Vitamin B_{12} (cyanocobalamin)
   (b) dietary fibre
   (c) Vitamin C (ascorbic acid)
   (d) Vitamin A (carotenes)
   (e) phytic acid
   (f) cholesterol.

CHAPTER 7

FOOD PROCESSING

7.1 INTRODUCTION

The whole foods described in Chapter 6 are mainly *raw* and *unprocessed*, with the exception of the *dried* legumes and fruits; *parboiled* rice; cheeses; fruit juices, sugar syrups and alcoholic beverages, which are *partly-processed* foods, or treated in some way by the application of human or other energy forms.

Most raw, unprocessed, whole foods can be digested in a healthy human digestive system. Many fruits and vegetables, milk, milk products and eggs can be consumed raw, but the majority of raw meats, offal, fish, shellfish and poultry, starchy vegetables and cereals are unpalatable raw. In the wealthy, developed countries there is a trend of serving many foods, including meat and fish, very underdone - *nouvelle cuisine* - such foods must be completely free of contamination as described in Chapter 11.

Processing foods by various energy-consuming processes, mainly the *cooking* processes, improves the *palatability* of food, changing its *flavour*, *colour* and *texture* (the three main palatability factors) and making food easier to digest.

Other important food processes include: *preparation* (cleaning, mixing, etc.) *preservation* (protection from spoilage) *packaging*, *storage* (see Section 11.2) and *transport*.

Processing is performed in the *home* by traditional methods on a small scale, and in *industry* by technology methods on a large scale. Industrial *food-processing technology* is based on a knowledge of applied food science, whilst traditional food-processing in the home is dependent mainly on the education and other influences which the person preparing the food has experienced from the family or the communication media.

7.2 FOOD PRODUCTION

Food production in many of the lesser-developed countries occurs at two levels: local traditional production or home-grown or reared foods on small farms, or settlements. The food is produced near to the home in sufficient amounts to feed a small group or family. Staple products with little variety are produced by mainly non-scientific methods, with a variable yield liable to severe loss by pests and drought during growth, harvesting and storage. The quality and flavour of the food product is frequently variable.

By contrast the second level of production by *agricultural technology* in many of the more developed countries using a knowledge of science, produces by methods of monoculture and intensive agriculture (see Section 3.13) a *uniform* product often with the same quality and flavour, subject to *contamination* by the same *pesticides*, *antibiotics* and *hormones* used to protect and maintain the health of the growing food crop.

Intensive monoculture production is used for chickens, eggs, fish such as trout, rabbits, pigs, calves and most vegetables, providing a product with a flavour which contrasts with free-range-produced chickens, eggs, game, and other wild stock foods.

Losses in food production

The *energy loss* in the different food chains (see Section 3.10) is *least* in a *short* food chain to produce food for human beings from plant sources. For example only about 15 per cent of the energy is lost when cereals are fed *directly* to human beings; whereas only 10 per cent of the energy in the *feed* fed to livestock becomes food energy for human beings.

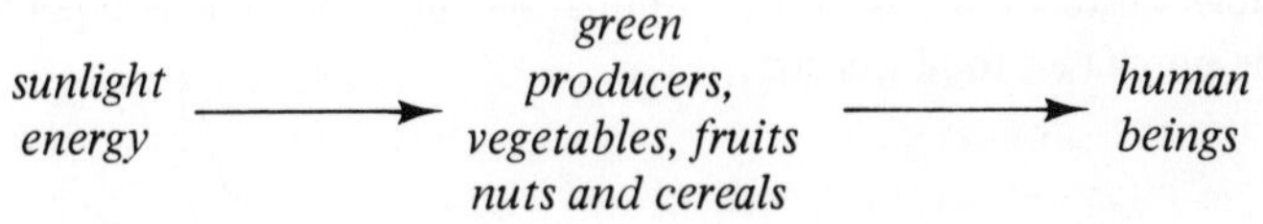

sunlight energy ⟶ *green producers, vegetables, fruits nuts and cereals* ⟶ *human beings*

In comparison the energy loss in the food chain to produce food from animal sources is *greater* in *longer* food chains. Over 90 per cent of the primary energy is lost at each feeding level. This provides support for alternative methods of producing *protein* from plant sources rather than from expensive animal sources (see Section 7.10 – textured vegetable protein). The world food supply experiences tremendous losses through spoilage, inedible waste, pests, processing, cooking and in distribution, which could amount to over 50 per cent of the world production. [See Sections 10.5 and 11.2.]

7.3 FOOD PREPARATION

Food preparation processes in the home and industry include: *cleaning* - removal of inedible waste, shells, bones, skin, guts - and other *physical* processes of slicing, mincing, mixing, grating, or chopping aimed at increasing the *surface area* of the food; or producing an *homogeneous mixture* of even composition throughout the whisking, blending and beating. Additional physical processes include *extraction*, *separation* and *expression* of juices or oils.

Industrial processes use special machinery to process pork *skin or rind* and *bones*, to produce *protein extracts*, and to process poor quality meat to form meat *slurry* or mechanically-recovered meat. Similarly fish is *minced*, and meat (fat, gristle and lean) is finely processed into a *meat mince*. These minces can then be reformed or shaped to resemble fish steaks, fish fingers and fish cakes or meat cubes or chopped meat.

Meat *paté* and *pastes* are made from meat slurry, and soups contain bone protein, whilst pork-skin or rind is a component of sausages and meat pies. In this way edible foods formerly discarded as waste in the preparation process are being *recovered* and their protein nutrient content *added* to other traditional meat and fish products, or to produce *re-formed* meat and fish products.

Inedible waste

The *inedible waste* includes the outer dead leaves, shells and skins of vegetables, nuts and fruits, together with the shells of eggs, molluscs and crustaceans.

In the home the inedible waste includes rinds, bones, gristle and fat, which is recovered by methods previously described in industry. The inedible waste of foodstuffs is summarised in Table 7.1 as a percentage of the purchased food weight.

7.4 LOSSES IN FOOD PREPARATION

Useful or valuable food nutrients are *lost* in certain preparation processes. Substances which are regarded as of *no* value as nutrients, for example, nut and shellfish shells, are considered as inedible food *waste*.

Outer leaves, peelings, skin and certain bones generally considered as waste in affluent countries, are more correctly nutritional food *losses*, since outer leaves and peelings are rich in certain vitamins, and methods of recovery can make them useful nutritionally in less affluent countries.

The main nutritional losses in food preparation are due to exposure

Table 7.1 *summary of inedible food wastes*

Food	Percentage inedible waste
Vegetables	
Broad bean	75 (pods)
Cabbage, cauliflower	30 (outer leaves and stalks)
Potatoes, parsnips	27 (peelings)
Lettuce, watercress, cucumber, spinach	20–25
Runner beans and peppers	15
Carrots, onions	5
Fruit	
Bananas, melon, grapefruit	40 (skin)
Rhubarb	35 (leaves)
Apples, oranges, pears	25–30 (skin)
Plum	10 (stones and skin)
Fish	
Herring	35 (bones)
Chicken	30–35 (bone)
Eggs	12 (shell)
Meat chops	20–25 (bone)

to *air oxygen*, light, certain metal knives and containers, or prolonged soaking in water, or by enzymes. The physical preparation process should be as *short* as possible before cooking.

1. *Air, oxygen*

   Exposure of prepared finely-divided foods to oxygen of the air reduces the ascorbic acid (vitamin C) content by oxidation.

   Vitamin A carotenes fade in colour and thiamin, vitamin B_1 and folic acid are also affected. Freshly-cut raw meat turns *bright* red (*oxymyoglobin*); on standing it turns *brown* (*metamyoglobin*) on exposure to air.

2. *Light*

   The ultraviolet content of daylight affects most vitamins excepting nicotinic acid and vitamin D. Lipids may begin to turn rancid.

3. *Metals*

   Copper and iron metals affect vitamin C (ascorbic acid) content. Vitamin B_1, B_2 and nicotinic acid are also affected to a lesser extent.

4. *Water leaching*

   Prolonged soaking or washing prepared foods will result in loss of *water soluble* mineral ions and vitamins B and C. Similar losses will occur in juices escaping from finely-divided or macerated foods.

5. *Enzymes*

   (a) *Blanching* Finely minced, chopped or shredded vegetables and fruits release an enzyme *ascorbic acid oxidase* which rapidly *destroys* vitamin C (ascorbic acid). This enzyme like most enzymes is heat sensitive (Section 8.6) and is destroyed by plunging the fruit or vegetables into boiling water for 1–5 minutes in the *blanching* process prior to cooking, canning or freezing.

   (b) *Enzymatic browning* Certain fruits and vegetables turn brown when the cut surfaces are exposed to air; this is caused by the combined action of oxygen and certain cell enzymes. It is prevented by blanching, or by addition of *acids* (lemon juice or vinegar) or covering with sugar, or keeping in boiled and cooled water (from which air and oxygen are expelled) or in solutions containing vitamin C (ascorbic acid). Potato *whiteners* are sulphite and tartarate solutions which keep peeled potatoes white.

   (c) *Autolysis* This is a process of *self-digestion* of cells; it is prevented by blanching vegetables and fruits. In animal cells of meat, poultry and game, the process of important in *conditioning* the meat in 'hanging' (Section 6.15).

   (d) *Meat tenderisers* Meat can be tenderised by hammering and beating to separate the muscle fibres (Fig. 6.3). When meat is hung, certain cell enzymes called *cathepsins* attack the connective tissue *perimysium* and help to separate the meat fibres. Plants produce protein-splitting enzymes; fresh pineapples give *bromelin*, fresh figs give *ficin*, and papaya (paw-paw) fruits give the enzyme *papain*. These can be sprinkled or forked into raw meat; alternatively sterile papain is injected into cattle before slaughter.

6. *pH* (Section 2.11)

   The use of *alkali*-producing reagents, sodium hydrogen carbonate (baking soda) and certain alkaline *whiteners* for potatoes will destroy vitamins of the B group and vitamin C.

Cassava preparation

Cassava starchy roots develop *hydrocyanic acid* by enzyme action in tissue beneath the skin; this is removed by grating followed by sun drying. Similarly when potatoes turn green they also produce a naturally poisonous substance solanine removable by carefully peeling.

7.5 MILLING

Milling is a preparation process of separating or extracting different components from a cereal grain or oil bearing seed. Plate 7.1 shows a boy grinding millet.

Plate 7.1 *a boy grind millet: part of a daily ration provided by the World Food Programme (WFP) which encourages resettlement from overpopulated areas to rural areas of Upper Volta, Western Africa (FAO, UN)*

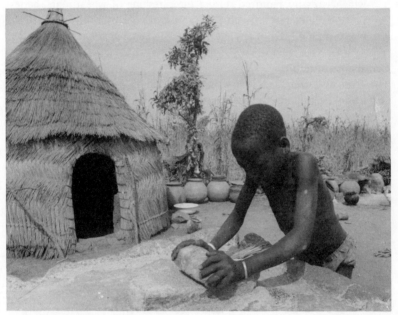

(i) *Oil milling*

A range of oil-bearing seeds - cottonseed, maize or corn, sunflower and groundnut are crushed in steel rollers then partly cooked by steam to release lipids from the plant cells.

The expressed oils are *refined* to remove free fatty acids and flavours, and *clarified* by filtration or centrifugation to remove suspended matter. The oils may be *winterised* or cooled to 7°C to crystallise solid alkanoic (fatty) acids which could cause vegetable cooking oils to *cloud* in cold weather.

The remaining material, rich in protein and carbohydrates, is called seed *cake* and is a useful cattle food. *Peanut butter* is a form of seed cake with a high lipid content; it is made by grinding a mixture of precooked peanuts of Spanish and North American origin.

(ii) *Cereal milling*

The cereal grains (Section 6.9) all have a similar structure being dry fruits or berries, botanically called a *caryopsis*, with a tough outer fruit skin (pericarp) closely joined to the seed coat (testa) both forming the outer layers called the *bran*, which forms 12 per cent of the grain.

Bran = fruit skin (pericarp) + seed coat (testa)

Around the grain are dry leaflike structures forming the *husk* which is easily removed during the threshing of wheat, oats, barley, rye and millet, but difficult to remove from rice other than by *dehusking*. Husk has little, if any, nutritive value being *inedible* waste.

Cereal grain structure

The fruit wall and seed coat - *bran*, surround an *embryo* composed of a *cotyledon* (scutellum) or seed leaf, plumule (future shoot) and radicle (future root); in effect a miniature plant, called the *germ*, forms 3 per cent of the grain. Figure 7.1 compares the structures of a pulse seed and a cereal grain.

Fig 7.1 *structural comparison of a pulse seed (broad bean) and a cereal grain fruit (maize)*

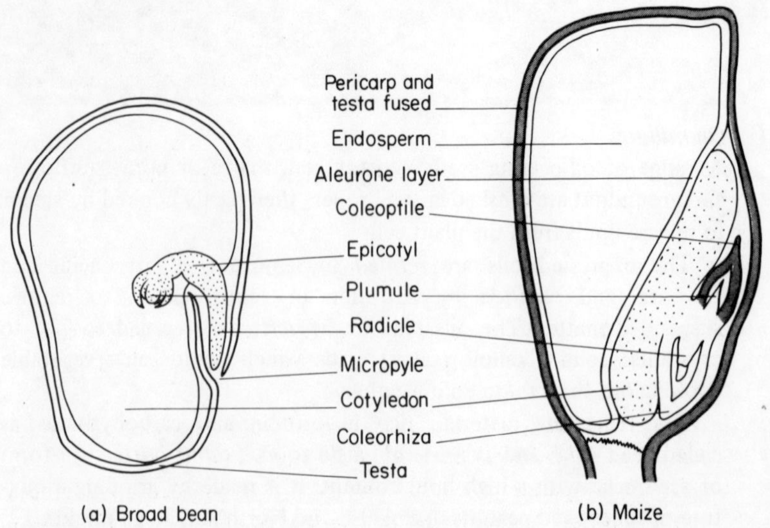

A reserve of food called *endosperm* consisting mainly of starch, and a surrounding *aleurone layer* rich in protein, provides nutrients for early growth in *germination*, this is the main component of the *flour*, and forms 85 per cent of the grain. Part of the aleurone layer may remain attached to the bran, and increase the nutritive content of bran (see Appendix).

Malt

If wheat or barley grains are allowed to germinate or sprout, the starch is changed into *maltose* by the enzyme diastase. Heating in a kiln stops the enzyme action and brown *caramel* forms. Water is used to prepare *malt extract* (Section 7.6).

Flour

The cereal grain bran coat resists digestion, consequently unprocessed cereal grains must be *crushed* and *ground* by the powerful masticatory action of teeth and jaws, to expose the grain nutrients to digestion in the human gut. Most cereals, dry legumes, and nuts can be ground or milled into *flour*. Soya beans produced soya flour, rice - rice flour, maize or corn - cornflour and maize meal, millet - millet meal, oats - oatmeal, and wheat a range of flours and wheatmeal.

Wheat milling

There are two main varieties of wheat:

(a) *Triticum vulgare* or common wheat used to make bread, cake and biscuit flour and breakfast wheat cereals.
(b) *Triticum durum* or durum wheat for making pasta, or alimentary pastes, spaghetti and macaroni. Semolina is used mainly in milk puddings.

Both are processed in the following similar manner:

(a) *Cleaning*, includes sieving and washing of previously threshed grain.
(b) *Conditioning* with warm moist air to allow the bran to peel away in *large* pieces during milling.
(c) *Breaking* the grain open by steel break-rollers to release the endosperm or semolina 85 per cent of the original grain.
(d) *Bran sifting* separates the bran or *wheat feed* into different grades called wheatings, depending on the amount of endosperm and aleurone

layer, clinging to the bran. *Germ* is also separated and sold as wheat-germ.

(e) *Reduction* is processing the endosperm between smooth steel rollers to produce *fine particles* of wheat flour.

Strong and soft wheat flours

The endosperm of a hard *Canadian*-grown wheat feels dry and is hard to compress, whilst the endosperm of weak English wheat is soft and mealy. Hard wheat gives *strong* flours containing 10–12 per cent protein whilst weak wheat gives a soft flour with 8–10 per cent protein (see Table 7.2).

Table 7.2 *different wheat flours and their uses*

Flour	*Uses*
Strong Canadian flour 10–12 per cent protein	Yeast-raised breads, batters, puddings, rich fruit cakes, puff and flaky pastries
Soft English flour 8–10 per cent protein	Light cakes, genoese and Victoria sponges, short crust pastry
Very soft low protein flours often with added rice, defatted soya flours or cornflour starch	Biscuits and shortbreads
Durum wheat flour is very strong, 8–15 per cent protein	Pastas or alimentary pastes; macaroni, farfals, noodles and spaghetti

Types of wheat flours

A wheat grain consists of 85 per cent endosperm, 12 per cent bran and 3 per cent germ. This will be present in the *wholemeal* flour or straight-run flour using *all* the wheat grain, that is, 100 per cent of the grain is in the flour. The figure 100 per cent is the *extraction rate*, whilst a flour or 72 per cent extraction rate show that 28 per cent of the grain is *removed* as bran, germ or outer aleurone layer (see Table 7.3).

Wholemeal flour 100 per cent extraction rate.
Brown flour 80–90 per cent extraction rate.
Wheaten and granary flour = brown flour + pieces of whole grain.
White flour 70 per cent extraction rate.
Patent white flour 45 per cent extraction rate.
Wheat germ flour = white flour + wheat germ.

Nutrient losses in milling

The general composition of whole grain cereals (Section 6.9) shows them to contain a range of useful nutrients of all kinds, with the exception of vitamins C and D, and in some cases vitamin A.

The nutrients are located in the grain roughly as follows (see Appendix for germ, bran and wheat flour compostion):

Endosperm and *aleurone layer*	Starch, protein, phytic acid.
Germ	Protein, lipids and most vitamins.
Bran and part of *aleurone* layer	Dietary fibre, protein, carbohydrates, calcium, iron, nicotinic acid, thiamin B1 and folic acid.

The effect of milling on the composition of wheat flours is shown as follows:

Wholemeal flour (see Appendix A) (100 per cent) contains *all* the nutrients and dietary fibre of the grain, so will other whole grain meals, rye meal, maize meal, millet meal and oatmeal.

White low extraction flour (45 per cent) (see Appendix A) will consist mainly of starch and some protein and lipid. the other valuable nutrients will all be *reduced*; vitamins of the *B* group (by 70–85 per cent) calcium (by 70 per cent) dietary fibre (by 70 per cent) and phytic acid (by 94 per cent). Similarly other cereals which have their bran and germ removed will suffer severe vitamin B groups losses. This is so in *rice* which has been *milled* or polished when up to 75 per cent of the B_1 (thiamin) content is removed. Further amounts are removed by washing polished rice. *Parboiling* rice involves boiling unhusked brown rice which drives the vitamin B group vitamins into the grain *interior*, thus less is removed in milling or polishing to produce white rice.

Flour enrichment

The following are added to 100g of white and brown flours in the UK to replace losses in milling: vitamin B_1 (thiamin) 0.24mg, nicotinic acid 1.6mg, iron salts 1.6mg, and calcium 0.028mg as calcium carbonate or pure chalk. In addition various additives are permitted in the UK to *bleach* flour making it whiter and to improve or strengthen flour dough. *Self-raising flour* includes sodium hydrogen carbonate and an *acid* salt, calcium phosphate or sodium pyrophosphate, added to a weak flour. The composition of white, enriched Canadian flour is shown in Table 7.3.

7.6 EFFECTS OF PROCESSING ON INDIVIDUAL NUTRIENTS

Processing in preparation, preservation or cooking can change certain food nutrients physically and chemically (Section 2.1). The physical

Table 7.3 *composition of white enriched Canadian wheat flour, 70% extraction rate (per 100g portion)*

Water	11%	*Vitamins*	
Energy	1525kJ	A carotenes	NIL
Carbohydrate	76g	B_1 thiamin	0.44mg
Protein	11g	B_2 riboflavin	0.26mg
Lipids	1g	Nicotinic acid	3.5mg
Phytic acid	low	C ascorbic acid	NIL
Dietary fibre	0.3g	Folic acid	22μg
		Minerals	
Calcium	16mg	Iron	2.9mg

changes are temporary and mainly reversible, whilst the chemical changes affect the food nutrients permanently and are *irreversible*.

Food nutrients are affected by the following processing conditions:

1. *Heat*, dry or moist
2. pH, acidity and alkalinity
3. Water solubility.
4. Oxidation
5. Reduction
6. Metals
7. Enzymes
8. Light or ultra violent radiation
9. Mechanical action – beating, etc.

Water

The water content of foods is affected by *dry* heat, causing it to evaporate, resulting in the drying and crisping of certain foodstuffs.

The high *specific heat capacity* of water (Section 2.4) makes it a heat reservoir in the food.

As a *solvent* it allows chemical reactions to occur, and provides water essential for *hydrolysis* (Section 2.12). It also enters living cells by osmosis, and dead cells by diffusion.

Carbohydrates

Carbohydrates undergo the following changes in processing:

Crystallisation is the physical process of forming crystals mainly from sucrose, this occurs in sugar confectionery products.

Hydrolysis is the chemical breakdown of polysaccharides, starches and disaccharides in the presence of *water* and dilute mineral *acids*, or *enzymes* into simpler monosaccharides.

Caramelisation is the chemical process of forming the brown-coloured substance from carbohydrates in the presence of certain acids by the action of heat. It is important as caramel colour and flavour.

$$\text{Carbohydrates} \xrightarrow{\text{Heat}} \text{Caramel}$$

Starch granules rupture under the influence of dry and moist heat, as is evident when making popcorn from maize grains. The burst starch granules allow the starch to dissolve more readily in water.

Dextrinisation is the chemical process of forming a mixture of soluble *dextrins* by the action of heat, acids or enzymes on starch. Dextrins form during bread-toasting, and in breadmaking.

$$\text{Starch} \xrightarrow[\text{and enzymes}]{\text{Heat, acids}} \text{Dextrins}$$

Gelatinisation is a process in which a suspension of starch granules *swell* up in water at the *gelatinisation temperature* of about 65°C to form a thick *paste*; as the paste cools it forms a *gel* (see Section 2.6).

(a) *Ordinary starch* from ordinary varieties of maize, rice, sorghum, wheat, tapioca and potato consists *mainly* of *amylopectin* (75 per cent) and 25 per cent of *amylose*. These starch sources form thick viscous *unstable* gels which on storage undergo physical *retrogradation* in which the gel breaks down, insoluble amylose particles form and water 'weeps' or is squeezed out by *syneresis*. Syneresis is also seen as oozing of water from jellies and baked custards on long standing. This retrogradation of starch gels happens when bread becomes stale, and when certain prepared puddings blancmanges or cornstarch preparations are stored.

(b) *Waxy starch* is mainly *amylopectin* and comes from *waxy* varieties of waxy maize, waxy rice, and waxy sorghum plants. This waxy starch forms *clear* mucilaginous *paste* which is stable and does not undergo retrogradation in stored products; it is used for sauces and puddings which may be stored and is unaffected by freezing.

(c) *Modified starches* are starches which have been chemically treated or heated, and include pre-cooked starch, phosphated and oxidised starches. These are used to make *instant* puddings, creams and soups and to thicken pie fillings.

Proteins

Proteins undergo the following changes in processing:

(i) *Water-binding* Proteins have a variable ability to take up or 'bind with' water. Flour proteins, glutenin and gliadin take up water to form elastic *gluten*, similarly gelatine swells in cold water.

(ii) *Denaturation* is a two-stage process affecting *natural proteins* causing a change in *physical* and *biological* properties and a disordered structure of the protein molecule.

When a protein is denatured the following may occur: loss of solubility, increase in thickness or viscosity, loss of water-binding ability, loss of enzyme activity, increased digestibility in the human gut.

The extreme effect of denaturation is its *second* stage called *coagulation*, seen also as gelation, curdling or flocculation.

The main conditions affecting denaturation are heat, pH changes, acids and alkalis, salts, poisonous metals, mechanical beating as the thickening of egg white and cream proteins on whipping; freezing also causes denaturation.

natural proteins

heat, acids, alkalis
beating, freezing, metal salts

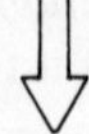

denatured proteins

insoluble, viscous, loss of water-binding ability, and enzyme activity

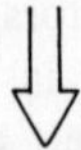

coagulated proteins

insoluble
visible as curdling, gelling,
and flocculation

(iii) *Hydrolysis* is an important process in the chemical breakdown of proteins into small molecules called peptides and amino-acids; the insoluble protein *collagen* in animal connective tissue is changed into soluble *gelatin* by moist heat.

(iv) *Enzymatic hydrolysis* of gelatin and certain other proteins can occur with bromelin (pineapple) papain (paw-paw fruit) and ficin (figs). These fresh fruits should not be added to gelatin jellies – their enzymes must be destroyed by heating the fruit (see also Section 7.4).

Amino-acids

Non-enzymatic browning (also called Maillard reaction browning) is the important process of browning *cooked* or *stored* foods due to the chemical reaction between proteins, amino-acids and reducing sugars. The amino-acids can be *free* amino-acids, or be the *functional* amino group of protein molecules.

amino-acids, or *protein amino group*	+	*pentoses,* *galactose* *glucose* *lactose* or *maltose* *sugars*	*cooking or long storage* ⟹	*brown coloured complex compounds*

The formation of this indigestible brown colour involves a nutrient loss mainly of the valuable essential amino-acids *lysine*, *tryptophan*, and *arginine* which readily participate in the change.

Experiment 7.1 *non-enzymic browning*

(i) Dip a one-third section of a clean filter paper in 1 per cent lysine solution, and dip another one-third section in 5 per cent glucose solution, and the remaining one-third section in *both* solutions.
(ii) Drain and allow to dry slightly, then deep fry in cooking oil until the first sign of browning is evident. Remove and compare the degree of browning of each section.

Lipids

Lipids are important in food processing because of the following properties:

Heat media

Lipid cooking oils and fats because of their lower specific heat capacity than water heat up rapidly and transfer their heat to food more rapidly in the cooking process.

Emulsion formation (Section 2.6)

The form *one* phase required in emulsion formation for sauces, creams and gravies.

Flavour

Certain lipids (for example, butter) are important in flavouring a food.

Textural qualities
The texture of baked cereal products (for example, shortbreads) is improved by certain lipids (for example, lard as *shortening agents*). The texture is due to the lipid fat crystal form and plasticity.

Lipid splitting
This is the decomposition of the lipids under the influence of heat, the lipid decomposing into propanetriol (glycerine) and alkanoic (fatty) acids. Further thermal decomposition of *propanetriol* (glycerine) products the unpleasant-smelling compound *propenal* (acrolein) associated with burnt fat.

Rancidity
This is the development of unpleasant tastes and odours in lipids though oxidation and enzyme action, and exposure to ultra-violet light (Figure 7.2), and is *catalysed* by copper and iron.

Fig 7.2 *types of radiation used with food: infra-red (radiant heat) and microwave (radar) for cooking; ultra-violet for food surface sterilisation, bread and cakes; gamma and X-rays destroy all micro-organisms – limited use in food sterilisation*

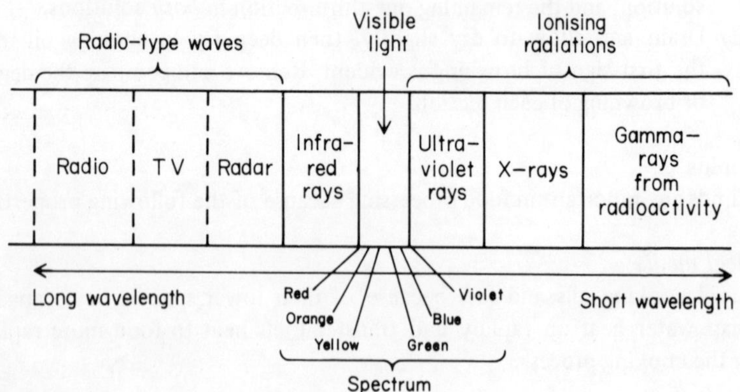

Dietary fibre
The components of dietary fibre are affected in food processing as follows:
(i) *Cellulose wall breakdown* The fibrous cellulose walls of plant origin foods are broken down by the action of moist heat to produce cellulose fibres allowing exposure of cell contents to digestive juices.

(ii) *Pectinisation* The *protopectins* cement the plant cells together in an *intercellular cement*, the moist heat of cooking weakens the intercellular cement separating the cells and tenderising the cooked vegetable or fruit. The process of *acid* hydrolysis brings about the formation of *pectins*, in the cooking and fruit ripening processes.

Mineral ions

The mineral ion components of food are mainly subject to *leaching* or dissolving in water used to process foods. They are mainly unaffected by other effects of food processing.

Ethanol

Ethanol is a *volatile* substance which rapidly evaporates from warm foods, has a lower boiling point than water (80°C) and is lost from heated foods. The use of wines in cooking is associated with the *flavours* they provide.

Vitamins

Processing has little effect generally on the *nutritive value* of carbohydrates, proteins, lipids and minerals. By contrast many vitamins are changed chemically to be of low or *no* nutritive value. Careless preparation, storage or cooking can cause considerable losses in food and vitamin content. Such vitamins as vitamin C (ascorbic acid) vitamin B_1 (thiamin), and folates undergo decomposition and are chemically *unstable*, whilst nicotinic acid is unaffected by processing conditions and is chemically *stable*.

The processing conditions which affect the *stability* of vitamins are heat, acidity, alkalinity, light, oxygen, milling and water-leaching. The *surface area* of the food exposed to processing, minced and grated foods, increases the losses. The effects of these conditions are summarised in Table 7.4.

7.7 COOKING METHODS

Cooking, the process of *transfer* of heat *energy* to foods, is the main process of food-preparation in the home or in industry. The following is a summary of the main methods used in the home and industry (see Section 11.6):

(a) Direct heat transfer

This includes grilling, broiling, salamandering, toasting and infra-red cooking. Heat travels as *radiant* heat energy from the source; temperatures reach 120-250°C.

Table 7.4 *effects of processing on vitamins*

Vitamin	*Effect of processing*
A retinol	Oxidised at high temperatures. Destroyed by exposure to sunlight – e.g. in sundried foods
D cholecaliferol	Stable to most conditions. Both are leached from roasted meat in lipid drippings because of their solubility in lipids.
E tocopherols	Very stable to heat
	The following are water-soluble and are affected by leaching in water
B_1 thiamin	Up to 40 per cent destroyed by heat cookery in neutral or alkaline solutions (baking soda – sodium hydrogen carbonate) – more stable in acid solutions up to 120°C. Milling cereals removes large amounts, and refining sugar reduces its concentration.
B_2 riboflavin	Up to 25 per cent destroyed by heat cookery in alkaline solutions, and also by exposure of fresh food, such as milk, to sunlight.
B_{12} cyanocobalamin	Stable in meats in most ordinary cooking conditions. Unstable in boiled, pasteurised or UHT treated milk.
Folic acid	Up to 90 per cent destroyed by heat-cookery in alkaline and neutral solutions; fresh foods affected by sunlight and air. Stable in acid solutions.
Nicotinic acid	The *most stable* of vitamins, unaffected by processing conditions.
C ascorbic acid	The *most unstable* of vitamins. Oxidised in alkaline and neutral solutions. Up to 75 per cent destroyed in cooking by heat, or exposure to sunlight, and the metals, copper and iron. Attacked by enzyme ascorbic oxidase. Stable in acid, and sulphite whitener solutions.

(b) Indirect heat transfer

This process involves heat transfer mainly by *convection* by different media – water, oil or air.

Air is the heat transfer medium in cookers or ovens used for roasting and baking. A circulating *fan* enhances the natural convection in forced-draught convection ovens. Temperatures up to 250 °C are reached.

Water with its high specific heat capacity is used as liquid boiling water or steam in a range of cooking processes from low-temperature slow-cooking, poaching, simmering and stewing, to boiling, casseroling and steaming at 100°C. Heat transfer is mainly by convection. Cooking water shoul dbe used for soups, sauces and gravies.

Pressure cooking is a process of steaming at a higher temperature, 110°C, under increased air pressure; this *increases* the rate of cooking and *decreases* the cooking time.

Oil, with its lower specific heat capacity, is used in small amounts as in shallow frying, sautéing, and fricassée, and involves heat transfer by *conduction*, whilst deep-fat frying is a process of heat transfer by *convection*.

Contact grills transmit heat by conduction to the food which cooks from the outside inwardly. Temperatures of between 150 and 230°C are reached.

Microwave ovens

The heat rays of radiant heat energy are also called *infra-red rays* and are situated beyond the red colour of the visible colour spectrum of light. By contrast the *ultra-violet* rays are situated beyond the violet colour of the spectrum.

Close to the infra-red rays are *higher* energy radiations called the radar or *microwaves*.

These microwaves are generated by special *magnetron valves* which are radiated in all directions within the microwave cooker and circulated by a *stirrer*.

The microwaves *penetrate* directly into food up to a depth of 5cm causing the good to heat up *rapidly*; this heat then passes into the food by *conduction*.

Function

The microwave oven has the following functions:

1. *Defrosts* ready-cooked or uncooked frozen foods.
2. *Reheats* previously cooked foods.
3. *Cooks* mosts foods very rapidly, for example, a meat joint weighing 2kg takes only 45 minutes to cook. Thin or sliced foods cook more quickly.

Table 7.5 *effects of cooking on foods from plant sources*

Plant source food	*Main cooking effects*	*Main losses*
Vegetables*	Cell wall cellulose softened, and cells separate. Starch gelatinises and granules break down. Colour intensifies. Some amino-acid/sugar browning (as in roast potatoes and chips).	Minerals, Vitamin C (60% loss) and B_1 (thiamin) (40% loss) by heat and leaching. Free folic acid (90% loss).
Fruits*	Cell walls softened and cells separate. Pectinisation releases gums and pectins. Syrups cause fruit shrinkage. Water swells fruits.	75% Vitamin C lost; minerals and sugars leached.
Cereals	Starch granules swell and burst and gelatinisation occurs. Baking causes dextrinisation, and amino-acid/ sugar browning. Gluten denatures and coagulates.	Vitamin B_1 (10% loss) with nicotinic acid loss of 40-80%.
Sugar Sucrose	Solubility in water increases with temperature. High temperatures cause *caramelisation* (Section 7.6). Fruit acids cause *inversion* of sucrose - glucose and fructose. *Crystalline* confectionery forms at *low* boiling temperatures below 150°C - fondant, fudge, creams. *Non-crystalline* confectionery forms at *high* boiling temperatures - boiled sweets, toffees.	

*Vegetables and fruits should preferably be cooked lightly and unpeeled, and served quickly.

Browning of the food by the amino-acid - sugar non-enzymatic browning process may not occur. This is achieved by browning with an infra-red grill.

7.8 GENERAL EFFECTS OF COOKING ON FOOD

The main effects of cooking are:

(i) *increased palatability* which affects *texture* or softens the food; *colour* in attractive browning and improved appearance; *flavour* and aroma are enhanced,
(ii) *increased digestibility* in correctly cooked food; *overcooking* frequently decreases the digestibility.
(iii) *destruction of enzymes* and anti-enzymes which prevent trypsin functioning in some foods.
(iv) *destruction of microbes* helps to sterilise the food.
(v) *decreased vitamin and mineral* content through thermal instability and leaching in water (Section 7.4).
(vi) *increased nutrient value* by addition of nutritive cooking fats.

Table 7.5 summarises the effects of cooking foods from *plant* sources.

Table 7.6 summarises the effects of cooking foods from *animal* sources, including oils and fats.

Table 7.6 *effects of cooking on foods from animal sources*

Animal source food	*Main cooking effects*	*Main nutrient losses*
Fish	Proteins denatured and coagulate rapidly. Connective tissue collagen rapidly forms gelatin. Less flesh shrinkage	Leaching of mineral ions in cooking water
Meat	Proteins denatured and coagulate slowly. Connective tissue collagen forms gelatin, and meat fibres separate. Gristle elastin unaffected. Flesh *shrinks* and meat juices squeezed out – these should be used for gravies and sauces. Red myoglobin turns brown. Some amino-acid/sugar browning also occurs. Lipid fats melt and turn brown in dry heat. Microbes destroyed.	Peptides, Amino-acids, Mineral ions, Vitamins of B group (30% loss). Dripping contains vitamins A and D.
Milk	Heat denatures and coagulates protein as 'skin'. Acids coagulate protein. Lactose caramelised. Milk fats softened. Calcium salts precipitated.	Vitamin C, B_1, B_{12} and folic acid (25% loss) Microbes destroyed

Table 7.6 *continued*

Animal source food	*Main cooking effects*	*Main nutrient losses*
Cheese	Proteins denature and coagulate. Colouring by carbonisation or slight charring. Solid lipids melt.	25% B_1 thiamin loss and folic acid partly destroyed.
Eggs	Proteins *denatured* by poaching at *low* temperatures, and coagulated by *high* temperatures of boiling and frying. Shrinkage occurs and custards curdle. Useful as binders and thickeners. Colour due to iron and sulphur causing blackening around yolk.	Vitamins B_1 (thiamin) B_2 (riboflavin) (25% loss). B_{12} partially destroyed.
Fats and oils	*Melting* of solids fats. *Rancidity* develops by oxidation of hot lipids. *Hydrolysis* of lipids to fatty (alkanoic) acids and propanetriol (glycerine) from water in foods. *Thermal breakdown* at high temperatures into coloured substances called *polymers* and propenal (acrolein)	Loss of essential fatty acids and vitamin E.

7.9 FOOD PRODUCTS

Industrial and home-processing of raw foods produces a range of fully and partly-cooked *food products*. Foods which have been processed industrially and include a considerable amount of preparation and cooking are called *convenience foods*. These convenience foods are ready to eat with or without heating or with minimum preparation following simple mixing. They include the following categories:

(i) *Cooked foods*, bread, cakes, cooked meats, breakfast cereals and fish and chips, or 'take away' foods.
(ii) *Canned and bottled foods*.
(iii) *Frozen foods* and *dehydrated foods* (see Chapter 11) together with a range of *instant* coffee, tea and soups, and ready-mixed cake and stuffing mixtures. Convenience *meals* can be frozen, dehydrated or tinned or as *mixtures* of foods for a meal, for example, rice and beef, vegetables and beef, stews and casseroles.

7.10 VEGETABLE PRODUCTS

An important vegetable product is *textured vegetable protein*, TVP.

Foods from all plant sources contain an average of 7 per cent protein, compared with foods from all animal sources which contain an average of 15 per cent protein. The yield per hectare of protein from *plant* sources is *four* to *six* times the yield from animal sources raised on the same area of land.

The *costs* and *time* needed to produce *animal protein* is much greater than for producing *plant* protein, and more wasteful in *energy transfer* through long food chains, compared with shorter food chains to feed human beings (Sections 3.12 and 3.13). With a correspondingly large increase in world *human population* (see Section 11.4) it is necessary to find and develop more economical sources of protein in the human diet.

Sources

The main source of plant protein for making textured vegetable protein is in soya bean (42 per cent protein); other sources include oil-seed protein from peanuts, coconut, sunflower, rape and sesame seeds. Protein can also be extracted from grass, plant leaves, wheat gluten and yeasts. Other useful but hitherto underdeveloped sources include certain micro-organisms, algae (Plate 7.2), moulds and bacteria.

Production

The protein in *fat-free* soya bean meal is extracted with alkali and spun into *fibres* by a process resembling the manufacture of man-made textile fibres. A meat-like colour and flavour and the essential amino-acid *methionine*, together with vitamins B_{12} (cyanocabalamin) B_1 (thiamin), B_2 (riboflavin) and iron are added to *enrich* the product as *nutritive additives*, to make it as nutritious as *real* meat. The *spun* fibres or *extruded* sponge-like protein can be bound with fat, flour and gelatinising substance to produce slices, cubes, chunks or granules imitating chopped and minced meats giving a product with not less than *50 per cent protein* in the dry weight (see Section 7.3).

Uses

TVP finds use as a meat *substitute* exclusively on its own in place of real meat in minces, stews, sausages, beefburgers and pies, or can be used as real meat *extenders* to be mixed with a certain amount of real meat in a mixture in various meat products. TVP is a very useful food and can provide an equally nutritious and more cheaply priced alternative to real meat, acceptable in vegetarian diets and in famine-relief foods.

Plate 7.2 *the experimental production of a green algae,* spirulina platensis, *as a source of protein to produce textured vegetable protein (FAO, UN)*

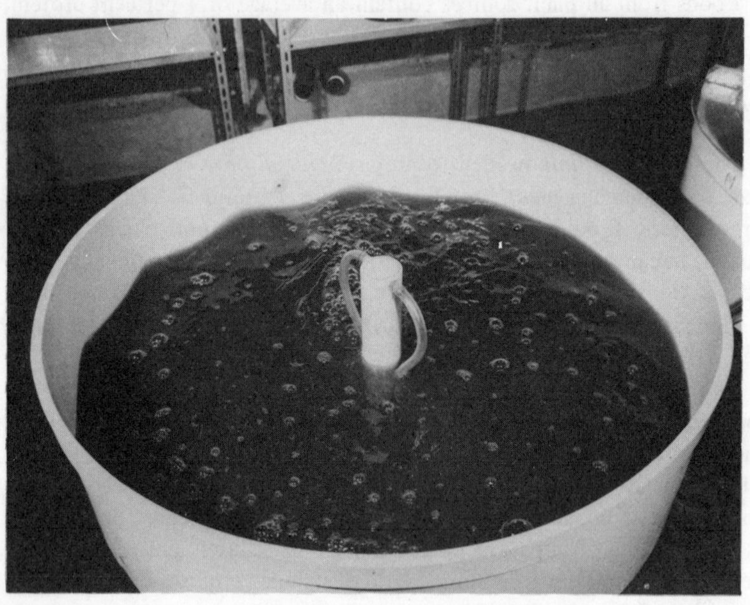

Nutritional Content (see Table 7.7)
Proteins from different plant sources *vary* in their essential amino-acid content (Section 4.9 and 10.9). Many are deficient in *methionine*, consequently this sulphur-containing amino-acid is added to TVP in a sympathetic or manufactured form. Since green plants do not produce vitamin B_{12} it is necessary to add this as well as vitamins B_1 and B_2 to fortify the TVP nutrient content.

Table 7.7 *general composition of dry, flavoured, spun protein (per 100g portion)*

Water	2%	*Vitamins*	
Energy	2600kJ	B_1 thiamin	5mg
Carbohydrate	3.5g	B_2 riboflavin	0.2 mg
Protein	48.0g	Nicotinic acid	7mg
Lipids	46.0g	B_{12} cyanobalamin	2μg
Cholesterol	NIL	Folic acid	4μg
		Minerals	
Calcium	27mg	Iron	11mg

7.11 CEREAL PRODUCTS

Breakfast cereals are prepared from clean whole grains by a cooking process which may involve rolling to produce flakes, or baking to produce swollen puffed, or shredded product. Nutrient *additives* include calcium, iron, and vitamins of the B group. Added *sucrose* and *protein* gluten is present in certain breakfast cereals.

A range of *baked* products are prepared from *flour mixtures* of varying composition, with or without certain *raising agents*.

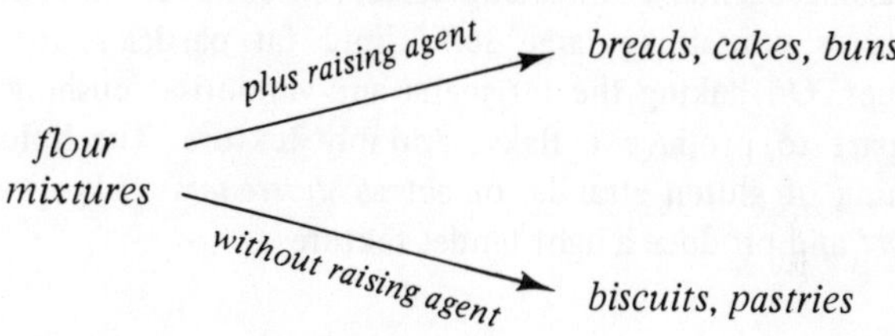

Flour mixtures

1. *Doughs* consist of about 65 per cent flour, and 35 per cent water and other components. Stiff doughs are used for bread, and soft doughs for buns.
2. *Batters* for cake mixtures and coating foods are 50 per cent flour and 50 per cent water and other ingredients.
3. *Pastes* are 80 per cent flour and 20 per cent other ingredients used for biscuits and pastries.

Raising agents

These serve to expand the flour mixture and reduce the density of the baked product or increase its lightness.

(a) *Yeast-leavened products* include breads, made from yeast and *strong* flour dough mixtures. Yeast (Sections 6.10, 6.12) produces carbon dioxide gas as by-products of anaerobic respiration (Section 5.6). On warming, the carbon dioxide and air mixture *expands*; this occurs when the bread dough *mixture* is *fermenting* – at the same time the *gluten* fibres are elastic and stretching as the dough rises. It continues in the *proving* process as gas collects in small pockets within the dough.

Baking in ovens at 230°C destroys the yeast enzyme activity causing the fermentation, and coagulates the gluten proteins, meanwhile the starches gelatinise and the crust forms dextrins and browns by the amino-acid and sugar process of non-enzymatic browning (Section 7.6).

Bread additives include vitamin C, caramel, preservatives, emulsifiers and also other cereal flours or defatted soya bean four and certain vegetable lipids.

(b) *Chemically-leavened products* include a range of cakes and batters containing either *baking soda* (sodium hydrogen carbonate) or *baking powder*, a mixture of sodium hydrogen carbonate and organic acids or acid salts, with starch. Both produce carbon dioxide gas by chemical reaction, and leave *alkaline* residues which can destroy vitamins B_1 thiamin, B_2 riboflavin and C aseorbic acid.

(c) *Unleavened products* are mainly biscuits or pastries without yeast or chemical raising agents. Pastries and certain biscuits are made from flour paste mixtures containing large *solid* lipid fat particles, for example, lard and suet. On baking the fat melts and vapourises pushing the flour mixture apart to produce a flaky, crumbly texture. The lipids prevent the stretching of gluten strands, or act as *shorteners* to keep the gluten strands *short* and produce a light tender texture.

7.12 MILK PRODUCTS

This section refers mainly to products from cow's milk.

1. Processed milk

Tuberculin tested milk is from cows which have been tested as free from tuberculosis, and the hygiene of the dairy and workers is of an approved standard. This milk can be sold as *untreated* TT milk, or as *pasteurised* TT milk. *Sunlight* destroys the B_2 riboflavin content of all processed milks.

Pasteurised milk is raw milk heated to 72°C for 15 seconds by the high-temperature short-time method. Pasteurisation destroys most harmful bacteria. The vitamin C (ascorbic acid) content is reduced by 25 per cent and B_1 (thiamin) by 10 per cent.

Sterilised milk is raw milk heated to 120°C in the bottle for 30 minutes with a space left above the milk in the bottle. The process is carried out in sterilisers or autoclaves resembling large pressure cookers.

UHT or ultra high temperature sterilised milk is raw milk heated at 150°C for *one* second and quickly cooled and sealed in special containers.

Both types of sterilised milk are completely free of *all* micro-organisms, and keep for long periods provided the containers are *not* opened. Between 60 and 100 per cent of vitamin C, 30 per cent of folic acid, 20 per cent of vitamin B_{12} (cyanocobalamin) and 10 per cent of B_1 (thiamin) are lost in processing.

Homogenised milk is heated (60°C) TT untreated or pasteurised milk forced through a small tube to break up the fat droplets into smaller globules, which remain suspended and do not separate into a creamline on standing.

Concentrated milks include:

(a) *evaporated milk*, evaporated under reduced pressure to 60 per cent of its original volume, it is sealed into cans and sterilised.
(b) *condensed milk*, which can be made from *whole* or *skim* milk; sugar is added (15–17 per cent) and the milks evaporated to 40 per cent of their original volume and sealed into cans or tubes.

Dried milks are made from *whole*, *half-cream* or *skim* milks and dried either by roller-drying or spray-drying. Losses of vitamins are similar to those occurring in pasteurisation.

Skim-milk or separated milk contains only 0.07 per cent of lipids - one fiftieth of the lipid content of fresh cows' milk (3.7 per cent); it also contains *less* of the lipid soluble vitamins A and D, but contains *all* the water-soluble vitamins, minerals, carbohydrates and proteins present in fresh cows' milk.

Skim-milk with its *lower* energy value (50 per cent that of fresh milk) and reduced lipid and saturated alkanoic (fatty) acid content, is a preferable source of nutrients for a healthful diet in *developed countries* (Section 11.3) in order to combat excessive body weight and its associated body disorders. Due to its lack of vitamins A and D it is unsuitable for baby-food unless accompanied by vitamin supplements.

Dried skim-milk powder is a valuable famine relief food (Section 11.6).

Cream

Cream is separated from whole milk in a spinner or centrifugal cream separator, the *skim milk* being a by-product. In the UK the following types of cream are available:

Cream type	*Lipid %*	*Protein %*	*Carbohydrate %*
Single	18	3.0	4.1
Double	48	1.6	2.4
Whipping	36	2.2	3.1
Clotted	63	3.0	2.5

The protein is *denatured* during the mechanical heating of whipping or double creams at 4°C. The creamy *colour* is caused by Vitamin A carotenes, associated with vitamin D cholecalciferol.

Butter is made by churning either *fresh* or *soured* creams. The butter vitamin A content is protected from destruction by sunlight by wrapping in light-proof foil-lined wrappings.

Ice-cream

Dairy ice cream is made from butter or milk fat (6–12 per cent) milk *solids*, dried or condensed milk, (10–12 per cent) and sucrose (11-15 per cent); other *additives* include flavouring, colouring and emulsifiers. *Ice cream* or 'non-dairy ice cream' can be made from *non-milk* lipids - vegetable oils instead of butter or milk fat.

In both products a large amount of *air* is incorporated which *doubles* the original volume of the ice cream mixture, amounting to 50 per cent air by volume.

Soured and fermented milks

Yoghurt is made by the action of *acid*-forming bacteria which change *lactose* into *lactic* acid (2-hydroxy-propanoic acid) in warmed homogenised milk or skim milk at 44°C; this acid the denatures and coagulates the *casein* milk proteins to produce clots with a texture similar to that of junket or custard.

Fermented milks can contain varying amounts of ethanol (1-3 per cent) in *kumiss* (fermented mares' milk) and *kefir*; the ethanol forms by yeast action on lactose.

7.13 MEAT AND FISH PRODUCTS

Raw meat and fish are sold as cuts, steaks or fillets of *recognisable* raw meat and fish.

A range of meat and fish *products* with a variable content of lean and fat meat content, which can also include textured vegetable protein as meat *extenders*, is available in cooked and uncooked forms.

In the UK these meat and fish products must have a *minimum* meat or fish content; the other ingredients can include non-meat cereal, soya bean flour, milk powder, fat, vegetables, flavourings, pastry, preservatives, colourings and water.

Fish products include fish paste (70 per cent fish) and fish cakes (35 per cent fish). Table 7.8 summarises the *minimum* amount of meat (lean and fat) in various food products.

Offal find limited use in the preparation of meat products; the following main products are *liver sausage*, *black pudding* (blood, suet and barley) and the *Haggis*, a tasty and nutritious product of protein (10 per cent) fat (20 per cent) carbohydrate (20 per cent) with useful amounts of mineral ions, calcium and iron, and vitamins of the B group. It is prepared from

Table 7.8 *minimum meat content of different meat products*

Minimum meat content (%)	*Meat product*
95	Canned meats, corned beef and ham
90	Minced meat, potted meat
85	Tinned mince with gravy
80	Hamburgers and tinned luncheon meat
70	Meat pastes and paté
65	Pork sausage
50	Canned meat, vegetables and gravy, beef sausage
35	Curried meat and meat pie filling
25	Meat pies, canned stew
12.5	Meat and vegetable pies or puddings

sheeps' liver, heart and lungs minced and mixed with oatmeal, suet and herbs and cooked within the sheep's stomach. Similar use is made of the sheep and pig's small intestine as a casing or container for sausage meat in sausages.

7.14 QUESTIONS

1. Briefly outline the main methods of preparation of raw vegetables prior to cooking. What are the main inedible wastes and which nutrients are lost in the processing?
2. Describe the structure of meat and fish flesh. What changes occur during the cooking process by moist heat?
3. Draw and describe the structure of a cereal grain and outline the process of milling to produce a flour. Which nutrients are lost in discarded cereal bran?
4. Briefly describe each of the following with examples of the type of change:
   (a) enzymatic browning
   (b) non-enzymatic browning
   (c) dextrinisation
   (d) denaturation
   (e) gelatinisation
5. What are the main types of processed liquid milk? How are they prepared and what nutritional loss do they experience in processing? What are dairy ice cream and ice cream?

7.15 EXPERIMENTAL WORK

A range of experimental procedures concerning food processing is contained in Chapters 8 (moisture loss in oven cookery) 9, 10 (fruit waste and pectin) 11, 12 (vegetable waste and cooking effects) 14 (cereal grains and flours) 16, 17 (baking and chemical raising agents) 18 (starches thickeners and gelatinisation) 19, 20 (sucrose sugar boiling and caramelisation) 23, 24 (lipids in cooking) 27 (egg custards and foams) 33 (meat) and 36 (food browning) of O. F. G. Kilgour and Aileen L'Amie *Experimental Science for Catering and Homecraft Students*.

CHAPTER 8

FEEDING

8.1 INTRODUCTION

Feeding is a complex process concerned with the provision of nutrients to all human body *cells* and their usage for different cell *functions*. The processes involved in feeding include:

(a) *intake* of foodstuffs into the gut or alimentary system
(b) *digestion* of foodstuffs within the gut
(c) *absorption* of digested foods
(d) *transport* of nutrients to cells
(e) *assimilation* or usage of nutrients within cells by metabolism
(f) *homeostatic balance* in maintaining the constant level of nutrients in the *tissue fluid* (Section 1.4 and Figure 8.6 later in this chapter).

8.2 FOOD INTAKE

The normal method of food intake is *oral* feeding by way of the mouth into the alimentary system. *Special* feeding methods include:

(a) *Tube* feeding by introducing a flexible tube into the stomach and connecting this to a drip-feed container of a fluid mixture of foodstuffs such as milk, egg, glucose, vegetable oil, mineral and vitamin supplements or a proprietary food mixture (*Complan*, *Casilan*, etc.).
(b) *Parenteral* or intravenous feeding involves the passage of a *sterile* solution of nutrients directly into a *vein*, from a drip-feed container. The sterile solution consists of a mixture of glucose, amino-acids, emulsified soya bean oil, ethanol, vitamins and minerals. This method of feeding does not require digestion or absorption since the nutrients are ready for transport to the body cells.

8.3 FOOD APPRECIATION

Hitherto emphasis has been placed on the *nutrient content* of foodstuffs towards an understanding of *eating sensibly*. Without this nutritional knowledge eating can be regarded as a *pleasant* experience of which we are made aware by the *sensory organs* of the human body, stimulated by different attractive or appetising foods. Nose, tongue, eyes and ears are all concerned with *food appreciation*.

Nose

Olfactory sense organs appreciate food odour or aroma, and bouquet (wines).

Tongue

Gustatory sense organs called taste buds, appreciate the *primary* tastes of sweetness (sugars and sweeteners) saltiness (sodium and potassium chlorides) sourness from fruit and other acids, and bitterness as from quinine in 'bitter-flavoured' mineral waters.

Tasting is only possible for substances in a solution of water as provided by saliva. *Dry* foods cannot be tasted unless they are moistened with water. Tasting is an important *protective* process in identifying unpleasant-tasting, bad or poisonous foods.

Flavour is a combined effect of food *smell* and food *taste*. The flavour of a food cannot be detected if the nose is blocked by a head cold; only the taste is evident. Warmth provided either by the mouth or warm food causes *volatile* components to reach the nose cavity and help in appreciating flavour.

Herbs and spices

Herbs are soft-stemmed plants which produce flavours attributable to various chemical components, such as *thymol* in thyme, *menthol* in mint and peppermint and *eugenol* in bay.

Spices are mainly tropical plant products – from bark, for example, cinnamon; fruits, for example, nutmeg and clove, flowers such as saffron or root, for example, aniseed.

Both herbs and spices are available as *dried* and *ground* preparations, and these are often contaminated with bacteria, soil and dust.

Purified essential oils and extracts in ethanol are available in *natural essences*. Dry-powder preparations include purified extracts *dispersed* and *encapsulated* in starch, glucose or gums.

Texture
The crispness, chewiness or *feel* of food, in addition to its *temperature*, is appreciated by the tongue, mouth lining, palate and teeth.

Eyes
Eyes appreciate the attractive appearance and *colour* of food (which also gives an indication of its freshness) as well as the pleasantness of the *surroundings* in which the meal is eaten.

Ears
Ears as auditory organs appreciate the chewing sounds, crispness or crackling sounds, in addition to sounds associated with *food preparations*: dinner gongs, dishes and cutlery clatter.

Apart from *sensory appreciation* of food, one may have a *psychological* appreciation based on likes and dislikes based on previous experience, or a refusal to eat in *anorexia nervosa*, or for other reasons such as religion, taboo or traditions.

Experiment 8.1 *fresh fruit juice flavour*
Obtain a sample of fresh fruit juice and divide it into two equal portions. Boil one portion for 5-10 minutes and allow to cool. Taste the fresh fruit juice and compare with the boiled and cooled fruit juice flavour.

Fruit juices have a *taste* because of their sugars and fruit acids; they also have a fruity *smell* given by volatile essential oils which evaporate easily in the warmth of the mouth but are completely lost from the juice on boiling.

8.4 FOOD INTAKE CONTROL

Situated at the base of the brain close to the pituitary gland is the region of the brain called the *hypothalamus*. It is the *main centre* for controlling a number of functions of the internal body organs. It regulates sleep, body temperature and water balance and in addition is responsible for food intake through two centres: the *feeding or appetite* centre, and the *satiety* centre. The latter centre is affected by changes in the blood sugar concentration.

(a) *Appetite* is a pleasant sensation in response to the sight or smell of food, or thoughts and sounds associated with food. Appetite causes the secretion of saliva and stomach gastric juice. It may be affected by *appetite stimulants* such as vitamin B_1 (thiamin) present in soups and meat extracts, also by alcohol or in medicinal preparations prescribed for debility. Appetite may be lost in illness and by the effect of certain appetite suppressant or anorectic drugs, used in anti-obesity or weight reduction treatments.

(b) *Hunger* is an unpleasant sensation caused by changes in blood sugar and alkanoic (fatty) acid concentration, and a feeling of rhythmically contracting muscles of an *empty* stomach. It becomes more unpleasant in cold surroundings.

(c) *Satiety* is the feeling of fullness because of having a full stomach containing food. A similar feeling of fullness can be produced using a synthetic preparation of dietary fibre *methyl cellulose* which swells up with water in the stomach. The satiety centre of the brain hypothalamus lowers the desire for more food, hence reducing or stopping the food intake in a healthy person.

(d) *Bulimia*. This is an abnormal condition of an increased or insatiable appetite associated with over-feeding or *hyperphagia* with consequent overnutrition and obesity (see Sections 9.4 and 9.5).

8.5 HUMAN ALIMENTARY SYSTEM

The human alimentary system consists of the *alimentary canal* or gut, and digestive *organs*, teeth, salivary glands, liver and pancreas. (See Figure 8.1.)

Structure

The alimentary canal is 9 metres in length from mouth to anus. The *mouth* with its *palate* helps to pass food into the *pharynx, oesophagus* and *stomach*. Linked to the stomach is the *small intestine* consisting of the duodenum and ileum. The *large intestine* connects with the small intestine by the *ileocaecal valve*, and consists of the caecum, colon and rectum and terminates in the anal canal. At different positions in the gut are located circular *sphincter muscles* - for example, the stomach has a sphincter muscle which periodically relaxes to release some of the stomach contents into the first part of the intestine, the duodenum.

Gut motility

Nerves control the contraction and relaxation of mainly involuntary muscle in the gut wall. This results in a *mixing action* of the gut contents, and also the *onward* propulsive transport of the contents through the gut by *peristalsis.*

Mucus, a slimy sticky fluid, is produced by the gut lining and helps to *lubricate* the gut contents and *protect* the gut epithelial lining from digestion by digestive juices.

fig 8.1 *main component parts of the human gut or alimentary system*

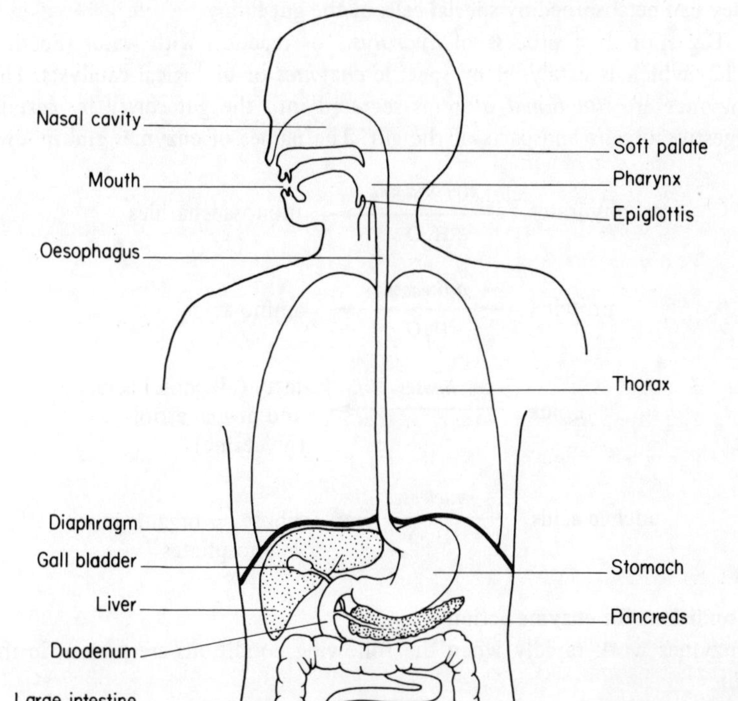

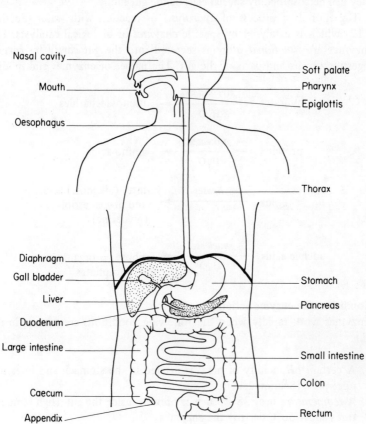

Gut epithelial cells are continuously shed and replaced by new cells every 48 hours; these loose dead cells forming the intestine lining may either be digested or collect in the *faeces.*

Bacteria

Bacteria are found mainly in the large intestine as natural symbiotic inhabitants; they are important in the synthesis of vitamins of the B group and Vitamin K.

8.6 FOOD DIGESTION

The *large* macro-molecules of certain nutrients - proteins, lipids, nucleic acids and certain carbohydrate starches and disaccharides, must be broken down into simpler and *smaller* component molecule units, in order that they can be absorbed by special cells of the gut lining.

Digestion is a process of *hydrolysis* or reaction with water (Section 2.12) which is catalysed by specific *enzymes* or biological catalysts. The enzymes are *functional* proteins secreted into the gut *cavity* by certain digestive organs and parts of the gut. The names of enzymes end in *-ase.*

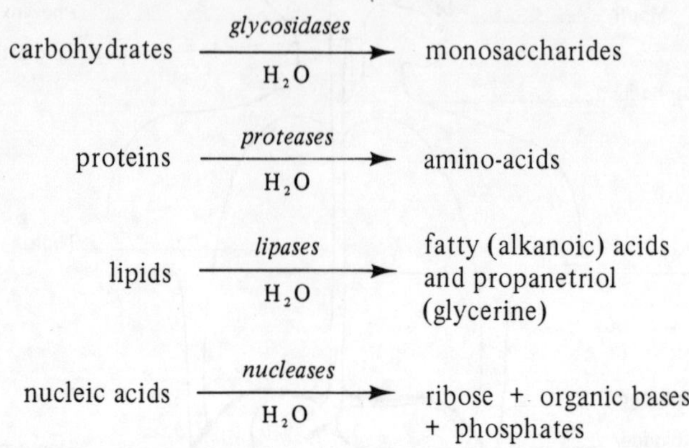

Conditions for enzyme action

Enzymes work rapidly when the following conditions are present in the gut:

1. A certain *pH*, acidity of pH 2 is needed in the stomach and intestinal juice pH 8 (Section 2.11).
2. A *temperature* near 38°C, such as prevails inside the gut. High temperatures above 50°C destroy the enzymes.
3. Certain minerals or vitamins may also be needed. (*Poisons* like lead, arsenic or cyanide destroy enzyme activity.)

Nutrients not requiring digestion include water, mineral ions, vitamins, ethanol, amino-acids, glucose and fructose together with other monosaccharides, all of which are ready for absorption.

Substances which cannot be digested include all the components of *dietary fibre* listed in Section 4.7, together with certain essential oils, flavourings and food colours.

8.7 DIGESTION OF CARBOHYDRATES

(a) Mouth

α-Amylase present in the *saliva* of most adults is secreted by three pairs of *salivary glands*; digests cooked starches containing dextrins to produce *maltose* and a small amount of *glucose*. Uncooked raw starch is changed into *dextrins.* Saliva is produced at the sight or smell of food, and by the feel of food on the tongue.

It consists of 99 per cent water and contains the lubricant *mucin* together with mineral ion *calcium* and several other minor components: 0.5-1.5 litres are secreted daily in adults.

(b) Stomach

The highly acid pH 1-2 of gastric juice halts the amylase activity commenced in the mouth.

(c) Small intestine

(i) Pancreatic juice from the pancreas contains small amounts of amylase which change starch into *maltose* (see Figure 8.2).

fig 8.2 *pancreas gland (gut sweetbread) produces insulin and pancreatic juice*

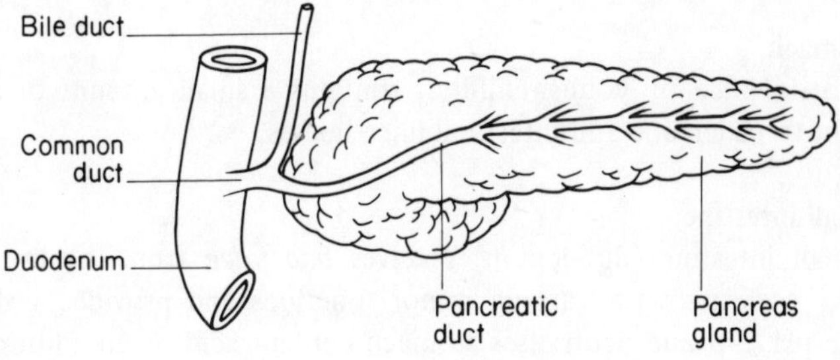

(ii) Intestinal juice from the cells lining the small intestine produce *disaccharidases* - maltase, sucrase, lactase - which are enzymes changing maltose, sucrose and lactose into monosaccharides.

Note: *Lactase* shows its maximum activity in babies, then decreases into adulthood. In certain African and Asian adults it may diminish entirely, to cause unpleasant digestive disorders on eating milk or milk products - this is called *lactose intolerance* (see Section 8.12).

8.8 DIGESTION OF PROTEINS

Large molecules of proteins are composed of over 100 amino-acid units; smaller molecules of proteins called *peptides* have *less* than 100 component amino-acid units.

(a) Stomach

The stomach of an adult secretes 2–3 litres of *gastric juice* daily and increases at the sight or smell of food; it contains the mainly protein-splitting enzymes and *hydrochloric* acid.

Pepsin enzymes commence the digestion of proteins into peptides. *Rennin* (produced only in babies) clots milk protein forming curds of *casein.*

(b) Small intestine

(i) *Pancreatic juice* from the pancreas is produced at a rate of 0.7–2.5 litres per day in adults and is rich in the *inactive* enzyme precursors trypsin*ogens* and chymotrypsin*ogens*. These are changed into the powerful and active *trypsins* and chymotrypsins by an ingredient of the intestinal juice (enterokinase). These enzymes convert proteins into smaller peptide and dipeptide molecules and into amino-acids.

(ii) *Intestinal juice* produces a mixture of enzymes (dipeptidases) called *erepsins* which converts peptides and dipeptides into amino-acids.

8.9 **DIGESTION OF LIPIDS**

(a) Stomach

The gastric juice of young children contains a small amount of *lipase*, different to pancreatic and intestinal juice lipases.

(b) Small intestine

The small intestine (duodenum) receives *bile juice* from the liver; this contains enzymes with varying minor functions and provides a slightly alkaline pH 7–8 and neutralises stomach content acidity. In addition the *bile acids* called cholic and chenodeoxycholic emulsify the lipids producing fine lipid droplets with a *large surface area* for action by lipase enzymes. Almost 700cm^3 to 1200 cm^3 of bile juice are secreted daily; this juice also contains 4 per cent cholesterol. Gallstones which can form in the liver gallbladder are 70 per cent cholesterol.

Lipases are secreted in the pancreatic and intestinal juices; these enzymes remove one fatty acid (alkanoic acid) unit at a time from the triester (triglyceride) to form propanetriol (glycerine), free fatty acids and simple monoester (monoglyceride) units.

Digestion of nucleic acids

Cells with large nuclei – yeast, brain, kidney and liver – contain nucleic acids (DNA). The enzymes required for their digestion are called *nucleases* and are present in digestive juices chiefly of the pancreas and stomach. Purines and pyrimidines are amongst the products of nucleic acid digestion.

Purines (Section 4.10) – adenine and guanine – are present in *large* amounts as components of nucleic acids found in brain, kidney, liver, sweetbreads, meat extracts, fish roes, herrings, sardines and mackerel. *Moderate* amounts of purines are present in pulses, meat, fish, whole grain cereals, spinach and cauliflower, whilst most other foods have a *low* purine content.

Purines are metabolised in the body and changed into *uric acid* (see Table 9.7). This can be deposited in different tissues causing gout, arthritis and kidney stones. Food rich in purines should be reduced or avoided to prevent these disorders arising.

8.10 DEFAECATION

The small intestine contents pass into the large intestine by way of the ileo-caecal valve. In the large intestine 70 per cent of the water is removed from the contents and they become *faeces* (also spelt *feces*). After temporary storage they pass into the rectum and by way of the external anal sphincter muscle are *defaecated* to the exterior.

Faeces are complex mixtures of undigested food remains, dead gut-lining cells and bacteria. They are mainly dietary fibre and in adults vary in amount from about 50g daily (on a mainly meat diet) to 370g (on a mainly vegetable diet).

Faeces consist of 75 per cent water, 8–10 per cent food residues (seeds, cellulose, lipids, muscle and keratin fibres, insoluble salts, nitrogenous substances, mucus, undigested nutrient protein and shed epithelial cells). The remaining 15 per cent consist mostly of dead bacteria, coloured by bile pigments.

The first faeces of a newborn infant are a soft, sticky, odourless, greenish brown to black mass called the *meconium.*

Intestinal gases

Gas or *flatus* can collect in the stomach or intestine causing *flatulence* and *indigestion.* The gas may be *swallowed air* through gulping food or *carbon dioxide* from carbonated waters, beers, sparkling wines or aerated bread and souffles. The gas can be passed out by way of the mouth by *eructation.*

Intestinal gas originates from swallowed air or by bacterial action on food residues in the intestine. This offensive-smelling gas mixture consists of nitrogen 64 per cent, carbon dioxide 14 per cent, hydrogen 17 per cent, methane 3 per cent and oxygen 1 per cent. Hydrogen sulphide and other substances including ammonia are responsible for the odour.

Between 400 and 2000 cm^3 of gas is expelled daily by the anus; *less* is produced on *high* dietary fibre diets, and *more* on meat and bean diets.

Experiments 8.2 *to show enzyme action*

(i) *Saliva amylase activity*

Rinse all traces of food from the mouth.

Collect a sample of saliva and place in a clean container.

Add a pinch of starch to boiling water; cook it for half a minute; cool the solution.

Add a sample of fresh saliva to the cooked starch solution and maintain it at 37–40°C in a warm water-bath for 10 minutes. Test samples for unchanged starch, and for glucose and maltose using the procedures in Experiment 4.1.

(ii) *Trypsin action*

Prepare a 2 per cent solution of trypsin in water at 40°C.

Cut up thin strips of photographic film negative and place some in the trypsin solution and some in plain water. Maintain these solutions at 37–40°C in a warm water-bath.

Carefully observe any changes in the appearance of the negative strips.

Film negatives are plastic films coated with the protein gelatine and impregnated with black silver metal. Trypsin digests the gelatine protein producing water-soluble peptides, leaving the plastic base unaffected by trypsin.

8.11 ABSORPTION

This is the process of *entry* of the products of digestion and other sub-substances: monosaccharides, amino-acids, fatty (alkanoic) acids, propane-triol (glycerine), monoglyceride (monoesters), ethanol, water, mineral ions and vitamins, into the *cells* of the gut-lining. These substances enter the cell by (a) *passive absorption* by diffusion or osmosis (Section 2.7) or (b) *active absorption* involving the use of cell energy by *active transport* or (c) *endocytosis*, a process by which a cell *engulfs* tiny solid particles or fluids by means of the brush border *microvilli*, to form pinocytes as shown in Figure 8.3. If mainly solids are engulfed, the process is called *phagocytosis*; if the material is mainly liquid it is called *pinocytosis.*

Intracellular digestion

The main process of digestion occurring within the gut *cavity* is called *extracellular digestion.*

Large particles or molecules can be digested into smaller molecules within the *cell* during *intracellular digestion* using digestive enzymes produced by cell organelles, the *lysosomes* (Section 3.3). This is an import-

fig 8.3 *small intestine lining cells showing the brush border microvilli and engulfment of food particles by pinocytosis and phagosytosis*

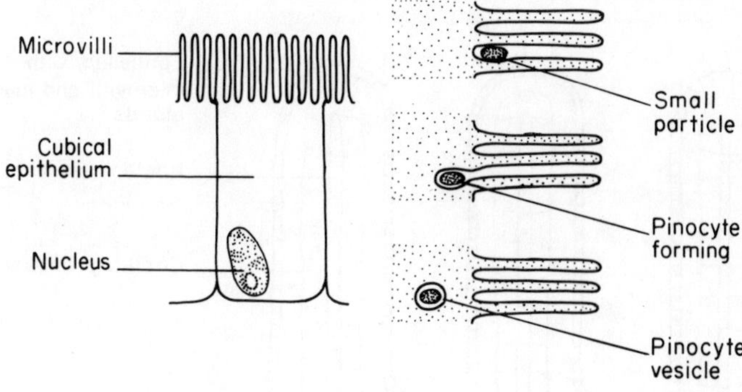

ant process for digesting peptides, di- and monoglycerides (di- and mono-esters) and tiny fragments of protein material or droplets (micelles) of lipid substances, which enter cells by endocytosis.

Intestinal villi

The main region of the gut concerned with absorption is the *small intestine*. Its inner surface has a large *surface area* because of numerous finger-like projections called *villi.* Each *villus* has a central core of *blood* capillary vessels around a *lacteal* lymph vessel. The surface of the villus is covered with absorptive epithelium cells of the brush border *microvilli* which provides a tremendous surface area for absorption, as shown by Figure 8.4.

Each villus continuously shortens and lengthens; this rhythmic pumping action helps to move the absorbed nutrients in the blood and *lymph vessels.*

Between certain villi are the *intestinal glands* secreting *intestinal juice* mainly in the gut duodenum region.

Experiment 8.3 *the small intestine*

(i) Examine either microscope slides showing transverse sections of the small intestine or 35mm photomicrographs.
(ii) Examine museum-mounted specimens showing the digestive systems of a small mammal.

A. Carbohydrate absorption

Glucose and galactose enter the small intestine cells and blood capillary vessels rapidly by *active transport* using cell energy; fructose being a larger molecule enters more slowly.

fig 8.4 *structure of small intestine wall showing intestinal villi providing an enormous surface area for absorption of digested food and for secretion of intestinal juice*

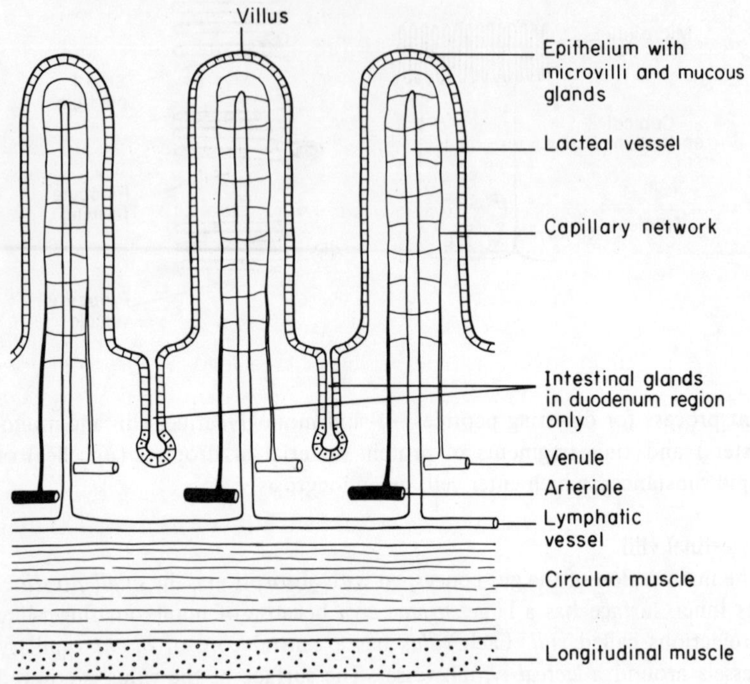

B. Protein absorption

Amino-acids and peptides are absorbed by way of the microvilli of the small intestine cells mainly by active transport, the smaller peptides undergoing further intracellular digestion.

C. Lipid absorption

The bile salts *emulsify* the lipids, then the pancreatic lipase and alkali splits *some* triglyceride (triesters) into free fatty (alkanoic) acids and monoglycerides (monoesters) together with propanetriol (glycerine). Further *physical* action by bile salts causes the lipids and digestion products to form very tiny particles called *micelles.*

The *micelles* enter the cells of the duodenum and upper small intestine lining by way of the microvilli by diffusion and active transport. Once within the absorptive cells and the lacteal vessel the fatty (alkanoic) acids and monoglycerides (monoesters) recombined to *reform* lipid *tri*glyceride (*tri*esters).

The re-formed lipids are then immediately coated with a *lipoprotein* coat and become particles called *chylomicrons.*

D. Absorption of other substances

Water, ethanol and small amounts of certain minerals and vitamins can be absorbed in the *stomach* by osmosis and diffusion. Absorption of water and mineral ions also occurs in the large intestine colon region. The main region of absorption for most nutrients is the small intestine.

Calcium

About 20 per cent of calcium available in foods is absorbed in the small intestine by active transport using cell energy, which is assisted by vitamin D. Calcium can be rendered *insoluble* and unavailable for absorption by phytic acid in vegetables, oxalic acid, and fatty (alkanoic) acids (Section 4.4).

Iron

Iron from animal origin food for example, blood *haem* is absorbed more easily than iron from vegetable origin food. The absorption occurs in the duodenum and first part of the small intestine. The iron Fe^{+++} must be *reduced* chemically by a reducing agent namely vitamin C (*ascorbic acid*) to the iron Fe^{++} form before it can be absorbed. (See Section 2.12.) Iron enters the absorptive cell by way of the microvilli either as ions or as a complex possibly by active transport.

Iron from *different foods* is absorbed to *different extents.* Iron absorption is dependent on the *amount* of iron already *stored* in the body. When body iron stores are *normal*, only 6 per cent is absorbed from the iron available in liver, 8 per cent from meat, and 28 per cent from pork. When the body iron stores are *low*, 24 per cent is absorbed from the iron available in liver, 18 per cent from meat, and 43 per cent from pork.

Generally people in developed countries on a balanced healthful *mixed* diet absorb only 10 per cent of iron in their food when iron stores are *normal*; this rises to 20 per cent when iron stores are *low*.

Water soluble vitamins

Most water-soluble vitamins of the B group, vitamin C and folic acid are absorbed in the *upper* part of the small intestine by passive diffusion, whilst vitamin B_{12} (cyanocobalamin) is absorbed in the *lower* part of the small intestine, assisted by the *intrinsic factor* provided by the stomach gastric juice.

Lipid soluble vitamins

Vitamins A and D become part of the *micelle* mixture, and later are part of the chylomicrons within the cells.

Table 8.1 summarises the process of digestion and absorption in human beings.

Table 8.1 *summary of digestion and food absorption in human beings*

Region of gut	*Gland and secretion*	*Enzymes and optimum pH other activity*	*Food digested, products and other activity*
Mouth Mastication by jaws and tongue	Salivary gland - saliva, 0.5–1.5 litres daily	(i) pH 5–7, slightly acid in adults, slightly alkaline to neutral in children (ii) Amylase	(i) Mucin lubricates food bolus (ii) (a) Starch (amylose) dextrins (b) Cooked starch maltose (+ trace glucose)
Oesophagus	None	None	Food bolus moves by peristalsis
Stomach Churning action. Temporary storage, 1–3 hours	Gastric gland, stomach wall - gastric juice, 2–3 litres daily	(i) pH 1, strongly acid (ii) Rennin (in young children) (iii) Lipase (in young children) (iv) Pepsin from pepsinogen (v) Nucleases	(i) Hydrochloric acid is *bactericidal* (ii) Clots milk protein → casein (iii) Lipids → fatty acids (alkanoic acids) and glycerine (propanebrial) monoglyceride (monoesters) (iv) Proteins → peptides + dipeptides *Absorption*: water, salts, vitamins and ethanol
Duodenum receives bile juice and pancreatic juice	(i) Liver - bile juice, 700cm³ 1.2 litres daily	(i) pH 7–8, slightly alkaline (ii) Enzymes with various minor functions	(i) Alters pH of stomach contents (ii) Bile, acids cholic and chenodeoxycholic emulsify or cream lipids
	(ii) Pancreas - pancreatic juice, 700cm³ daily	(i) pH 7–8, slightly alkaline (ii) Amylase	(i) Food as chyme propelled by peristalsis (ii) Starch (amylose) → maltose

		(iii) Lipase	(iii) Lipids → fatty acids and glycerine (propanetriol)
		(iv) Trypsinogens and chymotrypsinogens	(iv) Inactive, see below
		(v) Nuclease	(v) Nucleic acid → nucleotides → ribose, organic bases and phosphates
Small intestine and duodenum	Glands in intestine and duodenum wall - intestinal juice	(i) pH 7–8 (ii) Enterokinase changes trypsinogen into trypsin (iii) Lipase (iv) Glycosidases - maltase, sucrase, lactase	Proteins → amino-acids Lipids → fatty acids and glycerine (propanetriol) Disaccharides (maltose, sucrose, lactose) → monosaccharides (glucose, fructose, galactose) *Absorption*: large surface area, villi and microvilli, main region for absorption of vitamins, minerals, amino-acids, glucose, fatty acids, propanetriol (glycerine) and monoglyceride (monoester)
Large intestine	Lining with mucous glands	pH 6–8 No enzyme	(i) Mucus lubricates faeces (ii) Water absorbed from faeces (iii) Bacteria synthesise vitamin B group (iv) Faeces mainly: water, 75%; bacteria 15%; lipids, dietary fibre cellulose, other substances, 10%

8.12 DEFECTIVE ABSORPTION

Certain nutrients from the diet may *not* be absorbed for various reasons; this disorder of absorption is called *malabsorption.*

Cystic fibrosis is an inborn or hereditary disease which affects the pancreas which is unable to produce sufficient enzymes and some may be lacking entirely. It leads to severe digestive disorders. The lung mucous glands and skin sweat glands are also affects. Treatment with pancreas extracts helps to overcome part of this disorder.

Lactose intolerance. Milk sugar lactose requires the enzyme *lactase* present in the intestinal juice for its digestion. The disorder is prevalent among Asians and people from certain African countries. The symptoms on eating milk or milk products include various uncomfortable digestive upsets including pain, loose faeces and accumulation of gas in the bowel. A *lactose-free* diet overcomes the disorder (Section 8.7).

Coeliac disease is seen in children who have an abnormal small-intestine lining aggravated by the protein *gluten* component found in wheat, barley and rye. When the sufferer is fed on a diet which does *not* include gluten, the disorder is overcome and the intestinal lining returns to normal.

Bowel surgery. After surgical operations on the stomach and intestine in which parts are removed, the food is *partly* digested. For example, bile and pancreatic juice may be released *after* food from the stomach has already passed to the lower end of the small intestine. Iron is not absorbed when the parts close to the stomach are removed, and vitamin B_{12} may not be absorbed if the lower end of the small intestine is removed.

8.13 FOOD NUTRIENT TRANSPORT

Transport is the process of carriage of the absorbed nutrients from the gut *absorptive* cells to the *tissue fluid* (Section 1.4) surrounding all living cells in the human body.

(i) *Water soluble nutrients*, monosaccharides - glucose, amino-acids, ethanol, mineral ions and vitamins C and those of the B group and folic acid - leave the intestinal absorptive cell and enter the blood capillary network within the villus core. All these soluble nutrients dissolve rapidly in the *blood plasma* or *fluid component* of blood.

This blood collects from the gut in large blood vessels and is carried by a *hepatic portal vein* to the *liver*, and thence by the *hepatic vein* to reach the heart for circulation to every living cell via the *arteries* of the arterial system. . . . . (See Figure 8.5.)

fig 8.5 *the human liver, largest body gland, producing bile, store for iron and glycogen carbohydrate, amino-acid deamination, urea formation and with intimate contact with blood*

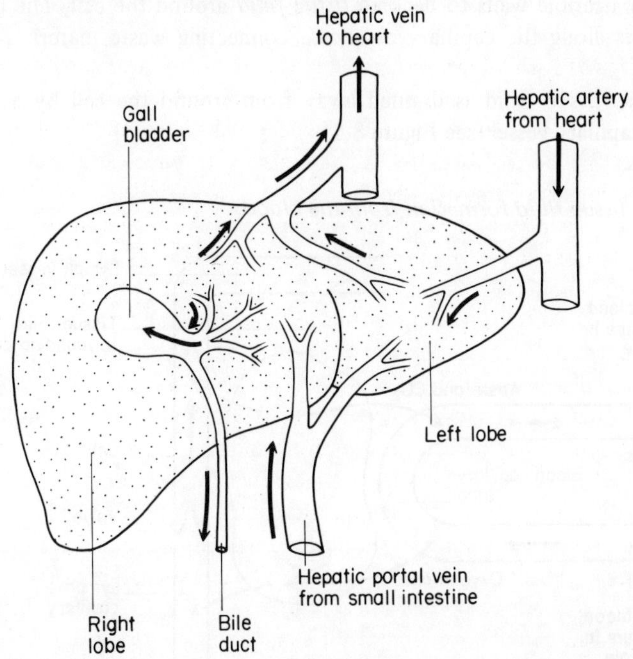

(ii) *Lipid soluble nutrients.* These include vitamins A and D, cholesterol, propanetriol (glycerine), free fatty (alkanoic) acids, and monoglyceride (monoester) *all* contained as a mixture in the *chylomicrons.* These tiny particles enter the central lacteal vessel in the villus core and are then collected in *lymph vessels* which empty into a *vein* near the heart, to mix with the blood and to be circulated to the living body cells by the *arterial* system (see Section 3.6 and Figure 3.3).

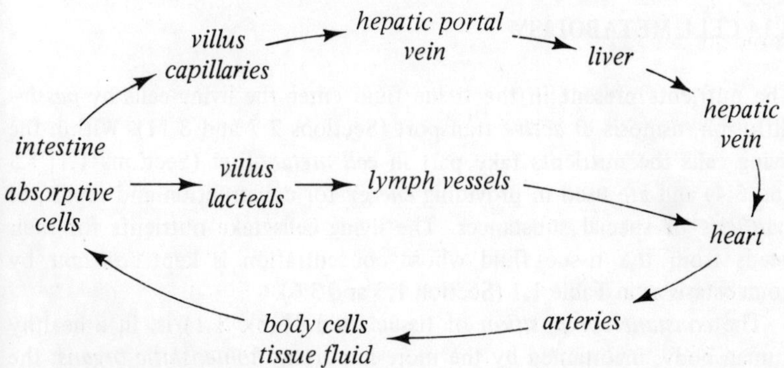

Tissue fluid formation

Every living cell is close to a blood capillary vessel. Blood reaches the cell through a tiny *arteriole*; the blood pressure causes *fluid* to pass through the thin arteriole walls to become *tissue fluid* around the cell. The blood continues along the capillary as *venule* connecting waste materials from the cell.

Excess tissue fluid is drained away from around the cell by a small lymph capillary vessel (see Figure 8.6).

fig 8.6 *tissue fluid formation from the blood*

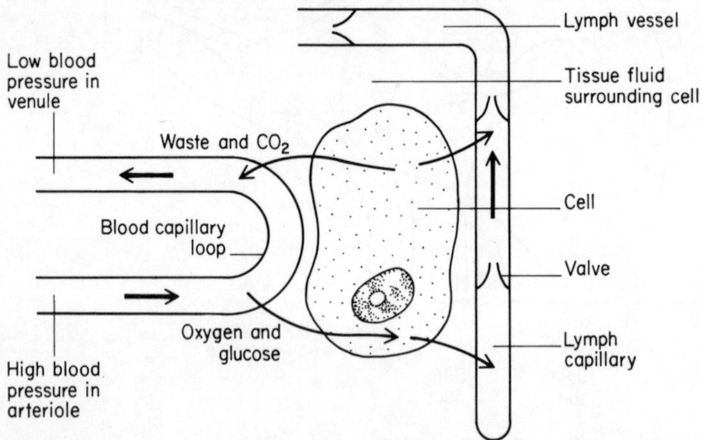

Physical exercise is a valuable and important means of promoting a good blood and lymph *circulation*, thus allowing nutrients to reach body-cells furthest away from the heart and the absorptive cells of the intestine. Physical exercise causes the skeletal muscles to act as a *muscle pump* acting on blood vessels.

8.14 CELL METABOLISM

The nutrients present in the tissue fluid enter the living cells by *passive* diffusion, osmosis or *active* transport (Sections 2.7 and 8.11). Within the living cells the nutrients take part in *cell metabolism* (Sections 1.1, 1.5 and 5.4) and are used in providing *energy* for construction and repair, or *synthesis* of special substances. The living cells take nutrients for their needs from the tissue fluid whose concentration is kept *constant* by homeostasis as in Table 1.1 (Section 1.3 and 3.6).

The *constant composition* of tissue fluid (Table 1.1) is, in a healthy human body, maintained by the more important *homeostatic organs*: the *liver, kidneys, pancreas* and *skin*, together with control centres in the *brain hypothalamus* (Section 8.4). These organs, supported by the *circulatory* and *respiratory* system, REMOVE *excess* nutrients from the blood plasma fluid or ADD nutrients from stores if there is a *deficiency*, hence controlling the important BALANCE of nutrients for a constant tissue fluid cell environment.

8.15 **FATE OF MONOSACCHARIDES**

All the absorbed monosaccharides are changed into *glucose* in the *liver* cells, which returns to the blood fluid plasma and tissue fluid to provide a blood sugar (glucose) *concentration* of around 0.1 per cent.

Glucose will be *removed* and *added* to the blood plasma by different processes; despite this the blood sugar concentration must remain around 0.1 per cent. It is *homeostatically controlled* by the liver and pancreas as *homeostatic* organs.

Glucose entry into cells

Glucose passes from the tissue fluid into the cell by the process of active transport; this is greatly affected by a *hormone insulin* produced by the pancreas and secreted directly into the blood.

(a) If the insulin blood concentration *falls*, glucose enters the cell *slowly*; meanwhile the blood-sugar concentration *rises* above 0.1 per cent. In a healthy person the pancreas is made to secrete *more* insulin by homeostatic controls or glucose is removed from the blood. If the pancreas is *defective* the disorder called *sugar diabetes* arises with the blood glucose concentration increasing and appearing in the urine and other symptoms such as thirst, hunger and weight-loss develop; it must be treated, usually by injections of insulin or special drugs taken by mouth.

(b) If the insulin blood concentration *rises*, glucose enters the cells *rapidly*; meanwhile the blood-sugar concentration *falls* to below 0.1 per cent. In a healthy person homeostatic controls slow down insulin production from the pancreas and glucose is added to the blood. If the pancreas is defective or too much insulin is injected, the brain cells are starved of glucose and the person becomes unconscious, in a *coma*.

The main use of glucose in the body cells is to provide *energy* by respiration (see Sections 5.4 and 5.5). This process occurs aerobically in the cell mitochondria, the glucose passing through several stages to form a substance *acetyl coenzyme A*. This substance enters the complex citric acid or Krebs cycle to produce 38 units of ATP energy-rich per mole of glucose substance, together with heat, carbon dioxide and water.

Surplus glucose

Surplus glucose not used for energy release can be *removed* from the blood and changed into either *glycogen* (animal starch) or made into lipids.

Glycogen formation

This occurs mainly in the liver cells and also to a lesser extent in the skeletal muscles.

$$\textit{glucose} \xrightarrow[\textit{(insulin)}]{} \textit{glycogen}$$

Certain enzymes, mineral ions and hormones including insulin activate the change. The glycogen then becomes a store or reserve of glucose or energy (Section 5.12 and Table 5.6).

Lipogenesis or lipid formation

This occurs when the intake of carbohydrates in the diet is *high*. Glucose is changed into lipids in the *liver, adipose cells*, heart and brain, together with the mammary gland cells in order to make *milk* fat in lactating females; elsewhere lipids are stored in the *reserves* beneath the skin, around the heart and kidneys and within skeletal muscle.

The liver is seen here as a major homeostatic organ for glycogen and lipid formation from glucose and thus *regulates* blood-sugar and tissue-fluid concentration by *lowering* blood-sugar concentrations.

Glucose formation

A. From non-carbohydrates – gluconeogenesis

Glucose can be produced in the *liver* cells from *non-carbohydrate* sources mainly amino-acids. The liver is also able to produce glucose from propane-triol (glycerine), fatty (alkanoic) acids, and lactic acid.

Amino-acids are *deaminated* by removing ammonia from the molecule; this becomes *carbamide* (urea) and glucose is formed.

B. From glycogen

Glycogen can be changed in *liver* cells into glucose by the effect of the hormone *glucagon* also secreted by the pancreas directly into the blood.

$$\textit{glycogen} \xrightarrow[\textit{(glucagon)}]{} \textit{glucose}$$

A similar conversion occurs in muscles by means of different hormones. The homeostatic function of the liver is seen here in its ability to *raise* blood sugar concentrations.

8.16 FATE OF LIPIDS

The *chylomicrons* break up within the *liver* cells to form fatty (alkanoic) acids and propanetriol (glycerine); they recombine and form lipid triesters (triglycerides). These reformed lipids can be stored in adipose tissue, or other lipid depots.

Propanetriol (glycerine) and fatty acids can be changed into *acetyl coenzyme A* (Section 8.15) and used to provide energy in the citric acid Krebs cycle.

8.17 FATE OF AMINO-ACIDS

1. *Protein synthesis* is the main process in which amino-acids are made into *structural* and *functional* proteins in the cell ribosomes under the influence of RNA (ribonucleic acids).

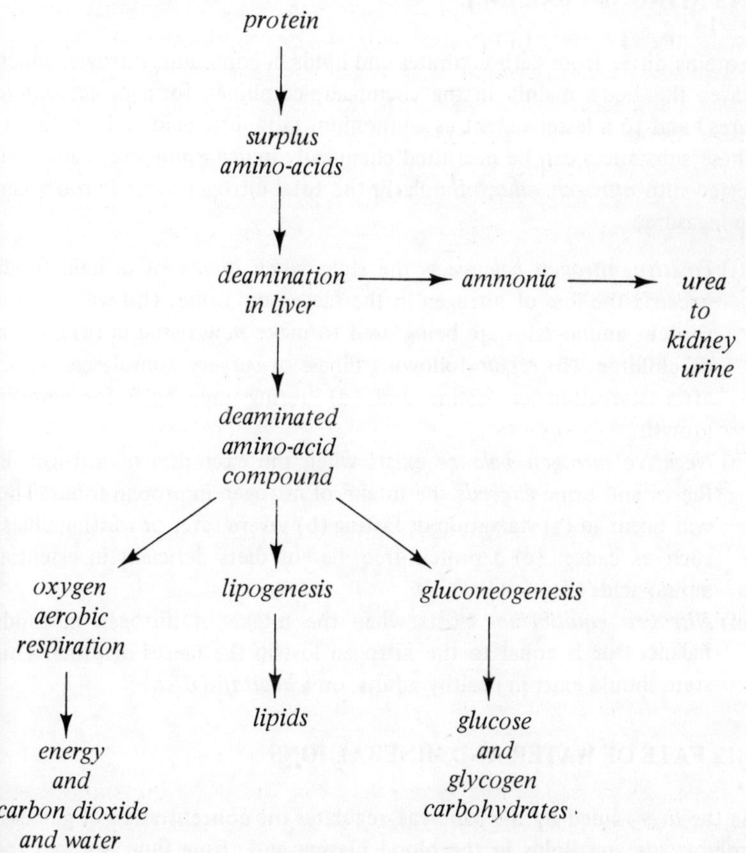

2. *Deamination* is the process occurring in the *liver* where surplus amino-acids have ammonia (NH_3) removed from their molecule – this poisonous substance is changed into harmless carbamide (urea). The remains of the amino-acid molecule then enter the *Krebs citric acid cycle* (Section 8.16) to produce energy, carbon dioxide, water and heat. Alternatively the deaminated amino-acid compound is changed into glycogen or glucose by *gluconeogenesis* or is made into propane-triol (glycerine) and in some cases fatty alkanoic acids to form lipids by lipogenesis.
3. *Transamination* is an important process of passing on an *amine* group (Sections 2.9 and 4.9) molecule parts derived from glucose or fatty acids, to form *new* amino-acids mainly of the *non-essential* amino-acid type. The ones that *cannot* be made in this way – *essential* amino-acids – must be present in the diet (Section 4.9).

8.18 NITROGEN BALANCE

Proteins differ from carbohydrates and lipids in containing *nitrogen* which leaves the body mainly in the chemically-combined form of *carbamide (urea)* and to a lesser extent as ammonium salts, uric acid and creatinine. These substances can be measured chemically in *urine and faeces* and converted into *nitrogen values.* Similarly the total nitrogen value in foods can be measured.

(i) *Positive nitrogen balance* is the state when *intake* of protein foods *exceeds* the loss of nitrogen in the faeces and urine. This will occur if protein amino-acids are being used to make *new* tissue in (a) *growth* of children, (b) *repair* following illness or surgery convalescence, (c) after starvation or fasting and (d) during pregnancy for embryo growth.

(ii) *Negative nitrogen balance* exists when the excretion of nitrogen in faeces and urine *exceeds* the intake of nitrogen in protein foods. This will occur in (a) starvation or fasting (b) severe fever or wasting illness such as cancer (c) a protein-free diet or diets deficient in essential amino-acids (Section 9.3).

(iii) *Nitrogen equilibrium* exists when the intake of nitrogen in foods balances or is equal to the nitrogen lost in the faeces or urine. This state should exist in healthy adults, on a *healthful diet.*

8.19 FATE OF WATER AND MINERAL IONS

As the *liver*, aided by the pancreas, regulates the concentration of glucose, amino-acids and lipids in the blood plasma and tissue fluid, so does the *kidney* function as a homeostatic organ to regulate the *water* and *mineral ion content* and *pH* of blood and tissue fluid, as shown by Figure 8.7.

The *skin* is the homeostatic organ regulating the temperature of blood and tissue fluid. Together these organs maintain the constant internal environment of the body by *homeostasis.*

fig. 8.7 *the excretory system of a human female, maintains the balance of water, salts and ions in the body at correct levels*

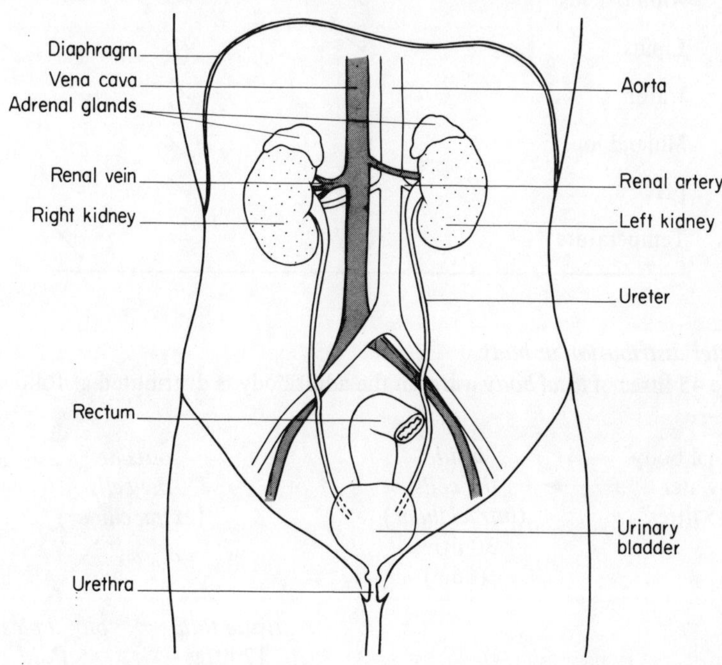

Water balance

The adult human body contains about 45 litres of water forming up to 62 per cent of the body weight (see Table 2.3).

Water in diet

Water in the body comes from three sources: (a) water in beverages and drinking water (b) water component of foods (c) *metabolic water* – the product of cell respiration (Section 5.5). One hundred grammes of pure lipids, proteins and carbohydrates produce $100cm^3$, $40cm^3$ and $60cm^3$ of metabolic water respectively, during cell respiration.

Table 8.2 *summary of homeostatic function of liver, kidney and skin*

Tissue-fluid component controlled by organ (See also Table 1.1)	*Liver*	*Kidney*	*Skin*
Glucose	✓ (Pancreas)	✓	–
Amino-acids	✓	–	–
Lipids	✓	–	–
Water	–	✓	✓
Mineral ions	✓	✓	–
pH	–	✓	–
Temperature	–	–	✓

Water distribution in body

The 45 litres of *total body water* in the adult body is distributed as follows:

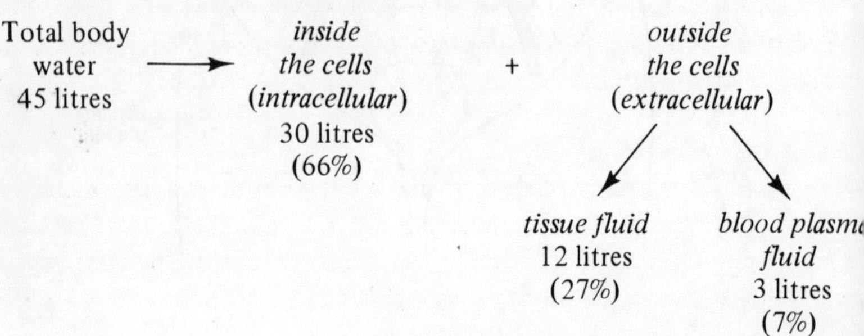

Water balance

The daily water intake must equal the daily water loss for the body to remain in a healthy state of *water balance*.

WATER INTAKE = WATER LOSS

The disorder of *dehydration* will occur if water loss exceeds water intake, the tissue fluid being made *more concentrated.* This occurs in excessive sweating and diarrhoea (Section 10.8 and Plate 10.2). Similarly *over-*

hydration, or collection of water around the cells in dropsy (oedema) occurs if water intake exceeds water loss, the tissue fluid being made *more dilute*. This can occur by *water intoxication* through obsessive water drinking.

The dangers of the dehydration which accompanies infantile diarrhoea are referred to in Section 11.8 and Plate 11.2.

The daily water balance for an adult man in good health, at rest, in a *temperate* climate is shown in Table 8.3.

Table 8.3 *water balance in human beings in temperate climate*

Water loss (cm^3)		=	*Water intake* (cm^3)	
Skin sweating	500 (20%)		In drink	1500 (60%)
Lung evaporation	400 (16%)		In food	700 (28%)
In faeces	100 (4%)		Metabolic water	300 (12%)
In urine	1500 (60%)			
Totals	2500 cm^3			2500 cm^3

Lactating mothers produce about 850cm^3 of breast-milk daily. This requires an additional intake of water of about 1 litre to replace the water used in milk formation.

Thirst and water intake

The *water homeostatic control centre* is located in the brain hypothalamus near to the appetite and satiety centre (Section 8.4). This centre activates the pituitary gland to produce the *antidiuretic hormone* (ADH), which stops the process of *diuresis* or urine secretion.

The kidney

This homeostatic *organ* made up of units called *nephrons* is in close contact with the blood and functions to separate blood *plasma* from the blood *cells.* The blood plasma filters through the thin-walled capillaries of the *glomerulus* contained in the cup-shaped *Bowmans* capsule (see Figure 8.8).

This filtered *fluid* contains (a) *excretory waste*, mainly carbamide (urea) and other nitrogen compounds; (b) *mineral ions* - sodium, potassium, calcium, sulphate, chloride and phosphate and (c) *water*. It also contains small amounts of other nutrients such as glucose (0.1 per cent). Some of these components - water, glucose and certain mineral ions - of the kidney

fig 8.8 *sectional view of a human kidney showing the location of its component nephron units*

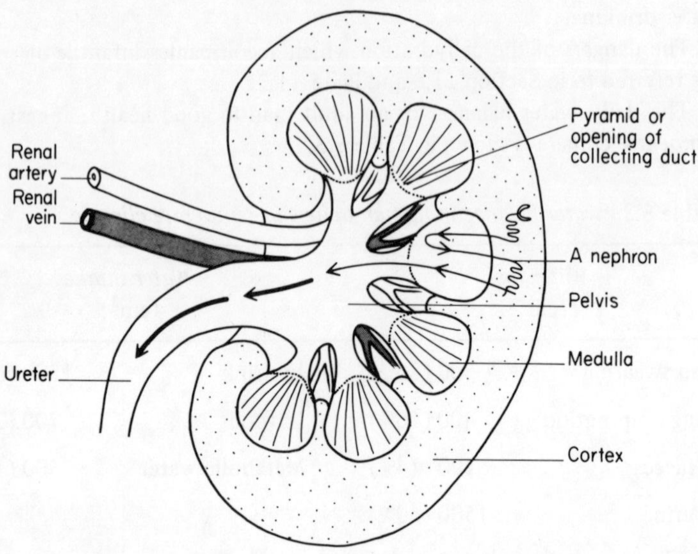

filtrate are reabsorbed for further use in the tissue fluid; this *reabsorption* process occurs by active transport in the kidney nephron *convoluted tubules*, as shown in Figure 8.9.

Of the total volume of blood which passes through the kidney daily only 1 per cent becomes *urine* amounting to 500–2000cm^3 daily. When excessive amounts of water are consumed the ADH secretion is *stopped*, allowing urine to pass freely by *diuresis.*

Urine composition

Urine has a variable composition being mainly water (96 per cent) with varying amounts of the nitrogen-containing substances carbamide (urea), uric acid and creatinine (2 per cent); these are products of amino-acid deamination.

The mineral ions include *phosphates* from proteins and nucleic acids, *sulphates* from the sulphur-containing amino-acids methionine, cysteine and cystine in the diet. Urine *colour* can be due to beetroot, carrot or rhubarb food pigments or added *food dyes*, rhodamine B and indigo carmine.

Salt balance

Salt, *sodium chloride*, is an important component of the tissue fluid and blood plasma, being *taken into* the body in foods or added to foods.

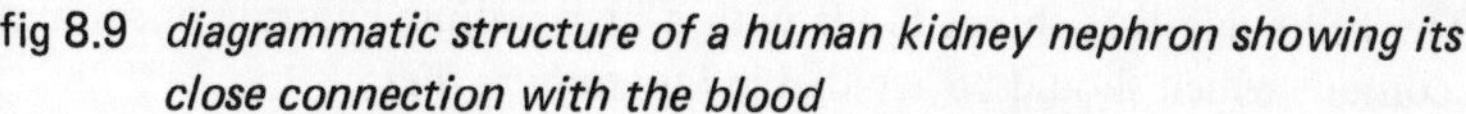

fig 8.9 *diagrammatic structure of a human kidney nephron showing its close connection with the blood*

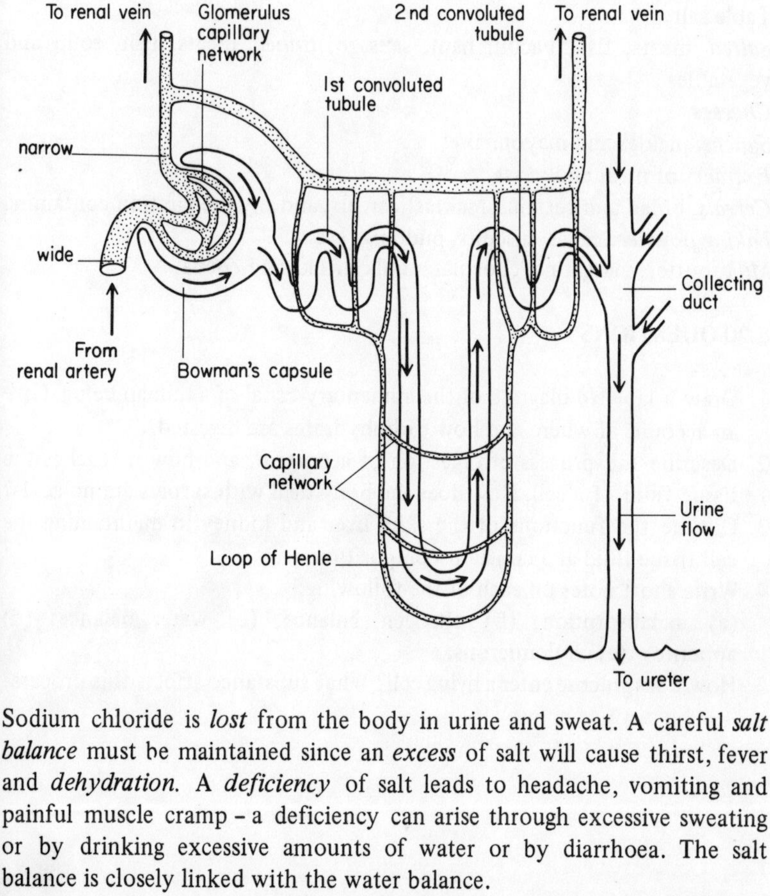

Sodium chloride is *lost* from the body in urine and sweat. A careful *salt balance* must be maintained since an *excess* of salt will cause thirst, fever and *dehydration.* A *deficiency* of salt leads to headache, vomiting and painful muscle cramp – a deficiency can arise through excessive sweating or by drinking excessive amounts of water or by diarrhoea. The salt balance is closely linked with the water balance.

Experiments with *animals* have shown that a *high* salt intake causes an increase in blood pressure. An increase in blood pressure in human beings is a risk factor in causing *heart disease* (Section 9.6). It is believed that individuals may be *salt-sensitive* and react with high blood pressure, others may be less susceptible.

Present intakes of salt in the UK diet from all sources is about 12 grammes daily; this originates from (a) table salt (b) salt in cooking and (c) salt in processed and preserved foods. The recommended daily intake should be reduced by 3 grammes, that is, a 25 per cent reduction on present intake.

An *alternative* to sodium chloride is a salt substitute, *potassium chloride.*

The following lists shows foods with a high sodium chloride or sodium ion content which should be avoided in *low sodium diet*:

Table salt
Salted meats, fish, bacon, ham, sausage; *tinned* meats, fish, soup and vegatables
Cheeses
Sauces, pickles and mayonnaise
Extracts of meat and yeast
Cereals, bread and certain breakfast cereals, and any preparation containing *baking powder*: cakes, biscuits, puddings etc.
Milk, butter, margarine, chocolate, milk drinks and cocoa.

8.20 QUESTIONS

1. Draw a labelled diagram of the alimentary canal of a human being. Give an account of where and how carbohydrates are digested.
2. Describe the process of digestion of a protein, and how it reaches the tissue fluid of a cell. How does the body deal with surplus amino-acids?
3. Outline the functions of the skin, liver and kidney in maintaining the cell tissue fluid at a constant composition.
4. Write short notes on each of the following:
   (a) malabsorption; (b) nitrogen balance; (c) water balance; (d) appetite; (e) chylomicrons.
5. How does glucose enter a living cell? What substance affects this process?

CHAPTER 9

DIET AND DISEASE

9.1 DIET

The *diet* is the daily food intake, or the average food intake over a certain period, of individuals, families or groups of people.

The *healthful* diet should provide a mixture of *nutrients* in selected *foods* served in planned *meals* with a *balanced* nutrient content to maintain the body in a state of *good health* throughout life.

The nutrient and energy content of a diet will vary according to the total number of meals taken daily, consequently it is important to calculate the nutrient content of a meal as follows:

(a) Determine the *portion* size in grammes of each meal component as served on the plate.

(b) Refer to the *food composition tables* in Appendix A for the nutritional and energy content corresponding to the portion weight. Since the food composition tables refer to 100g portions, the portion weight can be rounded up to the nearest values of 25, 50, 75 or 100g to simplify calculation.

(c) A *table* is constructed and nutritional values of the meal's food items arranged in it with the *total* values for each nutrient determined as shown in Table 9.1 which has taken the example of a meal of canned salmon, rice and peas followed by bananas and cream.

The *daily intake of nutrients* and energy of an individual can be calculted in a similar way by *weighting* every item of food and drink consumed throughout the day. This investigation is important when comparing the *actual* intake with *recommended* intakes discussed in Section 10.1.

Table 9.1 *nutritional value of a meal*

						Vitamins								Minerals	
Food item	*Portion size g*	*Energy kJ*	*Protein g*	*Lipid g*	*Carbohydrate g*	*A µg*	*D µg*	*B_1 mg*	*B_2 mg*	*Nicotinic acid mg*	*Folic acid µg*	*B_{12} µg*	*C mg*	*Calcium mg*	*Iron mg*
Salmon, canned	75	637	16.3	9.15	NIL	13	9	0.02	0.13	4.8	3	3	NIL	69	1.0
Rice, polished, cooked	100	460	2.0	0.1	24.2	NIL	NIL	0.02	0.01	0.4	3	0	NIL	10	0.2
Peas, canned, cooked	50	140	3.4	0.2	6.3	22	NIL	0.05	0.03	0.45	4	0	4	13	0.8
Banana	100	360	1.1	0.2	22.0	19	NIL	0.05	0.06	0.6	12	0	10	8	0.7
Whipped cream	75	900	1.6	22.8	21.2	187	0.5	0.01	0.12	0.05	2	0.15	1.0	56	0.07
Total		2497	24.4	32.45	73.7	241	9.5	0.15	0.35	6.3	24	3.15	15.0	156	2.77

9.2 DIETARY BALANCE

A healthful or *balanced diet* is a *varied* diet in which there is not great *excess* or *deficiency* of energy or any nutrient. Such a balanced diet will maintain the body in a state of *good* health throughout life.

Every individual person has his or her *own* particular requirement of energy and nutrients. The food intake and diet of most adults is usually related to maintain *an acceptable body weight* for the particular *height* and *build* as shown in Table 9.2.

When the dietary balance is *upset*, through a considerable *excessive* or *defective* intake of energy or nutrients over a long period of time, this can lead to various *nutritional disorders* also called *malnutrition*. [*Small* excesses and deficiencies of most nutrients are corrected by the body by homeostatic controls (Section 8.14)].

(a) *Dietary deficiency* disorders also collectively called *under nutrition* are: *starvation* because of insufficient food, or *malnutrition* caused by a deficiency of *one* or two nutrients, as in scurvy or rickets.
(b) *Dietary excess* disorders also collectively called *over-nutrition* are: *overweight* (obesity) resulting from too much lipids and sugar, in food intake, or an excess of *one* nutrient, as in vitamin D poisoning.

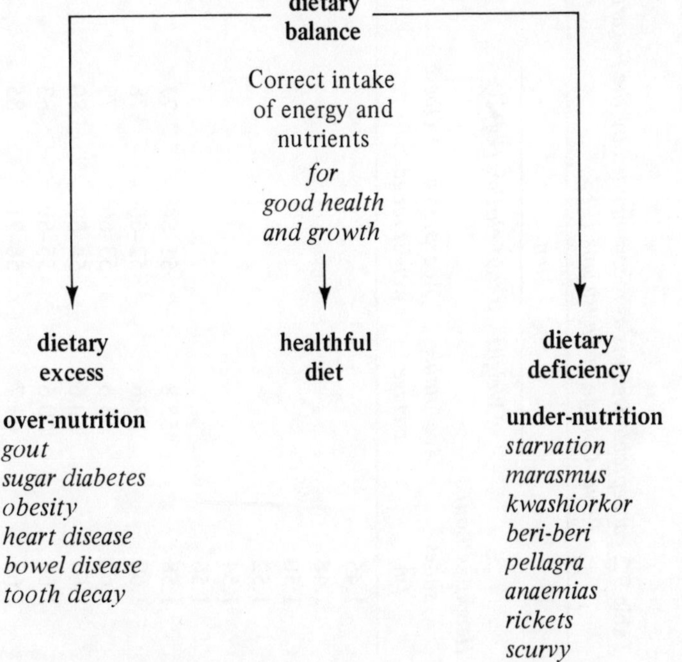

Table 9.2 *acceptable weights as recommended by the Fogarty Conference, USA 1979 and the Royal College of Physicians 1983*

Height without shoes (m)	*Men* Weight without clothes (kg)			*Women* Weight without clothes (kg)		
	Acceptable average	*Acceptable weight range*	*Obese*	*Acceptable average*	*Acceptable weight range*	*Obese*
1.45				46.0	42–53	64
1.48				46.5	42–54	65
1.50				47.0	43–55	66
1.52				48.5	44–57	68
1.54				49.5	44–58	70
1.56				50.4	45–58	70
1.58	55.8	51–64	77	51.3	46–59	71
1.60	57.6	52–65	78	52.6	48–61	73
1.62	58.6	53–66	79	54.0	49–62	74
1.64	59.6	54–67	80	55.4	50–64	77
1.66	60.6	55–69	83	56.8	51–65	78
1.68	61.7	56–71	85	58.1	52–66	79
1.70	63.5	58–73	88	60.0	53–67	80
1.72	65.0	59–74	89	61.3	55–69	83

1.74	66.5	60–75	90	62.6	56–70	84
1.76	68.0	62–77	92	64.0	58–72	86
1.78	69.4	64–79	95	65.3	59–74	89
1.80	71.0	65–80	96			
1.82	72.6	66–82	98			
1.84	74.2	67–84	101			
1.86	75.8	69–86	103			
1.88	77.6	71–88	106			
1.90	79.3	73–90	108			
1.92	81.0	75–93	112			

The healthy human body achieves dietary balance when there is an ample food supply, by the following dietary controls and regimen.

(i) *Brain* appetite and satiety centres and other undiscovered controls (Section 8.4).
(ii) *Psychological* control by will-power, habit; also affected by anxiety or unhappiness.
(iii) *Weight-watching* and obtaining an acceptable body weight (Table 9.2).
(iv) *Nutrition education* in planned meals of known nutrient and energy content related to *recommended daily intakes* as discussed in Section 10.1. Dietary imbalance and nutritional disorders will develop through the following causes:

(a) Famine or food shortage
(b) Gluttony and greed
(c) Food fads and diets, for example, vegan diet
(d) Digestive disorders, malabsorption (Section 8.12), loss of appetite because of disease, fever or surgery and in convalescence
(e) Alcoholism
(f) Unbalanced poorly planned meals deficient in nutrients
(g) Drugs, called anticonvulsants, reduce activity of vitamin D and folic acid
(h) Overmilling of cereals to remove valuable vitamins from wheat and rice
(i) Pregnancy and lactation demand nutrients and energy which must be met by increased intake (Section 10.1). Similarly infants, children and adolescents require increased intakes to prevent nutritional disorders.

9.3 DIETARY DEFICIENCY - UNDER-NUTRITION

Starvation, *marasmus* and *kwashiorkor* are dietary deficiency disorders mainly related to a shortage of *all* nutrients or to *protein* and *energy* deficiency when it is called *protein energy malnutrition* (PEM). (See Plates 9.1 and 9.2). These disorders are prevalent amongst children in poorer developing countries.

By contrast *anorexia nervosa* is a disease of psychiatric origin mainly amongst young women in affluent developed countries in which the person *refuses* to eat because of anxiety, depression or insecurity, and other reasons.

Table 9.3 summarises the main nutrient disorders caused by insufficient food and protein energy malnutrition (PEM).

The *vitamin deficiency* disorders which resulting from a deficiency of *one* particular vitamin are listed in Table 9.4 (see also Section 4.12).

Plate 9.1 *marasmus, a protein-energy malnutrition PEM, caused by early abrupt weaning onto dilute artificial feeds deficient in energy and protein, unhygienically prepared, with repeated infectious diarrhoeal infections. The child is usually less than 12 months old (WHO)*

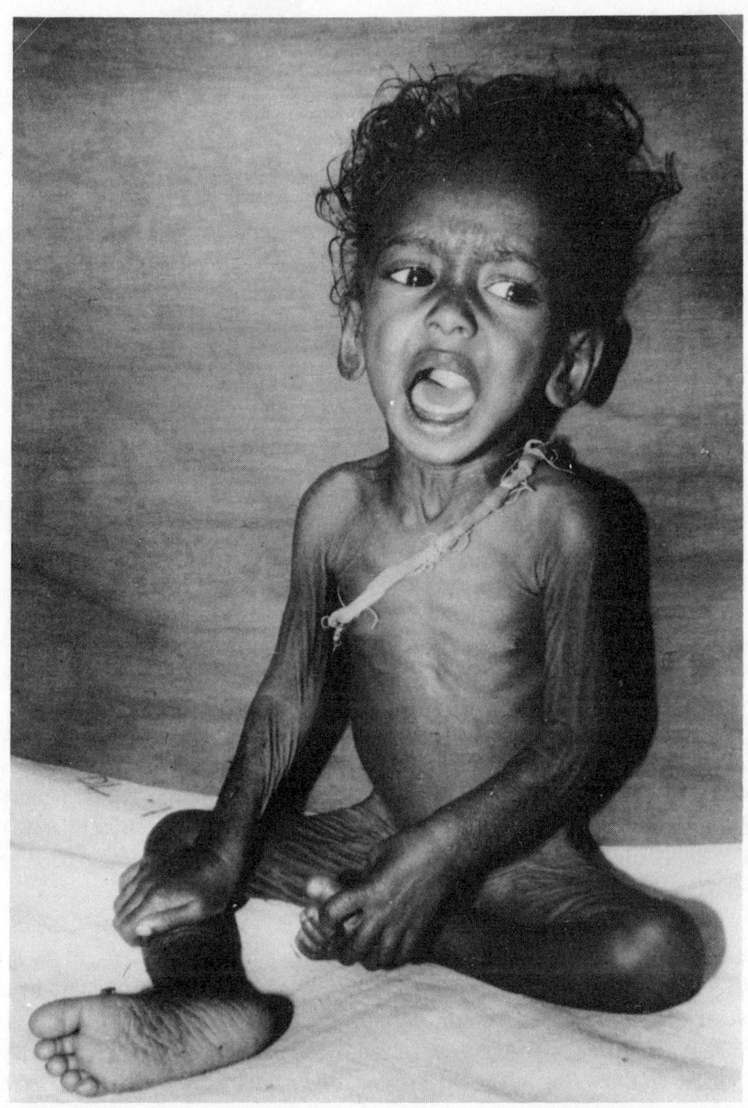

Plate 9.2 *kwashiorkor – a form of protein–energy malnutrition mainly caused by a deficiency of protein with adequate energy intake on a mainly starchy diet. The children are between 12 and 18 months old (FAO, UN)*

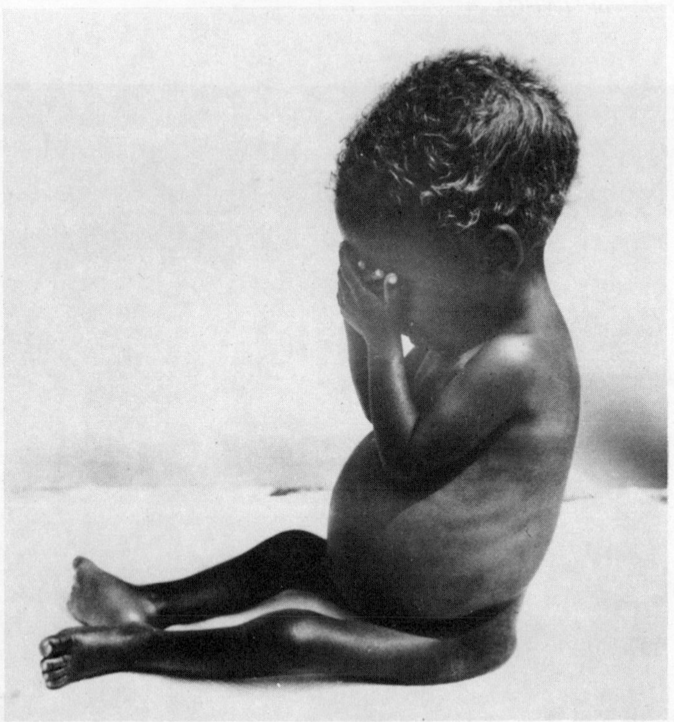

Certain substances which affect or destroy vitamins called *anti-vitamins* include certain *anti-cancer* and *anti-convulsant* drugs which destroy folic acid, and an enzyme in raw fish destroying vitamin B_1 (thiamin). *Alcoholism* causes a deficiency of vitamins of the B group, B_1 (thiamin), folic acid, nicotinic acid and vitamin B_6; certain minerals may become deficient also.

Anaemias

Anaemias are the result of *low* levels of haemoglobin in the blood and have several different causes; severe *bleeding* due to monthly menstruation or accident, insufficient *production* of red blood cells because of a *deficiency* of either *vitamin* B_{12} cyanocobalamin, *folic acid* or the mineral ion *iron*, these are nutritional causes of anaemias. Table 9.5 summarises the main nutritional deficiency anaemias (see Section 8.11).

Table 9.3 Protein and energy malnutrition (PEM) disorders

Nutritional deficiency and disorder	*Causes*	*Symptoms*	*Treatment*
Deficiency of all nutrients and energy. STARVATION, partial and total.	Famine, war, concentration camps, hunger strikes, cancer, inadequate care and feeding	Up to 75%, weight loss weakness, no growth in children, muscle-wasting, oedema, dry thin skin, damage to digestive system blindness and mental instability (see also Section 5.12)	Famine relief food as small amounts of sweetened bland staple cereal, milk, and lipids. Vitamin and mineral supplements.
Deficiency of protein and energy: MARASMUS starvation in children (Plate 9.1)	Early weaning from breast-milk onto unhygienic dirty, dilute, artificial foods causing starvation and repeated diarrhoea, gut disease and TB – i.e. gross underfeedling and general intestinal infection	Affects town children under one year old. Stunted growth, considerable weight loss, muscle-wasting, diarrhoea and irritability. Vitamin and mineral deficiencies	Fluid milk, corn, soya and dried milk mixtures with vitamin and mineral supplements. Warmth and convalescence on to balanced diet. Poverty relief. Education in child care and nutrition
Deficiency of protein KWASHIORKOR (Plate 9.2)	Prolonged breast feeding, then weaning onto *protein-deficient* diet of cassava, yam and plantain with high carbohydrate content.	Affects country children of 1–3 years old. Poor growth, muscle wastage, miserable and apathetic. Oedema of face, hands, feet. Swollen liver and abdomen. Hair changes colour and condition.	Similar to above. Relief of poverty. Education in child care and nutrition

Table 9.4 *vitamin deficiency disorders*

Deficient vitamin	*Causes*	*Nutritional disorder and symptoms*	*Treatment and Prevention*
A Retinol and Carotenese (Note: *Six* parts by weight of carotenes are needed to form *one* part by weight of retinol)	Insufficient lipids, poor absorption because of digestive and liver disorders	*Night blindness* *Xerophthalmia* dryness of eyeball. *Keratomalacia* softening of eye cornea causing permanent *blindness* in 0.1 m children each year. Occurs in South-East Asia, South America, Middle East and Tropical Africa.	Vitamin A dosage in fish liver oils. Improved nutrition and increase of yellow, orange fruits and vegetables, and red palm oil and margarine in diet.
D Cholecalciferol (see Plate 9.3)	Lack of sunlight. Calcium deficiency and digestive disorders	*Rickets* in children of minority Asian groups in UK. Bones soften and become deformed. *Osteomalacia* in adults – severe pain in limbs and back.	Sun-ray and sun bathing treatment. Ample calcium and fish liver oils in diet. Clean air and smoke abatement.
C Ascorbic Acid	Lack of fresh fruit and vegetables	*Scurvy*, swollen bleeding gums, with bleeding within body and beneath skin, bruising easily, death from internal bleeding. Occasionally seen in infants, elderly and alcoholics. Promotes iron absorption.	Orange juice and vitamin C essential in first two years of life, as treatment and in famine relief.

B_1 Thiamin	Refined sugar, overmilled and refined wheat and rice, vitamin removed in bran and embryo germ	*Beri-beri*, loss of appetite, vomiting, weakness and depression. *Wet beri-beri* with breathlessness, oedema, swollen legs and face. *Dry beri-beri* with muscle-wasting, weight loss, nerve inflammation and heart failure. Seen also in alcoholics	Thiamin dosage. Decline in disease noted when rice is parboiled thiamin added to bread, and general improvement of nutrition standards.
Nicotinic acid [*Sixty* parts by weight of essential amino-acid *tryptophan* can form *one* part by weight of nicotine acid	Deficiency of essential amino-acid, *tryptophan* and nicotinic acid in maize and sorghum staple cereals.	*Pellagra*, roughened skin, dermatitis on exposure to sunlight, inflamed mucous membranes, diarrhoea, weakness and mental confusion. Occurs in parts of Africa and India. (see Plate 9.4)	Nicotinic acid and nicotinamide dosage. Decline in disease brought about by improved living standards, addition of nicotinic acid to bread and maize meal; meat, milk and yeast in diet.
B_2 Riboflavin	Caused only as *experimental* deficiency in human volunteers	*Cheilosis* – sore, swollen, chapped lips *Glossitis* – swollen painful tongue *Stomatitis* – sores at mouth corners	Vitamin B_2 cures similar conditions in elderly malnourished people – cause otherwise not known

Plate 9.3 *rickets, mainly caused by a lack of exposure to sunlight when the child shown is kept indoors for five or six months during the rainy season. Human rickets was first cured in 1922 with Vitamin D (WHO)*

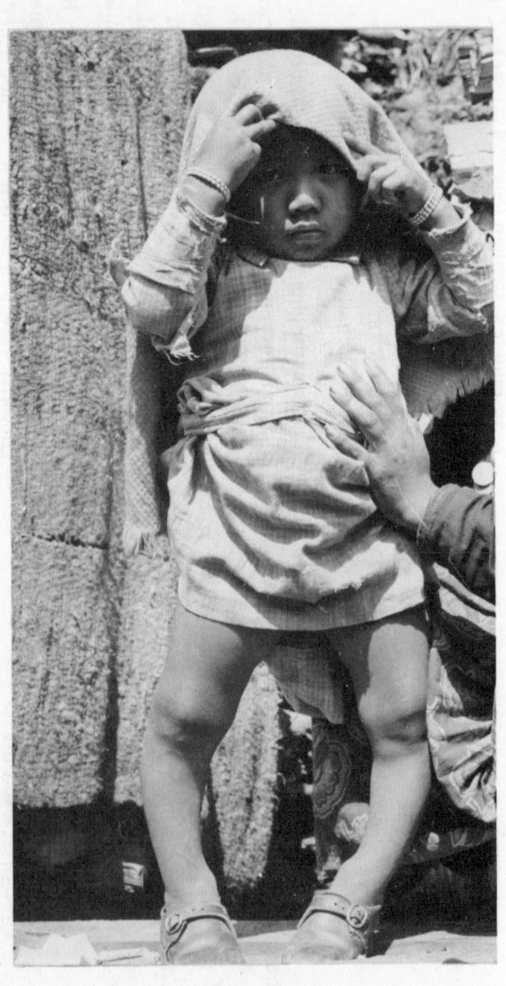

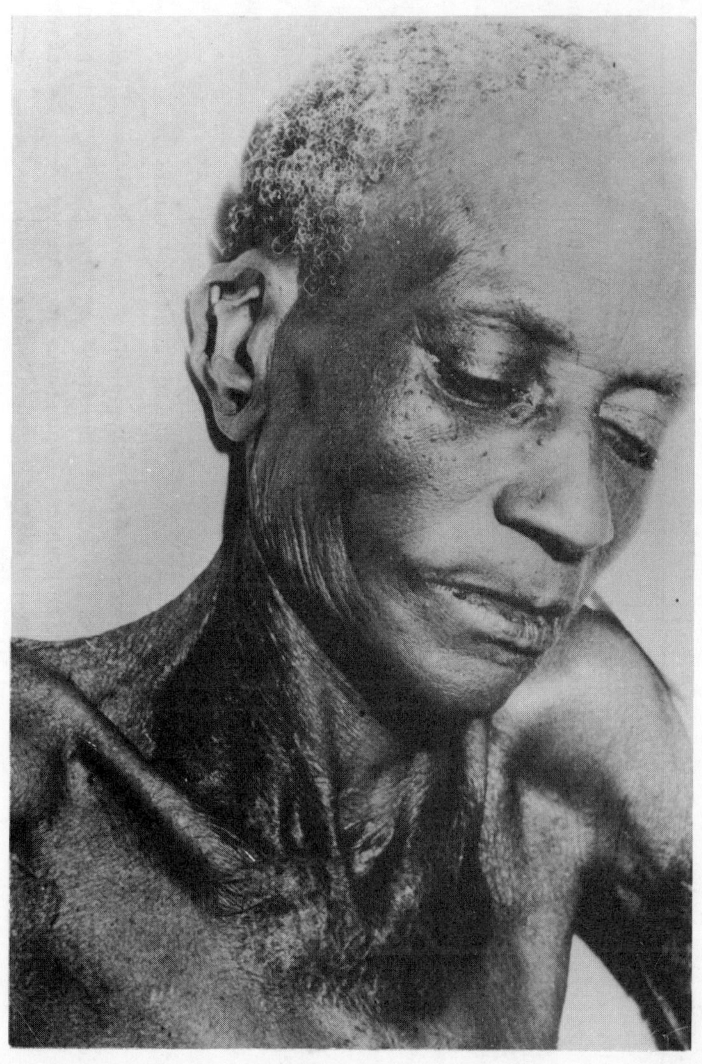

Plate 9.4 *pellagra: symptoms include mental deterioration, diarrhoea, underweight, together with dermatitis, the skin roughening and thickening. First treatment with nicotinic acid was in 1938 (WHO)*

Table 9.5 *types of anaemias*

Nutrient responsible	*Type of anaemia and cause*	*Symptoms*	*Treatment*
Iron Mineral ion.	*Nutritional iron* *Deficiency anaemia* caused by insufficient dietary intake, blood loss, or malabsorption following surgical removal of part of small intestine	*General to all anaemias* Tiredness, weakness, dizziness, headache, pale skin, loss of appetite, indigestion and breathlessness on exertion. Red blood cells *small* and pale coloured. Affects mainly young women and mothers, also infants and children.	Organic iron in meat and offal better absorbed than inorganic iron in tablets and bread. Vitamin C promotes absorption. Iron sulphate added to bread flour.
Vitamin B_{12} Cyanobalamin	*Addisonian pernicious anaemia* inability to secrete the *intrinsic factor* needed for Vitamin B_{12} absorption, because of stomach abnormality.	Symptoms as above. Red blood cells are *large*. It is a less frequent disorder than iron deficiency anaemia. Occurs in strict vegan diet, and sometimes in pregnancy.	Injections of vitamin B_{12} or feeding with *raw* liver. Treatment needed throughout life.
Vitamin Folic acid	*Folic acid deficiency anaemia* Caused by lack of folic acid in diet, effect of anti-cancer drugs and certain oral contraceptive pills. Up to 90% destroyed on cooking food.	Symptoms as above. Red blood cells are *large*. Seen in pregnancy and amongst underdeveloped countries with low intakes of meat and fresh green vegetables.	Folic acid with iron tablets in pregnancy and lactation. Leaf vegetables and yeast.

Other mineral deficiency disorders

Apart from the mineral ion iron, the following mineral ions – calcium, iodide and fluoride – can cause deficiency nutritional disorders, as summarised in Table 9.6.

Table 9.6 *mineral deficiency disorders* (see Plate 9.3)

Mineral ion deficiency	*Nutritional disorder and symptoms*	*Treatment*
Iodine	*Simple* or *endemic goitre* – enlargement of the neck thyroid gland, few if any symptoms. *Cretinism* is seen in thyroid-defective children showing mental and physical handicaps	Iodised table salt
Fluoride	*Dental decay* or *caries*, absence of fluoride from water encourages tooth decay	Fluoride added to toothpaste or drinking water
Calcium	*Osteoporosis* is the loss of calcium from bone with age; protein is also lost, and bones fracture easily. Also associated with decreased sex hormone production	Increased intake of milk, cheese, to replace calcium and and protein loss in the elderly

NOTE See also Plates 9.3 and 9.5.

Dietary fibre deficiency

A general deficiency of *dietary fibre* is evident in the diet of wealthy developed countries and in countries with excessive meat eating diets and where cereals are refined to produce white flours. The average daily intake in the UK is *less* than 20 grammes.

It is claimed that *low* dietary fibre diets are responsible for disorders of the gut including the following: constipation, piles or haemorrhoids, varicose veins, gallstones, appendicitis, diverticulitis and cancer of the large intestine. Similar unresearched and unproved claims indicate that dietary fibre deficiency contributes to heart disease, obesity and sugar diabetes.

9.4 DIETARY EXCESS – OVER-NUTRITION

The prefix *hyper-* means an *excess*, similarly *hyperphagia* is a term meaning excessive feeding. The prefix *hypo-* means a *deficiency* and the term *hypovitaminosis* describes vitamin deficiency, as explained in Section 9.3.

Plate 9.5 *goitre caused by a deficiency of iodine in food which causes the enlargement of the thyroid gland in the neck (WHO)*

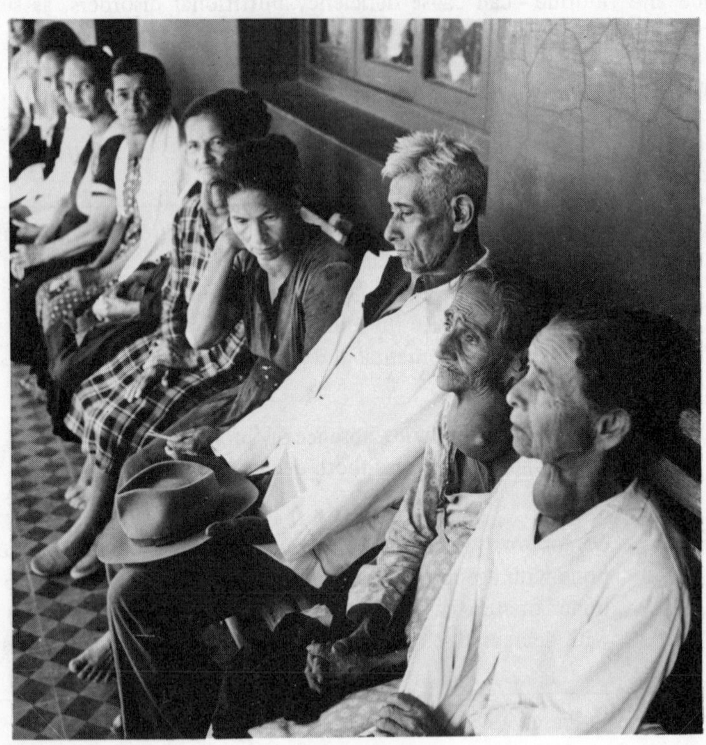

An excessive intake of nutrients in the diet will result in *increased concentrations* in the blood plasma or lymph and tissue fluid following *absorption* (Section 8.11). The excess nutrients are *removed* by the *homeostatic organs* (Section 8.14) in order to maintain a constant concentration or balance of nutrients for the tissue fluid.

When the homeostatic organs are *defective* the nutrient concentrations in the blood plasma become excessive, for example, when glucose levels are excessive *hyperglycaemia* occurs, leading to sugar diabetes (Section 8.15).

Table 9.7 summarises the main disorders which can arise through excessive intake of nutrients into the blood plasma.

Excess dietary fibre

People in rural parts of Africa consume between 50 and 120g of dietary fibre, whilst vegetarians in developed countries consume 42g daily. A *recommended* daily intake for adults is 30g.

Table 9.7 *disorders caused by excessive intake of nutrients*

Excess nutrient in blood plasma	*Related disorders*
Glucose	*Hyperglycaemia* leads to obesity and sugar diabetes (Section 8.15)
Uric acid	*Hyperuricaemia* from foods rich in nucleoproteins and purines; offal, liver, kidneys, sweetbread, sardines, fish, meat extract and certain vegetables - cause gout and kidney stones (Section 4.10, 6.16 and 8.9)
Lipids, triglycerides, alkanoic (fatty acids) and cholesterol	*Hyperlipidaemias* lead to heart disorders and obesity (Section 9.6). *Hypercholesterolaemia* associated with heart disease (Section 4.3, Table 4.1)
Vitamin A retinol and vitamin D cholecalciferol	*Hypervitaminosis* can cause poisoning and other disorders in the case of vitamins A and D and and calcium. (Water-soluble vitamins have no ill-effect since they are rapidly excreted) (Table 4.8)
Calcium	*Hypercalcaemia* with vitamin D causes chalk deposits in kidneys and heart
Sodium chloride or common salt	*Hypernatraemia* may cause increased blood pressure and oedema [Section 8.19 and 9.13]
Iron	*Siderosis* - the accumulation of iron in the liver and bone marrow. Arises by accidental poisoning with iron sulphate tablets causing vomiting, diarrhoea and death
Fluoride	*Fluorosis* is the mottling of the tooth enamel because of an excessive intake of fluoride. Occurs in parts of India and Southern Africa where water has a high fluoride content.
Ethanol	*Alcoholism*, intoxication, addiction, with associated malnutrition and liver disease (Section 9.8)

Excess dietary fibre has the following effects:

1. *Laxative* in speeding the passage of food and faeces through the bowel.
2. Reduces the absorption of sugars and lipid digestion products, through *rapid* intestinal transport.
3. *Lowers* the cholesterol level in the blood plasma (see heart disease - Section 9.6).
4. *Interferes* with *iron* and *calcium* absorption through its phytic acid content (Sections 4.4 and 8.11).

Disorders of the large bowel, appendicitis, irritable bowel syndrome, cancer and diverticulitis are rare in underdeveloped countries with a high dietary fibre content in a mainly cereal, vegetable, fruit and legume diet.

9.5 OBESITY OR OVERWEIGHT

This is a common nutritional disorder in affluent developed countries because of an excessive amount of body fat. It can be caused by an *excessive intake* of food energy over a long period from carbohydrates, lipids, proteins and ethanol, which is greater than the physical energy expenditure, the surplus being stored mainly as fat (Sections 5.12; 8.15; 8.16; 8.17).

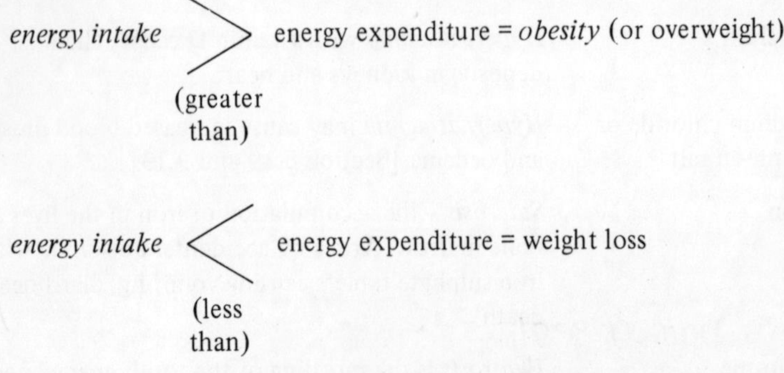

energy intake > energy expenditure = obesity (or overweight)
(greater than)
energy intake < energy expenditure = weight loss
(less than)

Obesity or overweight can also arise in a *minority* of people as a result of endocrine gland disorders, myxoedema (a thyroid gland disorder, or Cushion's syndrome (an adrenal gland disorder). When a person's weight exceeds the acceptable weight (see Table 9.2) by 10–15 per cent, he or she is considered *obese* or grossly overweight.

The percentage average of total body fat lipids in a healthy male adult is about 15 per cent, and about 25 per cent in a healthy female adult (Table 2.2) where it is distributed about the hips and thighs.

Skinfold thickness can be measured with special *calipers* (Plate 9.6); this

Plate 9.6 *skinfold caliper for measurement of subcutaneous fat layers beneath the skin in millimetres (Holtain Ltd)*

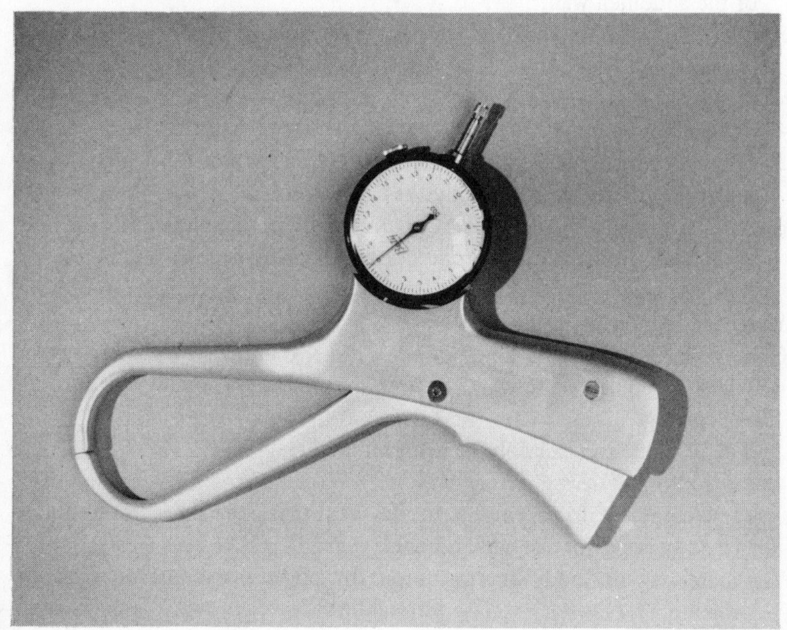

measurement in *millimetres* includes the thickness of the lipid fat layer beneath the skin and is taken at the back of the upper arm or other body parts. Reference of this measurement to special skinfold thickness *tables* gives the percentage fat in the whole body. For example, a 60mm thickness would indicate a 25 per cent body fat content in males and 31 per cent value in females, approximately an *excess* of 10 per cent and 5 per cent respectively.

Obestiy can be defined as a body weight greater than 10-15 per cent of those given in the height and weight tables (Table 9.2). The causes may be genetic, or a disorder of metabolism or psychological in origin. The treatment can be psychological or physiological, both requiring specialist advice by individual assessment.

Dangers of obesity and overweight

The human skeleton can only support a certain load, the effect of increasing this load can lead to the following disorders and complications:

1. *Life span* is shortened.
2. *Support* disorders are inevitable in flat feet, joint arthritis, ruptures of the abdomen wall.
3. *Digestive* disorders arise, gallstones, gall-bladder disease, sugar diabetes (Section 8.15), gout and hyperlipidaemias and cancer of the womb or uterus.
4. *Lung* function impaired causing breathlessness on exertion.
5. *Circulation* disorders include heart disease (Section 9.6), high blood pressure, varicose veins and piles or haemorrhoids.
6. Accidents occur by stumbling and tripping with consequent heavy falls and bone fractures. Surgical operations are made more difficult.

Weight reduction

Obesity developes over a long period of time, therefore weight reduction will take an equally long time, with an average target weight loss of 0.5–1.0 kg weekly.

Weight reduction can only be achieved by:

(i) reducing the food energy intake of lipids, certain carbohydrates (mainly sugar sucrose) and ethanol
(ii) increasing the body energy output by physical exercise or work, or maintaining regular exercise throughout life
(iii) reducing energy intake *and* increasing energy output.

Weight-reduction must be done under *strict medical advice*, since a weight-reducing diet suited to the *individual* must be constructed and prepared by a qualified dietician.

Essential nutrients must be included in the weight-reducing diet; this includes protein for nitrogen balance (Section 8.18) together with vitamins and minerals to prevent malnutrition disorders, and dietary fibre and water.

9.6 HEART DISEASE

Heart disease – also called coronary heart disease, CHD or 'heart attack' – is responsible for one in four deaths in populations of affluent developed countries. Heart disease occurs by the arteries of the heart becoming hardened and blocked, consequently reducing the heart's own blood supply.

There is no single cause for heart disease; several *risk factors* play a part in the development of heart disease. These factors are listed in Table 9.8, together with recommendations of how to combat the development of heart disease. It is possible that heart disease may be *inherited* and may

Table 9.8 *risk factors in heart disease*

Risk factor	*Recommended preventative measure*
Cigarette smoking	Stop the habit.
Lack of exercise, sedentary life	Increased regular physical exercise, maintained throughout life
Obesity	Avoid overweight by weight-watching
High blood pressure	Have regular medical checks. *Eat less salt*. Take caution with *salt* (sodium chloride) in diet and avoid salty foods. (Section 8.19)
Hyperlipidaemias	*Eat less fat*. Reduce saturated animal origin lipids in diet (Section 4.8); replace with plant origin unsaturated lipids (PUFA). *Reduce* high cholesterol content foods in diet (Section 4.3 Table 4.1). *Eat more fibre*. Increase fibre content of diet, through more cereals, vegetables and fruits in diet.
Sugar diabetes hyperglycaemia	*Eat less sugar*. *Reduce* consumption of *sucrose*, at present over 100g daily in developed countries.
Soft drinking water	Hard drinking water contains calcium and magnesium ions; the death rate from CHD is *lower* in hard water areas.

run in families. Males are more prone to it than are females, and *stress* may be another risk factor.

9.7 DENTAL CARE

Figure 9.1 shows the structure of a human tooth. Teeth become covered with a deposit of *plaque* consisting of bacteria and substances from food and saliva.

Sucrose enters the plaque and is changed into *acids* by the bacteria. If allowed to remain on the teeth the acid corrodes or demineralises the protective tooth enamel causing tooth decay or *dental caries.*

Gum disease or periodontal disease arises when plaque builds up around the edge of the gums, allowing more plaque and tartar to collect in pockets.

For good dental care:

1. *Reduce* and restrict the presently high daily intake (100g/d) of sucrose and soft sticky carbohydrate foods and sweet drinks.

Fig. 9.1 *structure of a human tooth showing the enamel layer that is attacked by sugar acids, and the gum, subject to inflammation and disease*

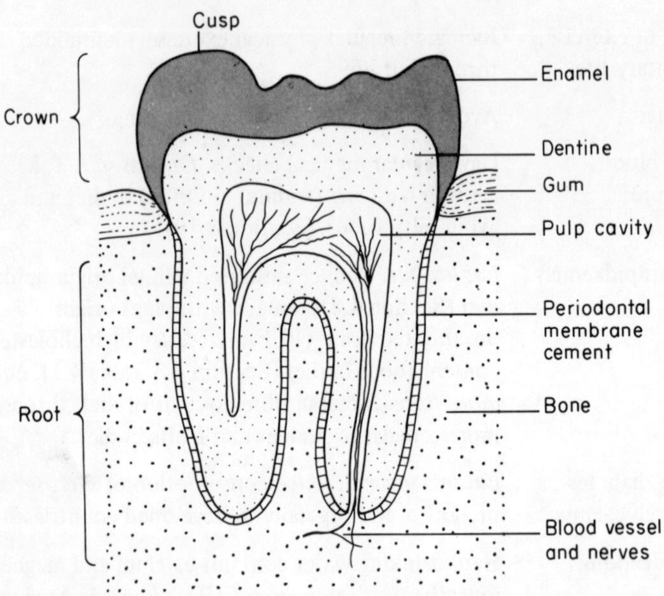

2. *Brush* teeth frequently and correctly after every meal.
3. *Fluoride* in toothpaste and drinking water reduces dental decay.
4. Have regular *dental* hygiene *treatment* by dentists.

9.8 ALCOHOLISM

Ethanol, or 'alcohol' (Section 4.3) alone as in spirits, is not an essential nutrient, although it has an energy value (Table 5.3) and can contribute to the total energy intake. Certain alcoholic beverages can provide limited amounts of minerals, vitamins, proteins and carbohydrates, but cheaper sources of energy and nutrients are available in other foods (Section 12.6). In certain developed countries ethanol or alcohol provides 4–9 per cent of the *total* energy intake; a recommended lower intake below 4 per cent is now advised.

Alcoholic intoxication is an excessive intake and starts when the blood alcohol level is over 0.1 per cent; *death* occurs when the blood alcohol is 0.5 per cent.

Alcoholism is an *addiction* caused by a high level intake over a long period. Apart from social economic problems, it causes physical disorders mainly affecting the liver – *alcoholic cirrhosis* and associated malnutrition.

9.9 QUESTIONS

1. Discuss the concept of energy balance to maintain a desirable body weight.
2. What are the main effects of protein and energy deficiency in a diet?
3. Describe the effects of an excessive intake and deficiency of one named vitamin and one named mineral ion?
4. Give a brief account of the value of diet in combating heart disease.

CHAPTER 10

DIET AND HEALTH

10.1 DIET FOR HEALTH–HEALTHFUL DIET

Since dietary excess or deficiency leads to ill-health as described in the previous chapter, doctors and nutritionists are able to estimate and recommend the minimum amount of nutrient or energy needed to prevent nutritional disorders developing and permit normal growth in groups of children. A *healthful* or *well-balanced* diet can be constructed using these minimum recommended amounts of nutrients; such a diet should then maintain good health in people.

International and national *committees* of nutritionists, physiologists, medical officers, dieticians and the like have prepared tables of *recommended daily amounts* (RDA) of nutrients and food energy to ensure health for a group of people.

Table 10.1 showing recommended daily amounts of nutrients is an international one prepared by the Food and Agriculture Organisation of the United Nations (FAO) and the World Health Organisation (WHO). It is intended to maintain the health of nearly *all* people in the *World*. It is intended for countries needing *improved* nutritional standards, and in some cases the values are much *lower* than RDA tables issued by affluent developed countries, UK, Europe and USA for example. RDA tables for the UK are obtainable by purchase from the Department of Health and Social Security or are included with other RDA tables in Geigy Scientific Tables, no. 1, 1982.

Since the dietary needs of individuals differ, the values given for nutrients are *averages* for a *group* of people and include a small excess called the *safety factor*, with the exception of food energy intakes which does not include a safety factor.

People suffering from *malnutrition* must first be restored to a state of good health by various *therapeutic diets*, and then *maintained* in good health by the RDA diet.

The RDA table is a very important guide to be used as follows:

1. To plan *future food supplies* for a country.
2. *Planning diets* for institutions, hospitals, schools, prisons and armed services.
3. *Labelling* packed foods to indicate the proportion of the RDA in average serving portions.

Example of using the RDA table

The nutrient composition of the meal given in Section 9.1 (Table 9.1), could be that consumed by an adult woman. By subtracting this meal's nutritional value from the recommended daily amounts given for an adult woman, the remaining *difference* in values would be used in constructing the remaining meals of the day to maintain *dietary balance*, as shown in Table 10.2.

10.2 **PROTEIN QUALITY**

The average daily intake of protein in affluent *developed countries* is over 90g; 60 per cent is from *animal* protein and 40 per cent from plant protein. In *less developed* countries the daily intake is below 50g; 20 per cent from animal protein and 80 per cent from plant protein.

The average *quantity* of protein recommended in the RDA table (Table 10.1) is estimated at 42g daily and this refers to *specific* milk or egg proteins. These *animal* origin proteins contain all the *essential* amino-acids (Section 4.9) needed in the human diet, and are called *high quality* or high biological value dietary protein.

Certain proteins–mainly of *plant* origin–are deficient in one or more essential amino acids, which are called *limiting amino-acids*, listed in Table 10.3 and are of *low quality* (or low biological value) dietary protein.

Table 10.3 shows how the *essential* amino-acid content of foods from plants and animals vary, and indicates which essential amino-acids are present in small amounts or are *limiting amino-acids.* Generally the protein from plant sources has an estimated 25 per cent deficiency of essential amino-acids compared with protein from animal sources. Note the high biological value of egg and milk proteins.

Gelatin, the water-soluble protein from meat, skin and bones, shows an exceptional 65 per cent deficiency of many essential amino-acids, and is of very low biological value or protein quality.

If one *low* quality protein containing a limiting amino-acid is eaten *alone* over a long period of time in a *staple* diet, it can lead to serious growth defects in children. If a *mixture* of low quality proteins from animal *and* plant sources is eaten, there will be *no* limiting amino-acid; for

Table 10.1 *recommended daily amounts of nutrients*

Age	*Body weight*	*Energy*		*Protein*	*Vitamin A*	*Vitamin D*	*Thiamin*	*Riboflavin*	*Nicotinic acid*	*Folic acid*	*Vitamin* B_{12}	*Ascorbic acid*	*Calcium*	*Iron*
		(1)		(1, 2)	(3, 4)	(5, 6)	(3)	(3)	(3)	(5)	(5)	(5)	(7)	(5, 8)
	kg	MJ	kcal	g	μg	μg	mg	mg	mg	μg	μg	mg	g	mg
Children														
1	7.3	3.4	820	14	300	10.0	0.3	0.5	5.4	60	0.3	20	0.5-0.6	5-10
1-3	13.4	5.7	1 360	16	250	10.0	0.5	0.8	9.0	100	0.9	20	0.4-0.5	5-10
4-6	20.2	7.6	1 830	20	300	10.0	0.7	1.1	12.1	100	1.5	20	0.4-0.5	5-10
7-9	28.1	9.2	2 190	25	400	2.5	0.9	1.3	14.5	100	1.5	20	0.4-0.5	5-10
Male adolescents														
10-12	36.9	10.9	2 600	30	575	2.5	1.0	1.6	17.2	100	2.0	20	0.6-0.7	5-10
13-15	51.3	12.1	2 900	37	725	2.5	1.2	1.7	19.1	200	2.0	30	0.6-0.7	9-18
16-19	62.9	12.8	3 070	38	750	2.5	1.2	1.8	20.3	200	2.0	30	0.5-0.6	5-9
Female adolescents														
10-12	38.0	9.8	2 350	29	575	2.5	0.9	1.4	15.5	100	2.0	20	0.6-0.7	5-10
13-15	49.9	10.4	2 490	31	725	2.5	1.0	1.5	16.4	200	2.0	30	0.6-0.7	12-24
16-19	54.4	9.7	2 310	30	750	2.5	0.9	1.4	15.2	200	2.0	30	0.5-0.6	14-28
Adult man														
(moderately active)	65.0	12.6	3 000	37	750	2.5	1.2	1.8	19.8	200	2.0	30	0.4-0.5	5-9

Adult woman														
(moderately active)	55.0	9.2	2 200	29	750	2.5	0.9	1.3	14.5	200	2.0	30	0.4–0.5	14–28
Pregnancy														
(later half)	+1.5	+1.5	+350	38	750	10.0	+0.1	+0.2	+2.3	400	3.0	50	1.0–1.2	(9)
Lactation														
(first 6 months)		+2.3	+550	46	1 200	10.0	+0.2	+0.4	+3.7	300	2.5	50	1.0–1.2	(9)

NOTES:
1. Energy and Protein Requirements. Report of a Joint FAO/WHO Expert Group, FAO, Rome, 1972.
2. As egg or milk protein.
3. Requirements of Vitamin A, Thiamin, Riboflavin and Nicotinic acid. Report of a Joint FAO/WHO Expert Group, FAO, Rome, 1965.
4. As retinol.
5. Requirements of Ascorbic Acid, Vitamin D, Vitamin B12, Folate and Iron. Report of a joint FAO/WHO Expert Group, FAO, Rome, 1970
6. As cholecalciferol.
7. Calcium Requirements. Report of a FAO/WHO Expert Group, FAO, Rome, 1961.
8. On each line the lower value applies when over 25 per cent of calories in the diet come from animal foods, and the higher value when animal foods represent less than 10 per cent of calories.
9. For women whose iron intake throughout life has been at the level recommended in this table, the daily intake of iron during pregnancy and lactation should be the same as that recommended for non-pregnant, non-lactating women of childbearing age. For women whose iron status is not satisfactory at the beginning of pregnancy, the requirement is increased, and in the extreme situation of women with no iron stores, the requirement can probably not be met without supplementation.

SOURCE:
Reproduced from *The Handbook on Human Nutritional Requirements* with the permission of the Food and Agriculture Organisation of the United Nations.

Table 10.2 *calculation using recommended daily amount (RDA) of nutrient*

			VITAMINS								*MINERALS*	
	Energy	*Protein**	*A*	*D*	B_1	B_2	*Nicotinic acid*	*Folic acid*	B_{12}	*C*	*Calcium*	*Iron*
	MJ	g	μg	μg	mg	mg	mg	μg	μg	mg	g	mg
RDA for moderately active adult woman	9.20	29	750	2.5	0.9	1.3	14.5	200	2.0	30	0.45	21.0
Amount in one meal (Table 9.1)	2.49	24.4	241	9.5	0.15	0.35	6.3	24	3.15	15	0.15	2.7
Balance to be included in remaining meals of day	6.71	4.6	509	NIL	0.75	0.95	8.2	176	NIL	15	0.30	18.3

*Protein being used for growth, maintenance and repair. It is wasteful to use protein for energy.

Table 10.3 *variable essential amino-acid content of food (g per 16g of nitrogen)*

Food	*Methionine*	*Lysine*	*Cystine*	*Leucine*	*Tryptophan*	*Phenylalanine*	*Threonine*	*Valine*	*Isoleucine*
Plant protein	1.6	5.0	1.4	6.4	1.11	4.0	3.2	4.3	3.5
Limited sources	Limited in most	Limited in cereals and nuts	Limited in most *except* cereals	Rarely limited	Limited in maize	Rarely limited	Limited in rice	Rarely limited	Rarely limited
Animal protein	2.6	7.9	1.4	8.55	1.43	4.6	4.6	6.2	5.2
Limited sources	Limited in most	–	Limited in most	–	–	–	–	–	–
Egg protein	3.2	6.2	1.8	8.3	1.8	5.1	5.1	7.5	5.6
Milk protein	2.9	8.2	1.0	10.2	1.4	5.4	5.0	7.4	5.6
Gelatin	0.8	4.0	Trace	2.9	NIL	2.1	1.9	2.2	1.4

SOURCE Abstracted from Ciba-Geigy Scientific Tables.

example lysine-*rich* legumes with lysine-*deficient* cereals provides a high quality or biological value protein mixture. Similarly, textured vegetable protein, TVP (Section 7.10) is *low* in the limiting amino acid *methionine*, consequently *synthetic* or manufactured methionine is added to TVP to increase its amino acid content and provide a *high* quality or high biological value protein equal to lean beef (Section 7.10). When two or more low quality proteins from different plant or animal sources are mixed to produce a mixture of higher quality or biological value proteins the process is called *protein complementation.* This is evident in traditional protein-mixture *meals* such as bread and cheese, bread and milk, fish and rice, fish and chips, cheese and spaghetti, meat and potato, milk and rice pudding, and cornflakes and milk.

Soya, peanut, maize flours mixed with skimmed milk powder gives a high quality protein complementation mixture used in *famine relief* foods for protein deficiency disorders (Table 9.3).

10.3 ENERGY REQUIREMENTS

The *metabolisable energy* (Section 5.8) corresponds to the *energy intake* of the body. This energy is used for *basal metabolism* (Section 5.13) and the *thermic or thermogenic effect of feeding* (Section 5.11); the remainder is used for work or body *physical activity* of different kinds.

$$\underbrace{\text{metabolisable energy}}_{\textit{intake}} = \underbrace{\text{basal metabolism} + \text{thermic or thermogenic effect of feeding} + \textit{physical activity}}_{\textit{expenditure}}$$

Practically all the metabolisable energy comes from carbohydrates and lipids; the amount of protein given in the RDA table is intended for growth in children and tissue repair and maintenance–it is *not* intended as a source of energy.

The energy expended in different physical activities depends on the person's sex, age, size, occupation or recreation activity.

In order to *compare* energy expenditure in different occupations or recreations, it is necessary to have a *reference man*–age 25 years and weighing 65 kg–and a *reference woman*–age 25 years and weighing 55 kg. (The woman is not pregnant or lactating).

Table 10.4 summarises average hourly energy expenditures of the reference man and woman in different occupations and recreations.

Table 10.4 *average hourly energy expenditure of the reference man and woman*

Level of activity	*Average hourly energy expenditure (MJ/hour)*		*Occupations*	*Recreation*
	Men	*Women*		
Light	0.58	0.41	Office workers, professional teachers, doctors, lawyers, shopworkers, housewives with appliances; unemployed	Sitting, standing, writing, walking slowly
Moderately active	0.73	0.51	Students, factory workers, fishermen, housewives without household cleaning appliances	Playing bowls, brisk walking
Very active	1.0	0.74	Heavy industry labourers, forestry workers, some farm workers, miners and bakery workers	Cycling, running, dancing
Exceptionally active	1.25	0.94	Lumberjacks, blacksmiths, construction workers, rickshaw pullers	Swimming (2.4MJ), football, skiing (3.6MJ), and walking upstairs (4.2MJ)

From FAO, *Handbook on Human Nutritional Requirements*

The *daily* expenditure of energy for reference man and woman in different levels of activity is given in Table 10.5(a) and 10.5(b).

The energy needs of infants, children and adolescents are summarised in the RDA table (Table 10.1).

10.4 PROTEIN AND ENERGY RELATIONSHIP

It has already been stated that protein *can* supply energy to the extent of 17kJ/g (Section 5.8). This will also occur when there is *insufficient* energy supply in a diet from carbohydrates and lipids, and will also occur in starvation when *tissue* protein is used. It is therefore very wasteful to use *expensive* protein as a source of energy, when *cheaper* sources are available in carbohydrates and lipids. The RDA of protein given in the RDA Table 10.1 apply only when the recommended energy is supplied fully from carbohydrates and lipids.

Thus a 10-year old boy requires a RDA of 10.9MJ of energy provided from carbohydrate and lipids in the diet, and a RDA of 30g of high quality protein (from milk or egg or other *mixed* protein source of high biological value) for the sole purpose of growth, tissue repair and maintenance of the body. If the daily *energy* intake is insufficient or less than 10.9MJ there is a danger of the daily protein being used to provide energy and consequently the boy suffers *protein and energy deficiency* malnutrition (PEM) affecting his growth (Table 9.3). The RDA of protein in Table 10.1 is *valid* only when the RDA of energy is fully met.

A protein intake in *excess* of the body requirements and in excess of the total energy intake is changed into lipid *fat* and is a contributive cause of obesity (Sections 8.17 and 9.5).

10.5 ENERGY AND PROTEIN REQUIREMENTS THROUGHOUT LIFE

World food protein and energy supply

If the *world's food supply* was *not* subject to tremendous *losses* (Sections 7.2, 7.3, 7.4 and 11.2) and was *equally* shared, it would provide *more* than the average daily requirements for everyone. Shared *equally* at the present level of food losses there would be *less* than the *average* daily requirements, as shown.

This shows that at *present* there is not sufficient food in the world to feed everyone properly.

The *present* world food supply is *unevenly* shared between the world population in developed and developing countries.

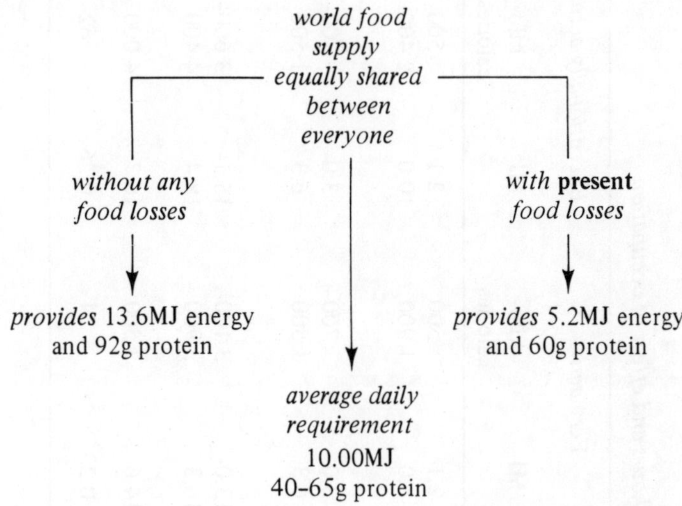

A. Protein requirements

The average daily protein requirements are shown in grammes of *high* quality protein (egg or milk) per kilogramme of body weight g/kg, in the graph for different people. These values have been derived from the RDA table (Table 10.1).

(i) *Babies, children and adolescents* need relatively greater intakes of protein than adults, for the purpose of *growth* and new tissue formation. Babies *double* their birth weight in six months and *treble* the birth weight in twelve months, and require almost *four* times the daily protein intake per kg body weight of an adult.

fig 10.1 *daily protein requirements throughout life*

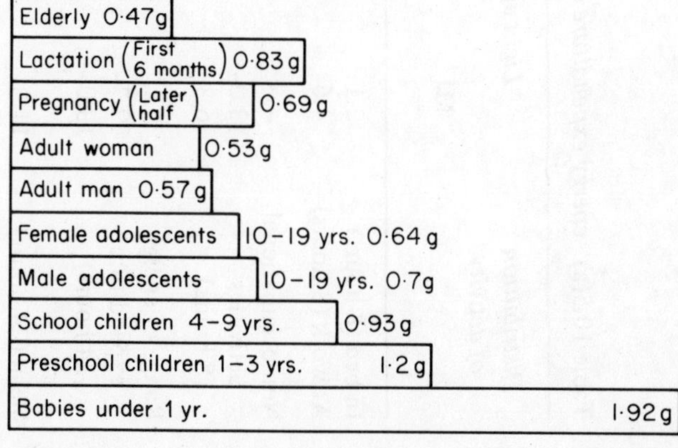

Table 10.5(a) *energy expenditure of a 65kg reference man distributed over 24 hours and effect of occupation*

Distribution of activity	*Light activity*		*Moderately active*		*Very active*		*Exceptionally active*	
	MJ	kilo-calories	MJ	kilo-calories	MJ	kilo-calories	MJ	kilo-calories
In bed (8 hours)	2.1	500	2.1	500	2.1	500	2.1	500
At work (8 hours)	4.6	1 100	5.8	1 400	8.0	1 900	10.0	2 400
Non-occupational activities (8 hours)	3.0–6.3	700–1 500	3.0–6.3	700–1 500	3.0–6.3	700–1 500	3.0–6.3	700–1 500
Range of energy expenditure (24 hours)	9.7–13.0	2 300 3 100	10.9–14.2	2 600–3 400	13.0–16.3	3 100–3 900	15.1–18.4	3 600–4 400
Mean (24 hours)	11.3	2 700	12.5	3 000	14.6	3 500	16.7	4 000
Mean (per kg of body weight)	0.17	42	0.19	46	0.23	54	0.26	62

Table 10.5(b) *energy expenditure of a 55kg reference woman distributed over 24 hours and effect of occupation*

Distribution of activity	*Light activity*		*Moderately active*		*Very active*		*Exceptionally active*	
	MJ	kilo-calories	MJ	kilo-calories	MJ	kilo-calories	MJ	kilo-calories
In bed (8 hours)	1.8	420	1.8	420	1.8	420	1.8	420
At work (8 hours)	3.3	800	4.2	1 000	5.9	1 400	7.5	1 800
Non-occupational activities (8 hours)	2.4–4.1	580–980	2.4–4.1	580–980	2.4–4.1	580–980	2.4–4.1	580–980
Range of energy expenditure (24 hours)	7.5–9.2	1 800–2 200	8.4–10.1	2 000–2 400	10.1–11.8	2 400–2 700	11.7–13.4	2 800–3 200
Mean (24 hours)	8.4	2 000	9.2	2 200	10.9	2 600	12.5	3 000
Mean (per kg of body weight)	0.15	36	0.17	40	0.20	47	0.23	55

From FAO, *Handbook on Human Nutritional Requirements.*

The increased protein intake continues into adolescence when growth stops after a *growth spurt* period.

Protein quality is important, and the intakes must be ***raised*** if the quality is less than milk and egg protein, and should be *mixed* protein preferably from cereal and vegetable and animal protein to ensure there is no deficiency of *essential* amino-acids (Table 10.3).

(ii) *Pregnancy and lactation* require higher intakes than for non-pregnant and non-nursing mothers. About 6g extra daily protein is needed to form body tissues in the foetus, and a greater daily intake of about 17g of protein is needed in nursing mothers to form the essential protein of breast-milk.

(iii) *Adults and the elderly* no longer need protein for growth and their reduced daily intake is required for tissue repair, and production of functional proteins, enzymes and hormones.

(iv) *Illness*, infection, surgical operations, fractures and convalescence require *increased* protein intake in *all* people for tissue repair and replacement.

B. Energy requirements

The daily energy requirements in *megajoules per kilogramme* body weight (MJ/kg) are shown in the graph (Figure 10.2). These values have been derived from the RDA table (Table 10.1).

The energy is required for:

(a) *basal metabolic rate* (Section 5.13);

(b) *thermic or thermogenic effect* of food (Section 5.11);

(c) *physical activities* (Section 9.9) which may need more than the average given in the graph.

fig 10.2 *average daily energy needs throughout life*

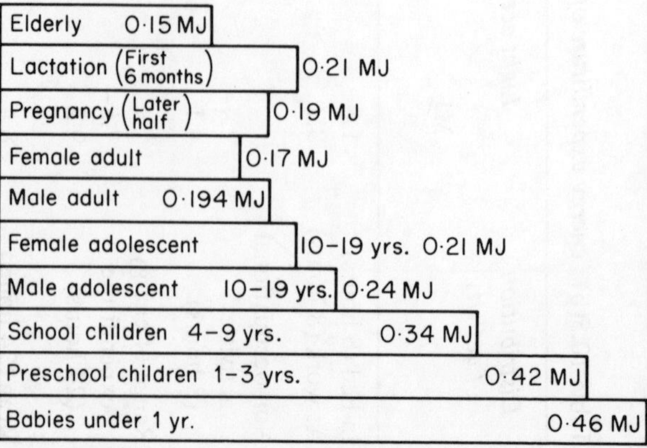

(i) *Babies, children and adolescents* all require a higher intake per kilogramme of body weight compared to adults. The physical activities *vary* amongst young people, making it difficult to measure their energy requirements accurately, and they generally satisfy their needs by hearty appetites and snacks between meals, these should preferably have a *low* sucrose content.

Male adolescents have a higher energy intake than that of *female* adolescents.

(ii) *Pregnancy* requires an additional intake of 1.3MJ energy daily to form new tissues and meet the requirements of the living *foetus*, and the *foetal membranes*, amnion and placenta. The increased body weight of the pregnant woman needs extra energy for her movement of her heavier body.

(iii) *Lactation*, the production of breast-milk amounting to 850ml daily requires about 3.8MJ energy daily for the carbohydrate and lipid content and for synthesis and secretion. Some of this energy comes from lipid fat *reserves* laid down during pregnancy and by additional intake of about 2.3MJ daily in the diet.

(iv) *Adults* require energy for various physical activities as shown in Section 10.3; Table 10.4. Male adults generally require more energy per kilogramme of body weight because of their increased muscle structure.

The elderly show a lower requirement since energy needs *fall* with increasing age because of *lesser* physical activity, a lower BMR (Section 5.14) and declining muscle, tissue and body weights after the ages of 55 to 60 years.

10.6 VITAMIN REQUIREMENTS THROUGHOUT LIFE

The average vitamin needs *per kilogramme of body weight* are summarised in Table 10.6.

(i) *Babies* require a higher intake of all vitamins compared with schoolchildren, adolescents and adults. Vitamins A, D and C are given as vitamin supplements in fish liver oils or orange juice. Care is needed that *hypervitaminosis* caused by excessive intake of vitamins A and D does *not* occur. Excess vitamins D can cause kidney and heart damage.

The need for young people to *sunbathe* is important in making their own vitamin D needs. Similarly minority groups of young Asians in the UK whose style of dress prevents sunlight reaching the skin need to give attention to vitamin D supplements. Female adolescents need slightly increased intakes of vitamins B_{12} and C and folic acid

Table 10.6 *summary of vitamin and mineral needs of the human body (per kg body weight)*

Group of people	*Vitamins*								*Minerals*	
	A	*D*	B_1	B_2	*Nicotinic acid*	*Folic acid*	B_{12}	*C*	*Calcium*	*Iron*
	μg	μg	mg	mg	mg	μg	μg	mg	mg	mg
Babies under 1 yr.	40	1.37	0.04	0.07	0.74	8.2	0.04	2.73	75	1.03
Pre-school 1–3 yr.	18	0.74	0.037	0.06	0.67	7.4	0.067	1.50	34	0.56
School 4–9 yr.	14	0.25	0.033	0.05	0.55	4.2	0.062	0.82	19	0.31
Male adolescent 10–19 yr.	13	0.05	0.022	0.034	0.37	3.3	0.039	0.53	13	0.18
Female adolescent	14.5	0.05	0.020	0.030	0.33	3.5	0.042	0.56	13	0.33
Male adult	11.5	0.04	0.018	0.027	0.30	3.0	0.030	0.46	7	0.11
Female adult	13.5	0.04	0.016	0.024	0.26	3.6	0.036	0.55	8	0.38
Pregnancy	13.5	0.18	0.018	0.027	0.30	7.2	0.054	0.91	20	0.38
Lactation	22.0	0.18	0.020	0.031	0.33	5.4	0.045	0.91	20	0.38
Elderly men	12.0	0.04	0.13	0.027	0.28	3.0	0.03	0.48	7	0.12
Elderly women	14.0	0.04	0.14	0.025	0.28	3.0	0.03	0.57	8	0.33

for healthy blood formation compared with male adolescents, because of blood losses through menstruation (Table 9.5).

(ii) *Pregnancy and lactation.* Pregnant women require increased intakes of vitamins of the B group, including B_{12}, folic acid, vitamins D and C. This increased intake is continued for nursing mothers to provide the essential vitamin content of breast-milk.

(iii) *Adults and the elderly* are at risk for vitamin deficiency if they are living alone and neglect to feed themselves correctly with sufficient meat, fresh fruit and vegetables, so that a deficiency of vitamins C, D, B_{12} and folic acid occurs with the consequent development of scurvy and anaemias. Vegans should take vitamin B_{12} supplements.

10.7 MINERAL REQUIREMENTS THROUGHOUT LIFE

The two main mineral dietary requirements are for *calcium* and *iron*; these needs are high in babies. The calcium requirements of women rise in pregnancy and increase further in lactation since calcium is an important component of breast-milk.

Iron in the form of *haem,* the organic component in blood cells from meat and fish is better absorbed than is inorganic iron from plant source foods, therefore a higher intake of iron is needed if the iron source is from plant foods (see Table 9.5). Similarly, vitamin C (ascorbic acid) promotes iron absorption; consequently adolescent girls, women, pregnant and lactating women need additional vitamin C together with their additional iron intake, compared with other people (Section 8.11).

10.8 INFANT FEEDING

Milk

Babies require milk either as human breast-milk, diluted cows' milk or artificial milk feeds.

Babies are seldom given cows' milk today; formerly it was used after being boiled and diluted with cooled boiled water, and sweetened with sugar.

Artificial milk feeds are made from modified cows' milk fortified with vitamin D, and some have the milk fat replaced by vegetable oils. The composition of human breast-milk, a made-up artificial milk feed and undiluted cows' milk are shown in Table 10.7.

Protein

Human milk protein is *different* from cows' milk protein. They both contain *different* amino-acid components in varying amounts, but the amino-acid *mixture* provides the same *essential* amino-acids. Breast milk has 60 per cent less amino-acids by weight than cows' milk.

Table 10.7 *composition of mature human breast-milk, undiluted pasteurised cows' milk, and artificial milk feed*

per 100cm³	*Human*	*Artificial*	*Cows*
Water	88g	88g	88g
Energy	300kJ	273kJ	280kJ
Carbohydrate (lactose)	7.0g	7.2g	4.6g
Lipid	4.4g	3.6g	3.7g
Protein	1.03g	1.5g	3.2g
Vitamins			
A retinol	58μg	80μg	30μg
D cholecalciferol	0.15μg	1.1μg	0.15μg
C ascorbic acid	5.0mg	5.8mg	1.0mg
Minerals			
Calcium	33.0mg	55mg	140mg
Iron	0.05mg	1.27mg	0.04mg
Sodium	17mg	25mg	70mg
Magnesium	3.0mg	5.3mg	13mg

Lipids

The two milks contain different fatty (alkanoic) acids, breast milk has 40 per cent *more* PUFA (polyunsaturated fatty (alkanoic) acids) than cows' milk. The *essential* fatty (alkanoic) acid in both milks is linoleic acid (see Section 4.8); breast milk contains 70 per cent more than cows' milk.

Carbohydrate

The main carbohydrate in both milks is *lactose* (see Sections 4.7 and 8.12) breast-milk having 33 per cent more than cows' milk.

Vitamins

All vitamins are present in useful amounts. Breast-milk contains 80 per cent more vitamin C than cows' milk, about 7 per cent more vitamin D and 50 per cent more vitamin A. The artificial feed milks are fortified with added vitamins A, D and C.

Minerals

Ample calcium is present in both milks, cows' milk containing 75 per cent more than breast-milk. The iron content is *low* in cows' and breast-milk, and a non-toxic iron salt is added to fortify artificial feeds. The amount of sodium ion in cows' milk is more than four times the amount in breast-milk – high sodium intake can be very harmful to babies (Section 9.4, Table 9.7).

A comparison of breast-feeding and bottle-feeding is made in Table 10.8. It is important to realise that some babies are unable to breast-feed through inability to digest the milk, or are too weak to suckle because of their premature birth. Similarly, some mothers, because of illness or medical conditions cannot or do not wish to breast-feed their babies. If it is at all possible all mothers who *can* breast-feed should do so for longer than three months, provided the baby thrives.

Table 10.8 *a general comparison of breast- and bottle-feeding of infants*

Breast feeding	*Bottle feeding*
The milk has the correct protein and amino-acid composition	Different protein and amino-acid composition
Free and ready prepared at correct temperature and of uniform composition; always clean and sterile	Must be purchased with money, and carefully prepared hygienically. Wrongly-prepared, weak or unhygienic feeds cause marasmus and intestine disorders (Section 9.3)
Contains natural protective substances providing *natural immunity* against disease	No protective substances
Less liable to obesity	Bottle-fed babies grow faster and become more liable to obesity
Non-allergic	Cows' milk protein may cause allergic reactions
Breast-feeding is a natural process establishing a psychological relation between mother and child	Bottle-feeding is an artificial process not requiring a mother-and-child relationship
Salt and sugar or other substances cannot be added to human milk to alter its composition	Substances can be added but this is *dangerous* and very *harmful*, since added excess salt can cause lack of appetite, irritability, convulsions and brain damage

10.9 A HEALTHFUL DIET FOR THE UK

The UK is an example of an *affluent developed country* with a *total diet* in energy terms at present composed of about 11 per cent *protein* (mainly from animal sources, meat and fish); almost 40 percent *lipid* fat (mainly from animal sources as *saturated* lipids); and about 50 per cent or more *carbohydrate* with excessive sucrose intake amounting to over 100g daily. In addition the *sodium chloride* intake is *high* at 12g per day, and the dietary fibre intake *low* about about 20g daily.

Suggestions for improving this *unbalanced* diet with its associated disorders of obesity, overweight, sugar diabetes and heart disease include the following:

1. *Protein* to form 11 per cent of the total diet mainly by lowering the animal protein intake and increasing *plant* protein intake; cereals, vegetables and fruits which at the same time increases the *dietary fibre* content to a daily intake of about 25g.
2. *Lipids* to form 38 per cent of the daily energy intake, a slight reduction in lipids from meat, dairy products and cakes, with a small increase in PUFA (polyunsaturated lipids) from vegetable sources.
3. *Carbohydrate* to form about 50 per cent of the total diet mainly by reducing *sucrose* intake and increasing *starch* carbohydrate intake with associated dietary fibre content, in bread, cereals, potatoes, fruit and vegetables.
4. *Salt* intake to be reduced.
5. *Vitamin and mineral* intake will be satisfactory and increased in certain cases by increase of food intake from plant sources.
6. *Alcohol* intake should not exceed 4–5% of the total energy intake.
7. *Cholesterol*, which is deposited within the arteries, is synthesised by the body from saturated lipids, and is a component of eggs, cheese, whole milk and other foods listed in Table 4.1. Various sources advise a moderate intake of these foods and less fatty red meat, replaced by poultry and fish, and polyunsaturated margarine (PUFA).

10.10 INDIVIDUAL DIETARY VARIATIONS

No two human beings are alike, even identical twins show slight differences from each other. The wide range of differences found amongst human beings is called *variation* and is seen in weight and height differences. Such variation is due to the different *gene* composition of cell nuclei (Section 3 3.4) and to effects of food and disease or to the *environment* described in Section 9.2. Dietary variations are found in individual human beings and mainly affect the intake and metabolism of certain nutrients. The dietary variations are of two kinds – discontinuous and continuous.

Discontinuous dietary variations

This type of variation is seen as distinct or sharp differences affecting nutrient metabolism, and is usually due to the effect of one changed or *mutated gene* (Section 3.4).

(i) Phenylketonuria

This is an extreme and rare dietary variation or disorder in which the *essential* amino-acid phenyl-alanine cannot be changed into the non-essential amino-acid *tyrosine*, because of a lack of the gene which produces the functional protein or enzyme *hydroxylase.*

$$\textit{phenyl-alanine} \xrightarrow{\textit{hydroxylase}} \textit{tyrosine}$$

As a result of this defect phenyl-alanine collects in the body cells, and another derivative, *phenyl-pyruvic acid*, collects in the blood fluid and urine. This substance can be tested for in the blood and urine of newborn babies.

If untreated the brain fails to develop and the child will suffer mental impairment. PKU-affected babies are bottle-fed on specially prepared milk with a *low* phenyl-alanine content. About thirty-five affected babies are born each year in the UK.

(ii) Galactosaemia

This is another extreme or rare dietary variation or disorder in which a baby is unable to change *galactose*, formed by the digestion of milk sugar *lactose* (Section 4.7) into *glucose* because of the lack of a gene to produce the functional protein or enzyme *transferase.*

$$\textit{galactose} \xrightarrow{\textit{transferase}} \textit{glucose}$$

Consequently galactose collects in the body cells and also in the blood fluid and urine. This substances can be tested for at the same time as the PKU test on a newborn baby's urine or blood.

If untreated the baby shows signs of weight loss, vomiting, jaundice and general difficulty with feeding. Ultimately the child will develop blindness and mental impairment.

Affected babies are bottle-fed on a milk preparation which does not contain lactose, and is prepared from malt and soya flour. About ten cases are reported each year in the UK. Many other dietary variations attributable to gene effects are known and include sugar diabetes (Section 8.15) and lactose intolerance (Sections 8.8 and 8.12) in addition to over fifty disorders of inability to metabolise certain amino-acids with symptoms ranging from severe to slight.

Continuous dietary variations

This type of variation is seen as *very small* differences mainly in the *amount* of certain nutrients, which are measured biochemically.

(i) Body fluid composition

The chemical analysis of the body fluids, saliva, gastric juice, urine and blood-plasma from different people shows a wide range or variation, for example, in the amount of protein present. Most people show an average or mean amount whereas others may have up to five times more than the lowest amount. Similarly, the range of vitamin C (ascorbic acid) in the blood of non-smokers is 1.75 times more than in heavy smokers.

(ii) Essential amino-acid intake

Measurements of the daily requirements of tryptophan, phenyl-alanine, lysine, and methionine amino-acids, determined by the nitrogen balance method (Section 8.18) showed that the amino-acid needs of different people varied. Tryptophan intake ranged from the highest intake which was three times the lowest intake; lysine ranged from the highest at four times the lowest intake to methionine which ranged from the highest at six times the lowest intake.

These four examples of dietary variation indicate that different individual human beings show different nutritional requirements, and it must be emphasised that the recommended daily amounts given in Table 10.1 are not necessarily suited for every individual. Between the examples of dietary variation there must be many more minor variations responsible for food 'likes and dislikes' or for particular food fads, and maybe the amount and frequency of feeding.

10.11 **POPULATIONS DIETARY VARIATION**

Populations of different countries show general variations in their carbohydrate, lipid and protein intake, depending on the availability of a staple food and the means to buy it.

Some countries Greenland, U.K., USSR derive between 30 and 50 per cent of their energy intake from *lipids*, whilst in Japan only 12 per cent of the energy need comes from lipid. Most countries derive 50–60 per cent of their energy needs from carbohydrates whilst by contrast Japan derives almost 80 per cent from this nutrient.

Protein intake is about 10 per cent of the total energy needs for most countries throughout the world with the exception of Greenland where it forms about 45 per cent.

Evidently some countries eat more fat than others, and some countries eat more carbohydrates, whilst some countries eat more proteins. The human body must therefore *adapt* to high lipid, protein or carbohydrate intake. This *adaptation* must result in increased enzyme secretion and increased metabolism to cope with the larger amount of nutrient – hence resulting in the dietary variation amongst the people of the World.

fig 10.3 *comparison of percentage of energy intake from different energy sources for different countries*

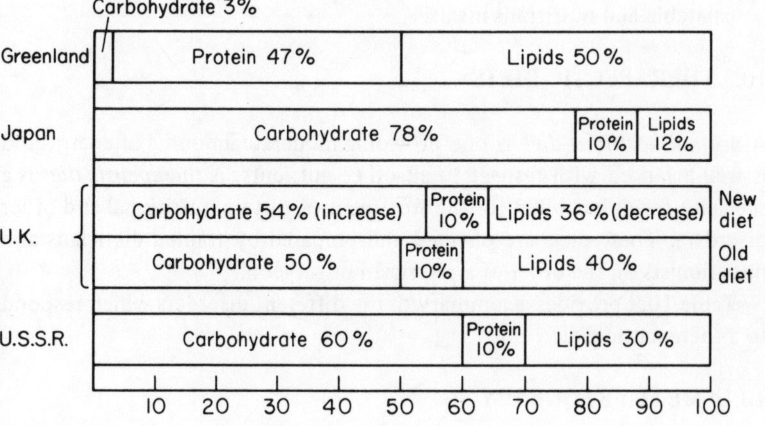

10.12 DIETARY MODIFICATION

The main influences which operate within a country or community in altering the diet are as follows:

1. *Government* and local authorities provide infant welfare foods and organise school meals. Food-rationing may operate in time of war and famine.
2. *Nutrition and health education* through schools and colleges, the media of television, magazines and books, and promotion by food-suppliers and marketing boards can result in recipes and menus for nutritionally suitable and palatable meals.
3. *Religious beliefs* influence the selection, preparation, and to some extent the time of eating and fasting.

4. *Home feeding* is of cardinal importance in establishing good feeding habits helped by the people who prepare food keeping themselves informed.
5. *Public feeding* in hospitals, schools, colleges, industrial canteens provides palatable food at reasonable costs in utilitarian circumstances. This contrasts with the increasing social habit of unrestricted intake feeding in hotels and restaurants, often at *exorbitant* costs in luxurious circumstances.
6. *Processed foods* require extensive promotion of their products through *advertising*. Many such foods are snack or junk foods or confectionery, together with alcoholic and non-alcoholic beverages, many of which are of very high *sucrose*, *lipid*, and *salt* (sodium chloride) content, intended as foods to be consumed *between* meals thus reducing the intake of palatable and nutritious meals.

10.3 THERAPEUTIC DIETS

A *normal healthful diet* is one providing moderate amounts of energy and is well-balanced with respect to all other nutrients. A *therapeutic diet* is a specially formulated diet for the treatment of certain nutritional and other disorders. These diets are planned and prepared by trained dieticians and nutritionists on the order of a physician or surgeon.

Table 10.9 provides a summary of the different disorders which respond to a therapeutic diet.

10.14 MEAL FREQUENCY

The number and size of meals taken in a day can vary for human beings. By contrast flesh-eating or *carnivorous* vertebrate animals take one large meal and vegetation-eating or *herbivorous* vertebrate animals feed continuously.

There are two kinds of feeding patterns in human beings:

(a) *Intermittent* feeding or the 'gorgers' pattern, seen in those who take in *one* large daily meal which consists mainly of a high *protein* content. This type of feeding was thought to be typical of primitive man and is still found in certain primitive societies.
(b) *Unintermittent* feeding or the 'nibblers' pattern, seen in those who take six or more meals spaced at 2- or 3-hour intervals. This pattern of feeding tends to have a high *carbohydrate* content.

An investigation into the *relationship* between meal-frequency and the incidence of *heart disease* amongst a large group of Czechoslovakians,

Table 10.9 *summary of the main conditions responding to therapeutic diet*

Disorder	*Dietary treatment*
Underweight, convalescence, and PEM (Section 9.3)	High energy, high protein, with adequate balance of other nutrients
Dehydration, diarrhoea, and gastro-enteritis (Section 10.7, Plate 10.2)	Low dietary fibre, semi-liquid, oral rehydration with sterile, hygienically prepared drinks 2% glucose, 0.3% salt in boiled and cooled water. Medium energy and protein intake
Overweight, and obesity	Low energy, medium protein intake with good balance of other nutrients
Heart disease	Low energy for the overweight. Low sodium, low-saturated animal lipid, with increased PUFA lipid intake
Sugar diabetes	Restrict carbohydrate intake and maintain normal protein intake, follow strict diet planning with insulin treatment
Kidney disorders:	
(a) Nephritis	(a) Low-protein intake with low to moderate energy intake
(b) Nephrotic syndrome	(b) High protein and low sodium intakes
(c) Kidney stones and gout	(c) Low purine diet (Sections 4.10, 8.9)
Gut disorders:	
(a) indigestion, stomach ulcer	(a) Bland, low dietary fibre, moderate energy and protein intake
(b) Colitis, large intestine colon inflammation	(b) High protein, low dietary fibre, increased vitamin B group intake
(c) Constipation	(c) High dietary fibre (Section 4.7 Table 4.3)
Liver disorders	Mainly a very low lipid fat intake, with increased carbohydrate intake in vomiting, jaundice, and liver inflammation
Genetic disorders	Galactosaemia – lactose-free diet Phenylketonuria – low phenylalanine diet Coeliac disease – gluten-free diet

showed that the people who were 'gorgers' tended to suffer more from heart disease than the people who were 'nibblers'.

The human *stomach* acts as a storage organ in which the food is held from two to three and a half hours; meat, poultry and lipids remain longest in the stomach. Evidently it is preferable to consume small meals at three-hourly intervals. In so doing the task of digestion and absorption is evenly spread compared with the overloading of the stomach after one meal taken by 'gorgers' which can cause discomfort and later unpleasant feelings of hunger when the stomach is empty. *Breakfast* which follows the longest time when the stomach is without food, should be a meal made of palatable or bulky cereal or other food which is not only high in dietary fibre, but also a ready source of carbohydrate to replenish low blood-sugar levels in the body.

10.15 NUTRIENT PORTION SIZE IN THE DAILY DIET

The recommended *daily total diet* measured as a percentage of the total daily energy intake is given as follows for the UK (see also Section 10.9); other developed countries make similar recommendations:

Protein 11 per cent, lipids no more than 36 per cent, and carbohydrate 53 per cent, (of this last, sucrose sugar should not exceed 12 per cent).

It is possible to *calculate* the portion sizes of protein, lipids and carbohydrates, from the foregoing percentage values, using the *recommended daily amount* of energy given in the RDA table (Table 10.1) and RDA tables for other countries.

Calculation

If the rda table shows that a person's daily RDA of energy is 10MJ, Table 10.10 will show how this energy allowance is distributed between the nutrients.

The portion size of the daily total diet will be made up of the following 100% pure nutients;

Protein 65g, lipids 95g, and carbohydrate 311g

This could be provided in the rather nauseating and unpalatable mixture of textured vegetable protein, glucose, and lard! This would be a food mixture providing only protein and energy and would *lack* essential vitamins, minerals, dietary fibre and water.

By reference to the food composition tables in Appendix A, the calculated recommended amounts of nutrients can be translated into more

Table 10.10 *distribution of total daily energy allowance (10MJ) among nutrients*

	Protein	*Lipid*	*Carbohydrate*
% pf total energy allowance	11	36	53
Proportion of daily energy allowance	1.1MJ	3.6MJ	5.3MJ
Portion weight in g of pure 100% nutrient	$\frac{1100}{17} = 65g$	$\frac{3600}{38} = 95g$	$\frac{5300}{17} = 311g$

dietarily acceptable and *appropriate* food items, with a wider nutrient content than the TVP, glucose and lard mixture!

Calculation

If it is decided that mackerel is to feature in the day's menu and this is to provide all the daily recommended amount of protein, viz. 65g as already shown, the portion size of mackerel providing this amount of protein is calculated by reference to the composition of mackerel given in the food composition tables in Appendix A:

100g of mackerel contains 19g of protein

Therefore the amount of mackerel containing 65g is calculated from

$$\frac{65 \times 100}{19} = 342g$$

Similarly the *lipid content* of this portion of mackerel is found knowing that:

100g of mackerel contains 12g of lipid

therefore

$$342g \text{ portion contains } \frac{342 \times 12}{100} = 41g \text{ lipid}$$

This leaves a remainder of the daily lipid allowance

$$95 - 41 = 54\text{g lipids}$$

to be accounted for in other foods featuring in the daily menu. (See also Tables 9.1 nutritional value of a meal and 10.2, calculation of the RDA).

10.16 MENU AND MEAL PLANNING

Deciding on what foods will form the daily healthful diet is the essential part of menu and meal planning. In addition to knowing the *recommended amounts* of nutrients, and the *portion size* of protein, lipids and carbohydrates it is necessary to have a knowledge of the *composition* of the appropriate foods (detailed in Chapters 6 and 7). Such food composition is conveniently summarised by classifying foods into the following *five food groups* listed in Table 10.11, together with their major nutrient contributions. A satisfactory daily planned menu can be constructed by selecting *two* components together with water from *each* group every day. This will provide a healthful balanced diet for a normal person. provided the nutrients are present in the amount given in the various RDA tables. The greater the *variety* of foods selected the more healthful and nutritious the diet will be. Needless to say, other factors such as availability and cost will affect the selection and menu planning.

Vegetarians and vegans will have a more restricted selection of foods, and strict vegans must guard against Vitamin B_{12} (cyanocobalamin) deficiency.

NOTE Sucrose, ethanol, and possibly sodium chloride (salt) are not included in the Food Group table, since these items have a relationship with various dietary and health disorders (Sections 9.2, 9.4, and 9.8).

The following lists basic courses for three daily meals, the combined courses will provide the selection of items from the five main food groups;

Breakfast	*Lunch*	*Dinner*
Fruit and tomato juices	Sandwiches	Soups
Cereals	Meat dishes	Fruit juices
Milk	Fish dishes	Meat dishes
Rolls or toast	Egg dishes	Fish dishes
Eggs	Legume dishes	Egg dishes
Bacon and egg	Vegetables	Cheese dishes
Sausages, kidneys	Salads	Legumes
Tomatoes	Cheese	Vegetables, salads
Grapefruit	Fruit	Puddings, ice cream, fruit

Table 10.11 *the main food groups and their major nutrient contributions*

Food group	*Major nutrient contributions*				
	Energy	*Protein*	*Vitamins*	*Minerals*	*Dietary fibre*
Meat, offal, fish, eggs, cheese, *also* beans, peas, lentils, and peanuts	–	Best source	B group, best source	Best source *Fe*. (Mg and P)	Legumes only
Milk and milk products	–	Best source	B group	Best source *Ca*. (Mg and P)	Nil
Fruits and vegetables	–	–	Best source vitamin C and Folic acid, also Carotene vitamin A	(Ca and Fe)	Good source
Bread, cereals and potatoes	Best source	Good source	B group	(Fe, Mg, P)	Best source
Butter, margarine, vegetable cooking oils	Good source	nil	Best source vitamins A and D	nil	nil

NOTE Best source of essential fatty acids and polyunsaturated lipids is in vegetable oils and derived margarines

THE RULE: TWO HELPINGS FROM EACH FOOD GROUP DAILY = A HEALTHFUL BALANCED DIET.

10.17 QUESTIONS

1. Explain what is meant by a nutritionally balanced meal and a healthful balanced diet?
2. What is meant by protein complementation?
3. Compare the nutritional requirements of two women of the same age, body weight and height, engaged in light physical activity - one being seven months pregnant and the other a breast-feeding mother.
4. Describe inherited conditions in which children are unable to metabolise an amino-acid and a monosaccharide component of their diet.
5. Briefly outline the components of the following therapeutic diets; (a) low protein (b) gluten-free (c) high dietary fibre (d) low sodium. Indicate the disorders for which these diets are produced.
6. By reference to Table 10.6, display the vitamin B_{12}, folic acid, ascorbic acid, and mineral ion iron requirements by means of a histogram.

10.18 EXPERIMENTAL WORK

A. *to determine the nutrient content of a daily diet*
Procedure

(i) Weigh carefully every food item consumed during a whole day.
(ii) Construct a table of nutritional content similar to Table 9.1, using the food composition table in Appendix A. At the end of the day *total* the values for all nutrients and energy.
(iii) Refer to the RDA table (10.1) and determine your personal allowance. Make an *estimate* for your physical activities for the day.
(iv) Compare your nutrient and energy intake with the RDA value to determine whether a dietary *deficiency* or *excess* exists.

B. *to calculate the percentage composition of your daily diet*
Procedure

(i) Find total individual weights of protein, lipid and carbohydrate consumed in a day.
(ii) Calculate percentage of each nutrient in diet from the following:

$$\frac{\text{Total weight protein}}{\text{Total weight protein, lipid and carbohydrate}} \times 100$$

= Percentage protein in daily diet.

Repeat the calculation for carbohydrate and lipid.

CHAPTER 11

FOOD CARE

11.1 INTRODUCTION

Human beings and animals as *consumers*, together with certain moulds and bacteria, the *decomposers*, *all* compete together for the ready-made organic food made for them by the green plants or *producers* (Sections 3.9 and 3.10).

Those organisms which compete *directly* with human beings for their food are called *pests* since they (a) threaten to *deprive* and *deplete* the food supply, or (b) *spread* certain harmful *diseases* by the food, or (c) cause the decomposition and *decay* of the food.

Consequently food must be *cared* for and *protected* from pests, parasites, decomposers and other harmful agencies. Food is kept edible until it is needed by food *storage*, mainly by keeping it cold and/or dry.

11.2 FOOD SPOILAGE

Food *spoilage* is a form of *food loss* which can be *avoided* and accounts for about 30 per cent of the total losses from *all* causes described in Sections 7.2 and 7.4. Most raw, *fresh* foods with a high water content (see General Composition Tables, Chapter 6 and Appendix A) are *perishable*, particularly meat, fish, milk, eggs, fruits and certain fresh vegetables. If fresh foods are *unprotected* and kept in *warm* surroundings they *deteriorate* which changes in *quality*; that is, their *appearance*, *taste*, *smell* and *texture*. Further deterioration leads to their complete *spoilage* when they become *unfit* and *harmful* to eat. Spoilt food becomes mouldy, slimy, rotten and putrid and finally *decays* to produce the end-product - a spongy, brownish-black, organic substance called *humus*.

Spoilage is partly prevented by methods of *food processing* described in Chapter 7; for exampled *dried* cereals, pulses, nuts, fruits, egg, milk, biscuits and flours with a *low* water content are almost *non-perishable*, whilst specific processing by *food preservation* methods of canning, freezing and curing produce non-perishable forms of food.

Causes of food spoilage

[Changes in *quality* due to deterioration have already been described in Chapter 6 with reference to the selection of different fresh food commodities.]

The main causes of food deterioration and decay are summarised as follows:

1. *Damage* may occur during harvesting, transport or rough handling in the shops or home, causing bruising and discoloration of fruits, cracked eggs and torn leafy vegetables.
2. *Enzymes* present in all food with a cellular composition cause *autolysis* or self-digestion of the cell contents or its surrounding materials by lysosomes. It is a process that occurs in dead cells and prior to cell death (see Section 3.3). Most foods become softened by autolysis as seen in ripening fruits and deteriorating vegetables (Section 7.4).

   Meat and game muscle tissues are *tenderised* by autolysis by enzymes called *cathepsins* naturally present in the autolysed cells, which break down certain proteins.

   Cut and otherwise damaged fruits and vegetables will also discolour due to *enzymic browning*.

   Blanching is a process of dipping fruits and vegetables in hot water at 82-93°C for 1½ minutes; it serves to prevent enzymic action and maintain quality before further preservation.
3. *Oxidation* is a chemical reaction between certain food nutrients mainly *lipids* and oxygen present in the air (see Sections 2.8 and 7.4). Foods containing *lipids* can develop unpleasant flavours and odours because of *rancidity* evident in sour milk, butter and cheese. Vegetable oils are protected to a certain extent by vitamin E, *tocopherols*, from developing rancidity. Once the vitamin E is used up, or destroyed as in repeated heating, the oil rapidly becomes rancid, particularly when exposed to sunlight, and in the presence of copper and iron metals.

   Oxidation also takes part in the enzymic browning process of cut fruits and vegetables. Blancing will expel dissolved oxygen and air from prepared fruits and vegetables.
4. *Chemical contamination* may occur by various methods by *exposure* to *pesticides* used to protect the crop such as *herbicide* paraquat, *fungicide* containing mercury, *insecticide* containing lead DDT, or Dieldrin.

   Cattle and poultry meats can contain *antibiotics* and added *hormones* to encourage growth and fattening. The polluted air can lead to the presence of lead and radioactive metals in meat and milk.

Plastic packaging can lead to contamination by certain hydrocarbons.

5. *Pests* An estimated 50 per cent of food grown and stored in tropical developing countries is consumed or spoilt by pests such as various *insects*, *rodents* rats and mice and *birds*. (See Plate 11.1).

Plate 11.1 *brown rats feeding on spilled grain; they can transmit many diseases to human beings by their urine and faeces (Rentokil Ltd)*

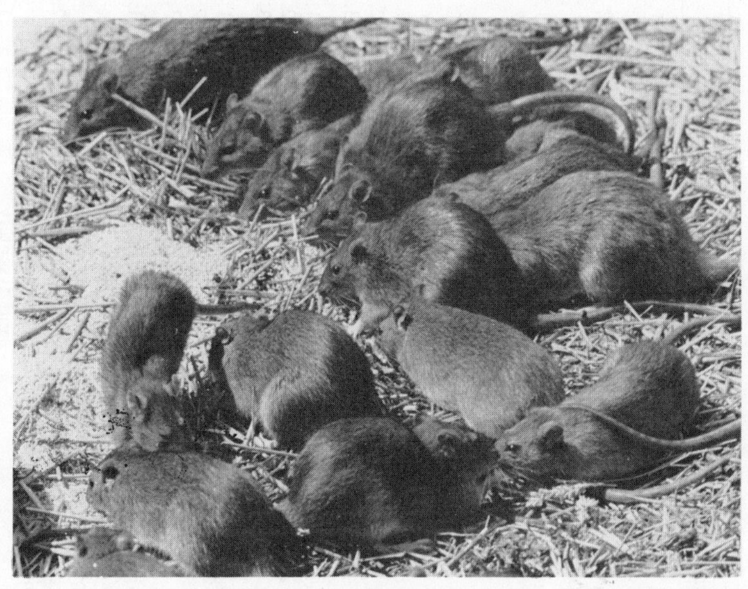

Food in *storage* will always attract pests which spoil the food by *physically damaging* it partly by eating it and partly by defaecating on it, causing *infection* by faecal micro-organisms. Table 11.1 summarises the common pests encountered in food storage and their effects and prevention.

6. *Micro-organisms* such as bacteria, fungal moulds or yeasts (Section 3.2) gain access to exposed food by means of soil, dust, insects, rodents, birds, pets or other animals and by unclean *handling* of food by human beings with unclean personal habits. Contaminated *water* is another means of entry.

The majority of micro-organisms are *harmless* as in the case of milk-souring bacteria or cheese moulds, only a small number of species are *harmful* and the cause of food poisoning or other food-borne diseases.

Table 11.1 *Common pests and their effects*

Pest	*Occurrence*	*Disease or harmful effect*	*Preventive measures*
Cockroaches of three types: 1. Black cockroach 2. Steamfly 3. Brown American cockroach	Warm places in kitchens, canteens, bakeries and food factories. Have a characteristic smell. Feed at night and hide by day.	Contamination and tainting of food by droppings causing salmonellosis.	1. Prevent accumulation of food debris with good hygiene 2. Insecticide, dusts, sprays or lacquers painted on floors
Mites: 1. Flour mite 2. Dried fruit mite	Dark, poorly ventilated food stores	Contamination of food with droppings	1. Fumigation 2. Insecticides, dust, sprays and lacquers 3. Good hygiene with frequent examination of stored goods
Larder beetle	In bacon, ham or cheese	Maggots contaminate food	1. Cool, clean stores 2. Frequent inspection of stock 3. Fumigation of store
Warehouse moth	Chocolate, cereals, dried fruit, spice and nuts attacked by grubs	Contamination by faeces	1. Stock inspection 2. Fumigation 3. Insecticides, sprays and powders
Biscuit beetles	Packed biscuits, flour, cereals and spices	Contamination by faeces	1. Stock inspection 2. Fumigation 3. Insecticides, sprays and powders
Common housefly and blowfly	Eggs laid in warm, moist refuse, decaying matter or faecal matter. Feed on any food containing sugar, or filth, excreta, decaying matter. Hairy bodies pick up microbes	1. Regurgitates saliva on to food, then sucks up soluble food 2. Contact of body and method (1) infects human food 3. Causes food poisoning, typhoid, and dysentery	1. Good hygiene, i.e. clean bins, no food debris; covering food, and use of clean utensils 2. Fly sprays and swatting 3. Insecticidal paints on walls and ceilings

			4. Spraying or destruction of breeding sites 5. Fly screens on windows and ventilators
Rodents: Rats are of two types: 1. Common rate or brown rat is large with a short tail 2. Ship's rat or black rat is small with a long tail	Brown rats found in drains, sewers or refuse tips. They stay at ground level Black rats are climbers and are found in warehouses and private houses	1. Gnawing habits cause destruction of wood, pipes, cables, boxes, and fabrics 2. Fouling of food and water causes salmonellosis, typhoid and dysentery 3. Rat fleas cause plague 4. Rat bites cause rat bite fever	1. Good hygiene with avoidance of food debris 2. Good storage and protection of food 3. Traps 4. Poison baits (Warfarin) 5. Sewer treatment
The common house mouse	Mice are found everywhere in Britain. Each colony restricts itself to a small area	1. Gnawing habits cause destruction of wood, pipes, cables, boxes and fabrics 2. Fouling of food and water causes salmonellosis, typhoid and dysentery	1. Good hygiene with avoidance of food debris 2. Good storage and protection of food 3. Traps 4. Poison baits (Warfarin)
Birds: Sparrows and pigeons	Warehouses and bakeries	Droppings foul exposed food – salmonellosis	Repellent strips

Microbial spoilage of food causes the decomposition seen as mouldiness, slime, rot or fermentation, with changes in texture, colour and smell caused by such gases as ammonia (rotten fish) and hydrogen sulphide (rotten meat and eggs). It is important to stress that the microbial-*spoiled* food has an *abnormal* and unattractive appearance, in contrast to bacterially *contaminated* food which causes *food poisoning*; such food often has a *normal* appearance.

11.3 MICRO-ORGANISMS

Micro-organisms are the microscopically small living organisms which can only be seen when magnified by either a light microscope or electron microscope (Fig 3.1 and Plate 3.1). They include:

1. *Viruses*, the smallest of all micro-organisms seen only by the electron microscope, enter *living* cells of plants and animals whre they *multiply* using the host cells resources, consequently causing the host cell's death. Many viruses cause diseases and are *pathogenic. Infectious hepatitis* is a disease, on the increase in Europe and the USA, caused by a virus transferred to food and water from infected *faeces*. This food-borne virus disease affects the liver causing its enlargement and symptoms of, fever, abdominal discomfort, generalised itching and jaundice.
2. *Algae* include one-celled green-coloured plants able to produce their own food by photosynthesis, and are found as the *plankton* in sea and fresh water. *Chlorella*, and *Spirulina* (Plate 7.2) are green algae found as a scum on pond water, have been used to provide an experimental source of *protein*. The *dry* algae contains up to 60 per cent protein (see Section 7.10). Most algae are harmless to human beings, but sea-mussels feeding on plankton may take in the algae called *gonyaulux*; this produces a harmful poisonous substance called a *toxin* which is unaffected by the heat of cooking and results in relatively rare *mussel poisoning*, causing vomiting, weakness and breathing difficulties.
3. *Protozoa* are simple one-celled animals living mainly in water and damp soil. The protozoa which cause a food-borne disease in human beings include the *Entamoeba histolytica* which enters the human gut from faeces-contaminated water and unwashed fruit and vegetables, causing *amoebic dysentery* with severe diarrhoea and internal bleeding. See Figure 11.1.
4. *Fungi* are a large group of plants without green colouring, and are mainly *saprophytes* and decomposers (Section 3.9). They are an important source of *antibiotics*, *proteins* and certain *vitamins*, and are also mainly responsible for food microbial *spoilage*; they are used

Fig 11.1 *protozoa entamoebae parasites in the human gut*

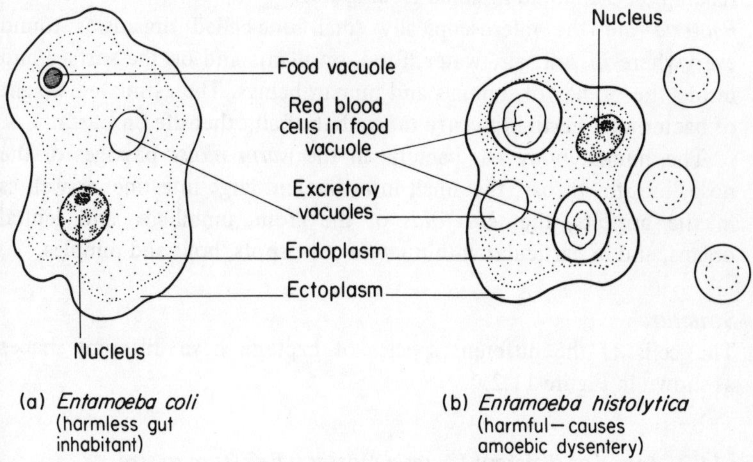

(a) *Entamoeba coli* (harmless gut inhabitant)

(b) *Entamoeba histolytica* (harmful—causes amoebic dysentery)

in the production of *ethanol* by fermentation and as raising agents in fermentated baked goods.

Yeasts are one-celled fungi, and are mainly saprophytes feeding on ready-made organic food nutrients (see Plate 6.3).

Moulds are visible to the naked eye as a growth on spoilt food, consisting of many threads or *hyphae*, interwoven into a body called a *mycelium*. They reproduce by small airborne *spores*.

Growth of moulds

Moulds can be grown artificially on a jelly-like *culture* medium; this contains the organic nutrients the saprophyte needs as food, mainly a higher proportion of *carbohydrate* as compared with proteins. This medium should have a pH of 5–6 slightly acid (see Section 2.11) and be sufficiently moist to provide essential water.

Warmth is required at an *optimum* temperature of 22–25°C to encourage maximum growth. Therefore microbial spoilage of food will be encouraged in *warm* and *moist* conditions.

Fungal poisoning

Certain species of toadstool called the Death Cap toadstool, *Amanita phalloides* is highly poisonous.

Rye cereal grain may become infected with a fungus disease called *ergot* and produces grain poisoned with *ergotamine*.

The mould *aspergillus flavus* can grow on groundnuts, cereals and other nuts stored in humid climates to produce poisonous toxins called *aflatoxins*, which are known to cause liver cancer in animals feeding on the mould-infected feeding stuff.

5. *Bacteria* are the microscopically small one-celled organisms found everywhere in soil, air, water, food, on plants and on the surface and inside the bodies of animals and human beings. The estimated weight of bacteria on Earth in *twenty times* that of all other life on Earth.

The human body has bacteria in the *warm moist* passages of the nose, mouth, throat, the small intestine and large intestine, as well as in the armpits, the *skin folds* of the groin, umbilicus, and genital organs, and in particular within *septic* cuts, spots, boils and pimples.

Structure

The cells of the different species of bacteria have different shapes as shown in Figure 11.2.

Fig 11.2 *forms of different bacteria mostly 0.5–3.0 μm in size*

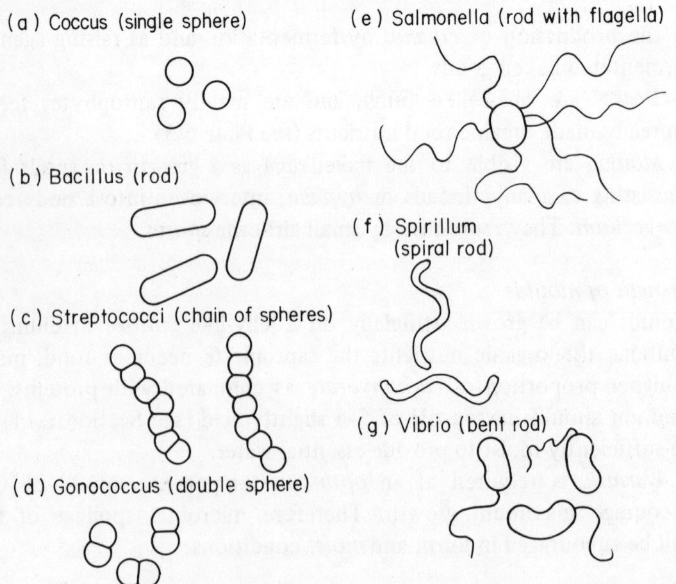

Bacteria names

Every species of bacteria has an *official scientific* name composed of two parts, the first name for the *genus* and the second name for the *species*. The names may come from Latin or Greek words, for example, *staphylococcus* from the Greek word *staphule* or bunch of grapes, and from *coccus* a berry. The names of eminent bacteriologists and doctors who discovered the bacteria can also be used; for example, Dr Salmon discovered the *Salmonella* family of bacteria and these were given species names according to the disease they caused, *salmonella typhi* for typhoid fever, or *salmonella dublin* after a type of food-poisoning first located in Dublin. Other eminent doctors gave their names to *Shigellae* (Dr Shiga), *Clostridium welchii* (Dr Welch), and *Shigella sonnei* (Dr Sonne).

Reproduction

Bacteria will reproduce or mulitply by dividing its cell into *two* daughter cells, this will take twenty minutes provided the *optimum* conditions are provided as described in Section 10.4. Within three hours one bacterium can produce over a quarter of a million (250 000) cells.

Certain bacteria of the genera *Bacillus* and *Clostridium* can produce special structures called *spores* when certain nutrients have been used up during times of food shortage. These spores are surrounded by *heat-resistant* coats of up to four layers.

Other bacteria genera which *do not* form spores are the *Salmonella*, *Shigella*, *Staphylococcus* and *Escherichia*.

11.4 BACTERIA GROWTH CONDITIONS

Since a majority of bacteria are *beneficial* to Man in the synthesis of *vitamins* of the B group in the human intestine, for synthesis of *antibiotics*, *fermentation* of cheese, butter and yoghourt, together with the decomposition of *sewage*, it is necessary to know how their growth can be encouraged.

1. Food nutrients

Bacteria secrete *enzymes* to digest the main nutrients sugars, proteins, lipids and in certain bacteria, *cellulase*. The cellulose-digesting bacteria are active in spoiling fruits and vegetables and in the intestine of cattle, sheep, goats. The simple products of digestion are absorbed into the bacteria cell for metabolism.

Bacteria can be grown in the laboratory on *culture media* which are mainly muscle or blood *extracts* in a firm jelly of agar in a small shallow dish – a *petri dish*. Culture media are available in tablet form or as a ready-made sterile agar sausage from which slices are cut with a sterile knife.

2. Water

Water is essential to all living organisms. It *transports* food into the bacteria and most raw whole foods contain between 55 and 98 per cent water, sufficient for bacterial growth, whilst culture media are almost 98 per cent water.

Dried foods contain 1–25 per cent water, insufficient to allow bacterial growth.

Humidity or moisture in the air encourages bacterial growth. *Wet* towels and dish-cloths allow bacterial growth.

3. pH

Most bacteria prefer a near neutral pH 7.4, whilst a *minority* need an acid pH 3 to pH 6.

4. Oxygen

Energy is released within the bacteria cell in some bacteria *aerobically* using oxygen, or *anaerobically* without oxygen (see Section 5.4); another group of bacteria respire with *or* without oxygen as *facultative* bacteria.

Clostridium welchii and *Clostridium botulinum* are both anaerobic bacteria. *Salmonella* and *Staphylococcus aureus* are both facultative bacteria, growing best in air or oxygen.

5. Temperature

Bacteria grow at different rates between a *minimum* low temperature 5°C and a *maximum* high temperature 45°C. Below the minimum temperature of 5°C in refrigerators and freezers their growth *stops* but they are *not* killed. Above the maximum temperature of 45°C their growth stops and they may be *destroyed*. Between the minimum and maximum temperatures there is an *optimum* temperature when growth is at the *greatest* rate and the bacteria thrive and multiply.

The *harmful* pathogenic bacteria which live in the human body and cause disease prefer an optimum temperature of 37°C – or near to blood-heat – normal human body temperature; consequently most bacteria can be grown on culture media at 35–42°C in special *incubators*.

There are *exceptions* amongst certain bacteria which prefer *lower* – 10–15°C – and in other bacteria *higher* – 30–65°C – optimum growth temperatures. *Clostridium welchii* has an optimum growth temperature of 43–47°C, *Staphylococcus aureus* 30–40°C, Salmonella 37°C.

6. Time and the bacteria population

A *population* is a group of individuals of the same species, therefore we can have a bacteria or a human population. The *number* of individuals in a population can be counted; bacteria using a microscope and tally counter and human beings by a *census*.

When bacteria reproduce under favourable conditions in an *enclosed* culture medium with a *fixed* amount of food and water, their rapid *increase* in numbers will be *seen* by the naked eye as coloured *colonies* composed of great numbers of similar bacteria clustered together. The different species of bacteria will produce different *shaped* colonies.

In time the *increasing population* of bacteria will have consumed *all* the food and water supply and their waste products will being to *poison* their surroundings or environment within the enclosed culture medium. Subsequent *overcrowding* occurs and bacteria begin to die off, until conditions within the culture medium are so bad that no living bacteria can survive at all. This extreme extinction can occur after a varying time of so many days or weeks.

This growth and decline of a bacteria population is shown in Figure 11.3 in which the *number* in the population is plotted against *time*. This particular growth graph has an equally important application to the *human population growth* described in Chapter 12.

Fig 11.3 *graph showing changes in a population of living organisms – for example, bacteria grown on an agar plate, or the human population on earth*

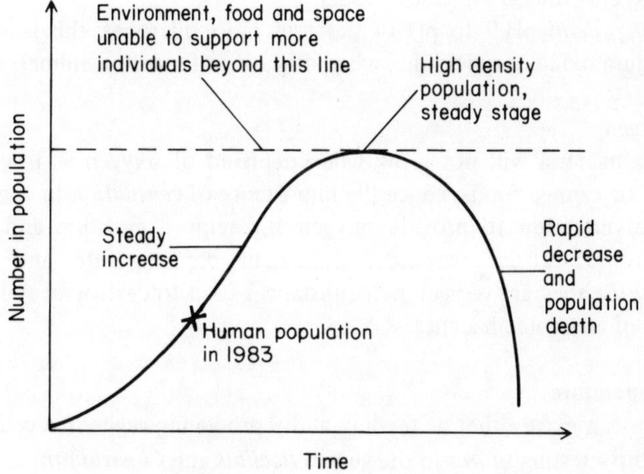

11.5 BACTERIA DESTRUCTION

Since certain bacteria are responsible for *food poisoining*, and other *food- and water-borne* diseases, and for the *spoilage* of food, it is necessary to know how to destroy them or how to curb their growth.

1. Food

Bacteria can be deprived of access to food by *covering* the food. Food remains must be removed from *equipment* and *working surfaces*, and also from the *teeth* by frequent cleansing and brushing.

Without food certain bacteria may survive as heat-resistant *spores* for long periods.

2. Water

In the absence of water, bacteria are unable to take in food and get rid of their waste products and therefore cannot multiply. *Dry* food and dry air will not support bacterial growth.

Strong solutions of *salt* (sodium chloride), and *sucrose* (sugar) used in salt curing and sugar preserves, withdraw water *from* bacteria cells by *osmosis* (Section 2.7) causing bacteria cells to die by *dehydration*. A few species of moulds, yeasts and bacteria *can* survive in dry, salty and sweet sugary conditions.

3. pH

Strong acid solutions pH 4 to pH 0 destroy most bacteria, with the exception of certain acid-liking bacteria which exist at pH 2.5–pH 6 in ethanoic (acetic) acid (vinegar - pickled foods).

Strong alkali pH 9 to pH 14 destroys most microbes; this is achieved by calcium oxide or quicklime, when disposing of infected animal carcases.

4. Oxygen

Aerobic bacteria will not grow when deprived of oxygen as in vacuum-packed or canned foods, hence the importance of *ventilation* in combating bacterial infection to provide oxygen and remove moisture and reduce humidity. Hydrogen peroxide, potassium permanganate and certain other *antiseptics* are oxygen-rich substances used to destroy or reduce the growth of anaerobic bacteria.

5. Temperature

Bacteria can exist either as feeding and reproducing *vegetative* cells, or as the inactive resting *spores* in the genera *Bacillus* and *Clostridium*.

Moist heat from boiling water, steam or pressure cookers, and *dry* heat from radiant grills, infra-red lamps and in baking ovens, are *sources* of heat which can affect bacteria.

(a) *Heat-sensitive bacteria* vegetative cells are those which can be destroyed if kept at temperatures of 60°C for thirty minutes. They include the *disease-causing Salmonella*, *Shigellae*, *Staphylococci* and *Clostridium welchii*. A *higher* temperature, 80°C, is needed to kill vegetative cells

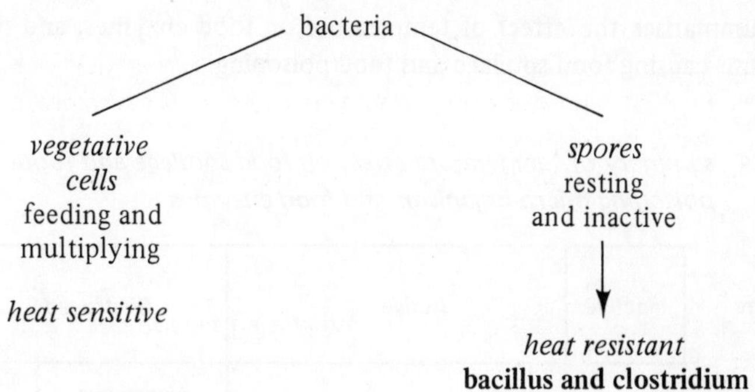

of *clostridium botulinum*. Many *food-spoiling* bacteria are destroyed at 60°C.

(b) *Heat-resistant bacteria spores* The *spores* of bacteria *Bacillus* and *Clostridium* have thick protective coats and are able to survive a temperature of 60–80°C which destroys most bacteria *vegetative* cells.

Higher temperatures of 100–121°C are needed to destroy *Bacillus* and *Clostridium* spores, by prolonged boiling for up to five hours, or pressure cooking at 121°C for 5–10 minutes.

(c) *Bacteria toxins* Toxins are the poisonous wastes produced by disease-causing or pathogenic bacteria. Toxins cause the unpleasant symptoms of many diseases, but the *presence* of certain bacteria vegetative cells can also cause disease symptoms. The bacterial toxins are of two main kinds:

(i) *Exotoxins* which diffuse out of the *living* bacteria cells into the host or culture medium; they are complex proteins *destroyed* by heat. *Clostridium botulinum* toxin is destroyed by heat at over 100°C.

(ii) *Endotoxins* are released with the *dead* bacteria cell breaks up by autolysis releasing into the host *or* culture medium complex substances, which are *heat resistant*. The toxins produced by staphylococci, salmonellae, and *Clostridium welchii* are *not* destroyed by boiling at 100°C.

(d) *Enzymes* The enzymes present in bacteria and those present in cellular food are destroyed above a temperature of 70°C (see Figure 11.4).

Low temperatures

Low temperatures below 5°C in refrigerators and freezers *do not destroy* bacteria vegetative cells, spores or toxins. They remain *dormant*, their metabolism is slowed down, and they do not multiply, but once the temperature is raised to the optimum they commence to multiply. Figure

11.4 summarises the effect of temperature on food enzymes, and micro-organisms causing food spoilage and food poisoning.

Fig 11.4 *summary of temperature effect on food spoilage and food-poisoning micro-organisms and food enzymes*

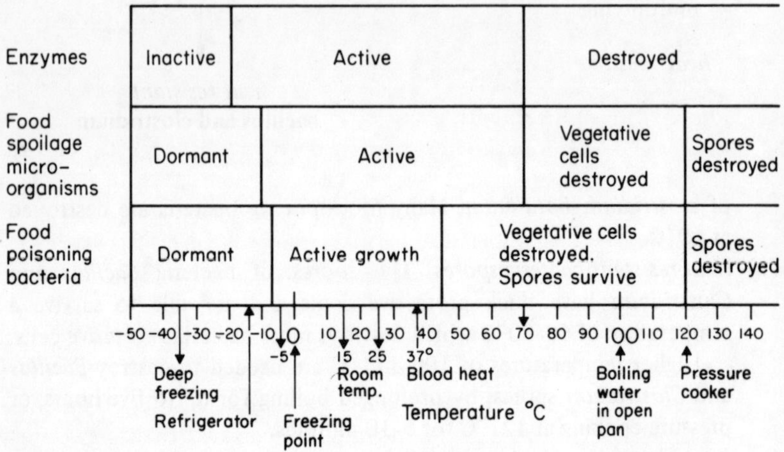

6. Irradiation

Visible light, ultra-violet rays, X-rays and gamma rays (Fig 7.2) are all components of the electromagnetic spectrum which radiates from the sun in various amounts. These different rays can be *generated* by different ray-producing machines such as ultra-violet lamps, and X-ray machines.

Sunlight slows down the growth of bacteria, consequently they flourish in *dark* places which are also warm and moist. Similarly bacteria culture media are incubated in the dark.

Gamma rays are the most powerful means of destroying bacteria cells, followed by weaker X-rays and ultra-violet rays.

7. Chemicals
Chemicals are used as components of *disinfectants* and *antiseptics*. Anti-sep

7. Chemicals

Chemicals are used as components of *disinfectants* and *antiseptics*. *Antiseptics* are also able to reduce the growth of bacteria. Some bacteria produce *antibiotics* which affect the growth of other species of bacteria. The bacteria *Streptomyces griseus* produces the antibiotic streptomycin and also produces *cyanocobalamin* (vitamin B_{12}).

Experiment 10.1 *Preparation of a culture media place*
WARNING The culture of micro-organisms can be *dangerous* and a source of *infectious diseases*. Experimental work and care of culture media should be supervised by a *qualified instructor*.

1. *Hands* Wash and scrub in hot soapy water, then sterilise by swabbing with cotton wool soaked in 70 per cent ethanol solution. This should be done before and after the investigation.

   Never eat, drink, smoke or touch the nose or lips with fingers when working with culture media.
2. *Benches* and table tops should be swabbed with a 5–10 per cent solution of strong disinfectant.
3. *Draughts* should be avoided by keeping doors and windows closed.
4. *Equipment* of glass and metal must be sterilised in an autoclave or pressure cooker kept for this purpose and *never* used for cooking. Plug test tubes with *non-absorbent* cotton wool, and leave tops of screw-cap bottles *slack*.

   Sterilise at 1.05kg/cm^2 pressure for 30 minutes at 121°C. Alternatively bake metal and glassware in an oven at 150°C for 30 minutes.

   Flame wire loops and glass bottle mouth openings by passing through the flame of a spirit lamp or bunsen burner.

   Disposal of culture media and contaminated equipment is by soaking in a solution of strong disinfectant or methanal (formaldehyde) for 2-3 days, followed by washing and sterilisation. Alternatively the material is wrapped in paper and burnt in a furnace.

Procedure

(i) Prepare a *nutrient agar* medium from proprietary tablet preparations, place one tablet in a sterile screw cap bottle together with 10cm^3 of water, and sterilise in an autoclave or pressure cooker.

(ii) *Pour* the molten culture medium into previously sterilised culture petri dishes. Replace the dish lids immediately and allow the media to set.

(iii) *Inoculate* the culture media by sprinkling a little quantity of dried mixed herbs onto the media and tape down and label the lid.

(iv) *Incubate* the culture media dishes in a warm place at 38–40°C for 2-3 days.

Observations
The *colonies* of bacteria will be visible as yellow, white and pink growths, together with fluffy growths of different coloured *moulds*.
CAUTION! Under *NO* circumstances are the taped down lids to be removed from the culture media dishes. The infected dish must be dis-

posed of by a qualified instructor by soaking the culture in strong disinfectant or methanol (formaldehyde) or by burning. Figure 11.5 shows the procedure and apparatus used in this experiment.

Fig 11.5 *procedure and apparatus for preparing a culture medium plate*

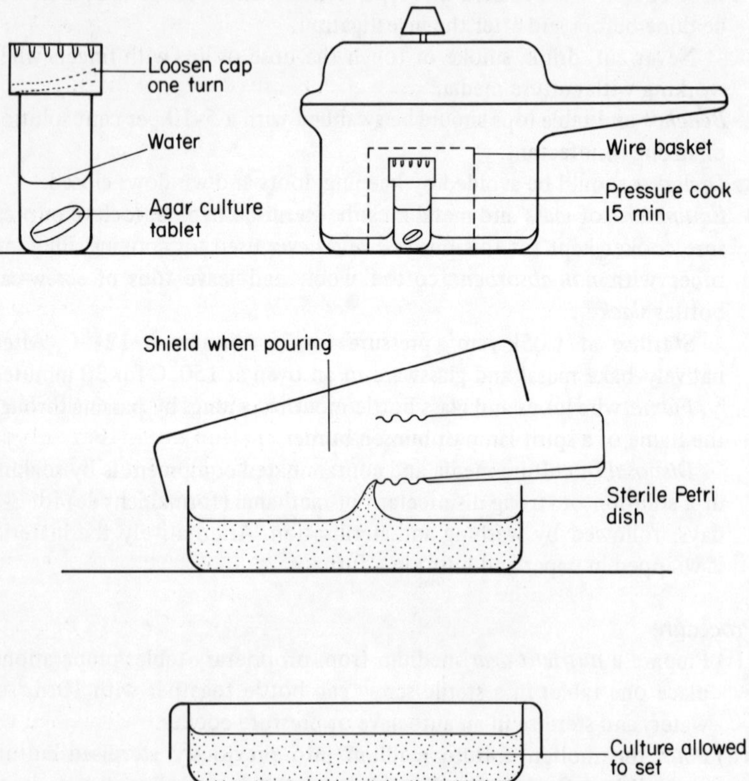

11.6 HARMFUL SUBSTANCES IN FOODS

Amongst the $1\frac{1}{2}$ million different plants and animals there are a small number of species which contain certain *non-nutrient* substances which are *toxic* or poisonous to human beings, in addition to many mainly micro-organisms which are *pathogenic* or *parasitic*, being a cause of *infectious disease* in human beings.

Poisonous plants include hemlock, deadly nightshade, henbane, laburnum seeds, in addition to poisonous fungi already described. Many plants contains poisonous *alkaloids* which, when extracted, are used in the preparation of useful therapeutic drugs.

Poisonous animals include many species of fish, known locally for their poisonous nature.

In addition, various disorders may arise by eating *excessive quantities* of broad beans (favism), bitter almonds (cyanide posioning), (cassava must be soaked in water to remove cyanides), rhubarb leaves (oxaluria). Cabbage seeds, peanuts, soya bean, and cassava also may cause enlargement of the thyroid gland (goitre) when consumed in *excessive* amounts (Plate 9.5). Green potato skins and sprouts can also cause intestinal disorders because of a toxic substance *solannine*.

Parasites in food

Parasites (Section 3.9) include different worms which can infect human beings, such as *roundworms* and *threadworms* which are transmitted by faecal contamination of salad foods. Many schoolchildren are infected with threadworms. Pork which is *undercooked* may be infected with the roundworm of *Trichinella spiralis*, this can enter human body tissues causing *trichinosis*.

Tapeworms may be eaten as cysts in pork and beef; these develop into tape-like adult worms up to 3m in length (pork) and up to 10m in beef tapeworm fixed to the wall of the human intestine by a head. The tapeworm absorbs *digested* food from the intestine causing loss in body weight and increased appetite. Between 25 and 75 per cent of African, Tibetan and Syrian populations may be infected with beef tapeworm. Figure 11.6 illustrates the life-cycle of the pork tapeworm.

The *fish* tapeworm can grow up to a length of 10m in the small intestine of humans who are infected by eating *raw* fish. The symptoms are anaemia due to the worm depriving the host of vitamin B_{12} (cyanocobalamin) and weight loss, together with abdominal pain. Tapeworms are eliminated by means of various drugs and certain plant products, including male fern extract and pumpkin seeds.

Meat inspection by qualified veterinary surgeons and meat inspectors reduces the incidence of parasite-infected foods reaching the consumer. Meat and fish should always be examined and cooked well to kill undetected cysts.

11.7 BACTERIAL DISEASES FROM FOOD

A number of diseases can arise by the intake of live bacteria or their toxins in food or water, causing mainly an inflammation of the stomach and intestine called *gastro-enteritis*. The ingested *live* bacteria may already be present in large numbers in the food, or may multiply within the

Fig 11.6 *life cycle of pig tapeworm, taemia solium, an endoparasite of human beings and pigs*

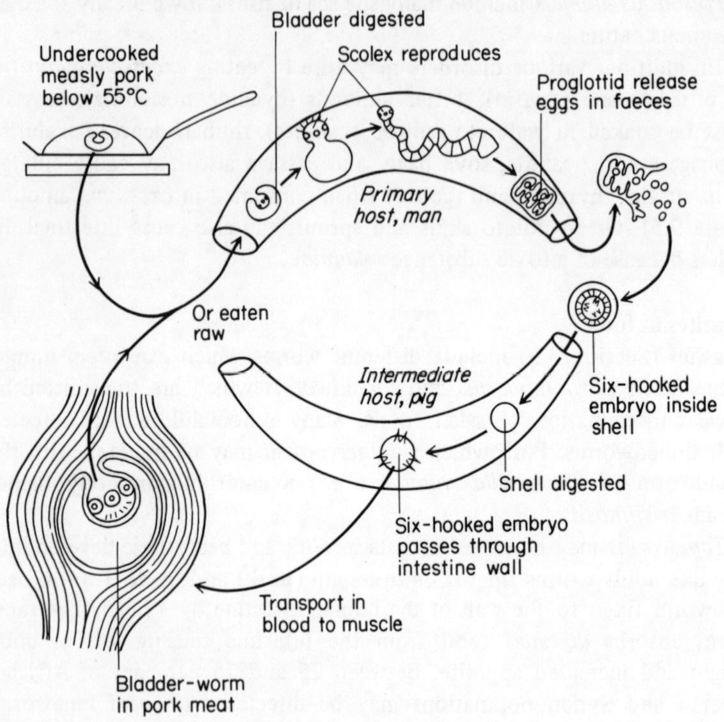

human gut, encouraged by the prevailing favourable growth conditions.

The pathogenic bacteria may *cling to* or *enter* the gut lining cells (see Section 8.11), or cause *irritation* by their toxins. This results in varying *symptoms* of gastro-enteritis which include: *diarrhoea* of a watery nature with or without blood, *vomiting* and abdominal *pain*, as in bacterial food poisoning by certain *Salmonella*, *Clostridium* and *Staphylococcus bacteria* (Section 11.10).

If the pathogenic bacteria or toxins enter the bloodstream, the symptoms may include *fever*, with or without diarrhoea, or gastro-enteritis as in typhoid, paratyphoid, or undulant fevers. The rare disease of *botulism* can cause paralysis of the *nervous* system and is often *fatal* because of the toxins of *Clostridium botulinum*.

The time of onset or the *incubation period* between infection and appearance of symptoms varies from half an hour to several days depending on the *kind* of bacterial infection.

11.8 MAIN INFECTIOUS DISEASES FROM FOOD

The main diseases caused by pathogenic bacteria in food and water are of two main types: *food poisoning infections* and *water- and food-borne infections*.

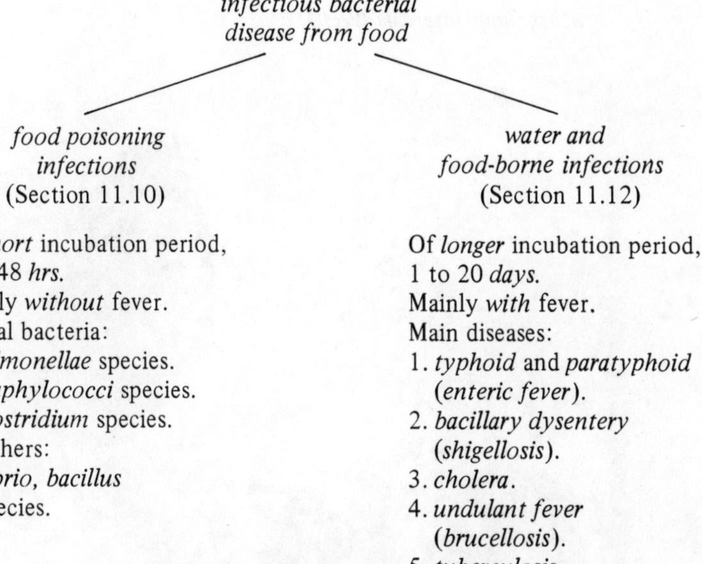

infectious bacterial disease from food
food poisoning infections
(Section 11.10)
Of *short* incubation period, $\frac{1}{2}$hr–48 *hrs.*
Mainly *without* fever.
Causal bacteria:
1. *salmonellae* species.
2. *staphylococci* species.
3. *clostridium* species.
4. Others: *vibrio, bacillus* species.
water and food-borne infections
(Section 11.12)
Of *longer* incubation period, 1 to 20 *days.*
Mainly *with* fever.
Main diseases:
1. *typhoid* and *paratyphoid* (*enteric fever*).
2. *bacillary dysentery* (*shigellosis*).
3. *cholera*.
4. *undulant fever* (*brucellosis*).
5. *tuberculosis.*

In addition there are intestinal infections which may be caused by more than one species of micro-organism, such as *Travellers diarrhoea*, and *infantile gastro-enteritis* causing diarrhoea and/or vomiting together with dehydration in children under 2 years in poorer developing countries, and cause the death of 5 to 18 *million* children each year. *Rehydration* by means of hygienically prepared water and drinks overcomes the problem of dehydration and thereby reduces the mortality rate (see Plate 11.2). *Breast-feeding* is more hygienic and affords some protection against infantile gastro-enteritis, since breast milk provides natural immunity against diseases with no risk of infection from contaminated, *dirty* and often dilute artifical milk bottle feeds.

11.9 DEATH AND DISEASE

The causes of death in wealthy *developed* countries of the world are *organic diseases* such as: *cancer*, and diseases of the *heart* or *blood* vessels (Section 9.6) which occur mainly in people over fifty, thus allowing a general life expectancy of 65–75 years of age. There are fewer deaths

Plate 11.2 *over 15 million children die from dehydration caused by infantile gastroenteritis each year. The former rehydration treatment was by intravenous drip. The number of child deaths is now reduced by giving a hygienically prepared drink by mouth consisting of boiled and cooled water containing 2% glucose and 0.3% common salt, in small doses at frequent intervals (WHO)*

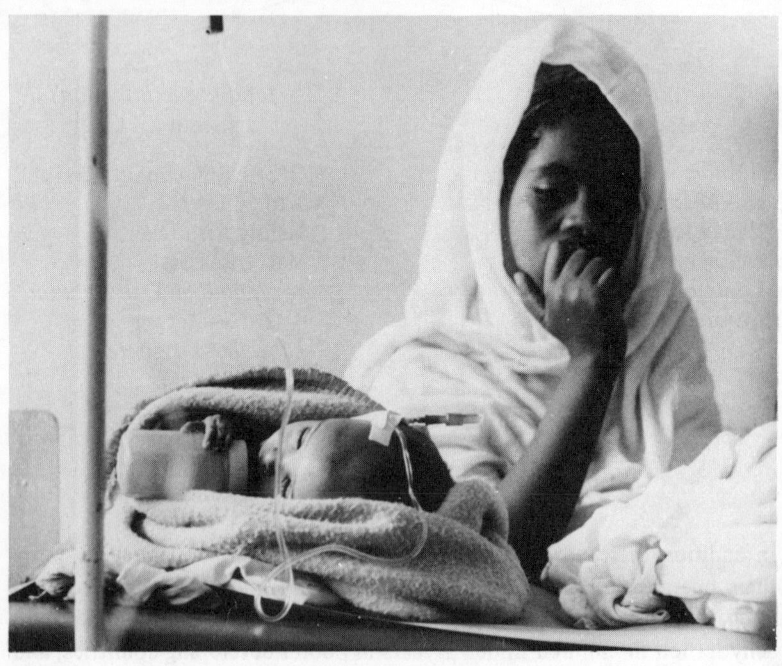

from *infectious* and *nutritional deficiency diseases* (Section 9.3) caused mainly by pathogenic micro-organisms because of less overcrowding, better hygiene and sanitation, nutrition, immunisation and availability of medicines (antibiotics etc.) to combat infectious disease.

In *poorer, developing* countries death also occurs from organic diseases, but more die *young* from *infectious* and *nutritional deficiency diseases* such as PEM, food poisoning, intestinal infections, and a range of *infectious* diseases such as malaria, yellow fever and trachoma. The higher death rate is the result of malnutrition, overcrowding, lack of hygiene and sanitation, parental neglect and poor medical facilities.

11.10 BACTERIAL FOOD POISONING

Bacterial food poisoning is a *sharp* outbreak of illness usually affecting more than one individual after *sharing a meal*.

Plate 11.3 shows *salmonella typhimurim* which is the *main* causal bacteria in about 80 per cent of food poisoning cases; the disease is called 'salmonella food poisoning' or *salmonellosis*. Other less common causes

Plate **11.3** *salmonella typhimurium magnified 6000 times: the cause of 80 per cent of food-poisoning cases (Unilever Organisation Ltd)*

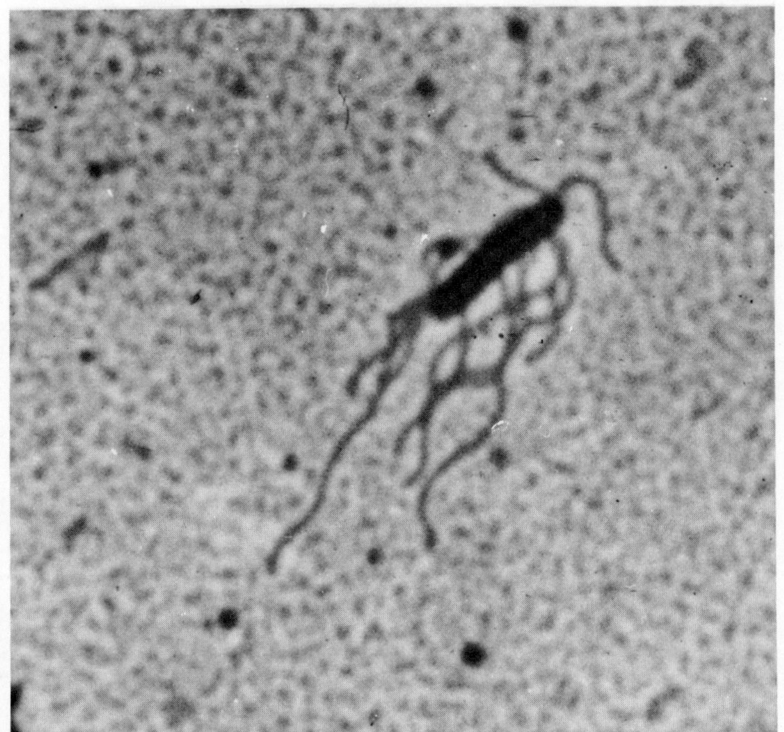

are other bacteria listed in Table 11.2, together with the main disease symptoms, incubation times, method of infection and foods involved.

11.11 REDUCING FOOD POISONING

Foods can become contaminated at their *source of supply*. Farm animals raised close together under intensive monoculture conditions can infect one another with *salmonella* species infections.

Table 11.2 *Bacterial food poisoning*

Organism, origin and its effect	*Food involved and contamination methods*	*Incubation time and symptoms*
Salmonella species, enter the gut-lining cells causing cell damage. Found in different *farm animal* intestine, and in human *carriers*.	Poultry, pork, ham, beef, cooked meats, sausages (50 per cent) and duck eggs (20 per cent), milk, and cream products (20 per cent). Infected faeces of humans, rats, mice, soil or dust contaminate *raw* or *cooked* food, by hands, surfaces or equipment. Rapid growth in food kept warm (37°C) or moist. Easily killed by *thorough heating* of food in cooking.	12–48 hours. Heavy infection needed to produce illness. Mainly *diarrhoea* also some abdominal *pain* and possibly fever. Duration several days. Can be fatal in young and elderly. [About 80% of cases caused by *Salmonella typhimurium*].
Staphylococcus aureus, the previously formed heat-resistant endotoxin irritates gut lining. Spread from the nose, hands and septic cuts, pimples and boils, of food handlers.	Infected pastries, custards, trifle, meats and pies, allow staphylococci to multiply when food is held in warm moist conditions. Cooking does *not* destroy the toxin, only vegetative cells are destroyed by heat.	½ to 6 hours. Mainly *vomiting*, with some abdominal pain and diarrhoea. Duration 8–12 hours.
Clostridium perfringens (welchii) Endotoxin released in the gut. Found in faeces, sewage, and soil.	Cooked meats, stews, pies, and poultry. Spores resist heat of cooking to survive and multiply in slowly cooling cooked foods, in anaerobic conditions *inside* stews, pies and rolled meat.	12–24 hours. Mainly abdominal pain, also some diarrhoea. Duration less than a day.
Clostridium botulinum An exotoxin already formed in the food enters the *bloodstream*. Found in soil and decayed *plants*.	*Home-preserved vegetables, meat or fish* – ineffectively sterilised. Spores resist heat, and multiply in anaerobic conditions, to produce *toxin* which can be *destroyed by heat* on boiling or cooking. NEVER CAN or BOTTLE VEGETABLES, MEATS OR FISH AT HOME	12–36 hours. FATAL in about half the cases. Vomiting, and rapid *paralysis* of limbs and chest muscles, and constipation.
Bacillus cereus Toxin preformed in cooked rice. Found in dust, soil and certain vegetables.	Aerobic bacteria multiply rapidly in previously cooked rice kept moist and warm.	1–6 hours. Diarrhoea, vomiting, abdominal pain for less than 12 hours.
Vibrio parahaemolyticus Endotoxin in bacteria found in tropical seawater.	Pacific fish, shellfish, and processed, raw, or undercooked, sea foods.	2–48 hours. Diarrhoea, vomiting, severe abdominal pain for up to 5 days.

Similarly vegetables and fruits can be contaminated with *soil* bacteria of the *clostridium* species.

Slaughter of farm animals may result in contamination of the meat carcase by intestinal bacteria *salmonellae*, or soil bacteria *clostridium*. *Staphylococci* can pass from septic cuts and skin infections of slaughter-house workers and butchers hands to infect exposed meat.

Further infection of *exposed* food may occur in shops, butchers and bakeries.

In the *home* there is a need for *cleanliness* or hygiene of the *person*, *equipment* and kitchen *premises* with the *exclusion* of infected cases or *carriers* of food poisoning bacteria, such as from certain infected people, or *pets* - cats, dogs, rabbits etc. - allowed in the kitchen or home.

Table 11.3 summarises methods of reducing and preventing food poisoning in the home.

Experiment 11.2 *to show the presence of greasy soils on crockery, glassware and metalware*

Procedure

(i) *Crockery*
Apply by means of a soft camel hair brush the *black disclosing powder* made from lampblack 70 per cent, graphite 20 per cent and acacia gum 10 per cent.
Blow away excess powder and note the *black* fingerprints or grease soil.

(ii) *Glassware and metalware*
Apply a *white disclosing powder* made from cornflower 43 per cent, china clay 43 per cent and acacia gum powders 14 per cent. Remove the excess and note the *white* fingerprints and grease soils.

Observations

Greasy food residues will cling to kitchen equipment and tableware; this grease film will also be associated with bacteria. The greasy soil should be removed in efficient washing with hot water and detergents.

11.12 FOOD- AND WATER-BORNE INFECTIONS

Over 25 per cent of the world population or 1000m people in the less developed countries lack a pure and adequate water-supply to drink or to maintain personal hygiene.

The following diseases - enteric fever, bacillary dysentery, cholera, campylobacteriosis, brucellosis, tuberculosis and *Escherichia coli* infections - can be transmitted to human beings either by infected or impure water, milk or food, contaminated by animal or human faeces. They are

Table 11.3 *Food poisoning preventative measures*

Location	*Hygiene practices*
Source: Farms and fisheries	Clean, disease-free *feeding stuffs*. Farmed trout can be starved for 3 days before slaughter in 'clean-up' ponds to reduce *Clostridium botulinum*. Veterinary care of animals. Eradication of rats and mice and other pests. Clean milking parlours and milk collection.
Processing	Hygienic slaughter and prevention of cross-contamination of carcases. Rapid and hygienic gutting of sea fish. Maintenance of high standards in food factories, bakeries and food processing plants.
Home and institutional catering	*Personal hygiene* 1. Infected people and carriers *not* to handle food. 2. Infected pets and other animal reservoirs to be *excluded*. 3. Personal habits must be CLEAN HABITS – WASH HANDS after visiting TOILET. NO smoking, spitting, sneezing, coughing or fingering of cooked foods. 4. Hair should be kept covered. *Cooking and preparation* 1. Thoroughly clean and WASH salads, vegetables and fruit. 2. *Raw* foods must be kept well APART from *cooked* foods. 3. COOKING should be *thorough* at a *high* enough temperature and for sufficient *time* to *penetrate* into the centre of meat and poultry. Cook stuffing separately. 4. Eat cooked food *hot* as soon as ready. 5. If not for immediate eating COOL RAPIDLY – slow cooling encourages bacterial growth. 6. COVER all cooked and raw foods to prevent infection by exposure to dust, and airborne micro-organisms. 7. HANDLE *cooked* foods, cakes, custards etc. with clean food TONGS.

Equipment

1. WASH in very hot water at 75 °C with detergent. Then rinse in separate water sink at 60 °C. Stack to air dry.
2. Use disposable napkins and towels, or sterilise kitchen cloths and tea towels *daily*.
3. WORK SURFACES should be free from cracks and crevices and be non-absorbent.

Refrigerators

BACTERIA, SPORES AND TOXINS *SURVIVE* IN REFRIGERATORS, only their growth is prevented.

1. Maintain at 5 °C.
2. Cool hot cooked foods quickly *before* storing in refrigerator.
3. Keep RAW and COOKED foods covered and well apart from each other.
4. Frozen foods must be *completely thawed* before cooking.
5. Never refreeze *thawed* foods.

mainly serious diseases of long duration and relatively long incubation periods, compared with 'bacterial food poisoning' diseases.

Plate 11.4 *sterilisation of a well-water supply with a chlorination compound reduces water-borne disease, cholera and typhoid (WHO)*

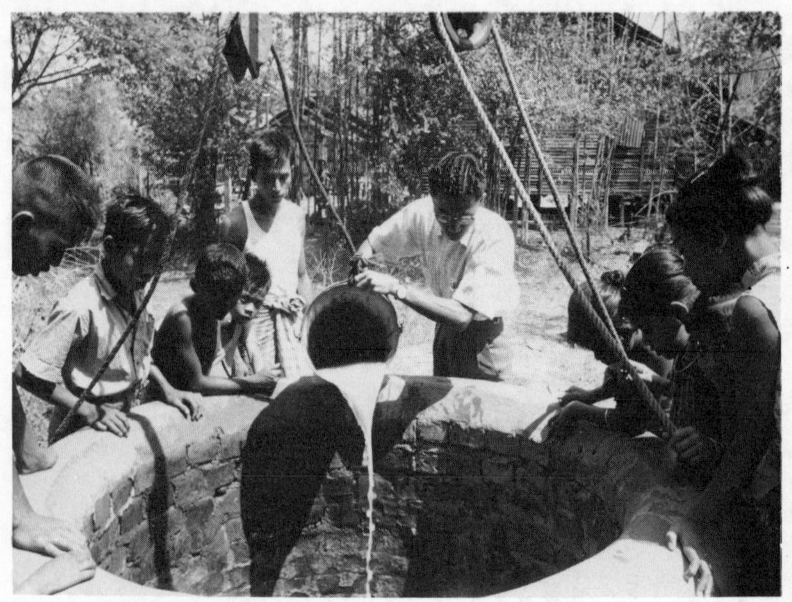

Many of these diseases can be prevented by purification and sterilisation of *water* supplies and the *pasteurisation* and *sterilisation* of milk as in Section 7.12.

Since only a *small dose* or injection of bacteria is required for most of these disorders, strict *personal hygiene* is needed to prevent cross-infection by other methods than food, as, for example, *contact*, *overcrowding* or spread by flies and pests. An adequate clean water supply is essential to maintain personal hygiene.

Protection against cholera and typhoid is given by *vaccination* for travellers to foreign countries. Revaccination is required after a certain period.

Table 11.4 gives details of the main food- and water-borne intestinal infections.

11.13 SHORT-TERM FOOD STORAGE

Perishable foods (Section 11.2) can be stored for short periods in:

(a) ventilated food *safes* or *cupboards*, cool ventilated larder or cellar *rooms*;
(b) domestic *refrigerators*.

Most *processed* foods are DATEMARKED on their labels with 'Sell by' or 'Best before' dates. Table 11.5 gives details of short term storage methods.

11.14 PRESERVATION – LONG-TERM STORAGE

Perishable food can be kept for very long periods provided:

(a) *micro-organism* growth is controlled or prevented (see Sections 11.3, 11.4 or 11.5) by various methods of cooling, heating, drying, chemicals, pH control etc.;
(b) *enzyme action* or autolysis is controlled or prevented (see Section 11.2) by *blanching*;
(c) *oxidation* of food components by oxygen in the air is prevented (Section 11.2) by excluding air as in vacuum-packing and canning, or by adding *antioxidant* chemicals.

Food preservation is also a form of *food processing* (Chapter 7). The various methods of preserving food are summarised in Table 11.6.

11.15 ADDITIVES

Additives are various chemical substances deliberately added to most processed foods in order to restore *losses* in *palatability*, flavour, texture, colour and nutritional composition arising from *processing* (Chapter 7); certain additives help food processing. *Preservatives* including sucrose, salt (sodium chloride), ethanol and certain *antibiotics* (for example *nisin*) are additives to combat spoilage by micro-organisms (Section 11.14).

Since food can also be *adulterated* or *contaminated* – for example, tea, pepper, and dried herbs mixed with *other* unrelated dried plant material; brown sugar with sand; flour with excess chalk; vegetable cooking oils with mineral hydrocarbon oils; milk with water – it is essential to protect the consumer legally by laws in different countries which control what may be permitted as food additives.

The permitted substances are rigorously tested for any harmful effects

Table 11.4 *Food- and water-borne intestinal infections*

Disease, bacteria	*Transmission and prevention*	*Incubation, symptoms*
Enteric fever, caused by *Salmonella typhi* (Typhoid) and *Salmonella paratyphi*.	Transmission by direct or indirect contact with *faeces* or *urine* of a *patient* or *carrier*, then by contaminated water and food and milk. Prevented by a CLEAN WATER supply and personal hygiene. Vaccination protects for up to 5 years.	10–20 days. Fever, headache, abdominal discomfort, maybe diarrhoea later. Paratyphoid has shorter incubation, 4–5 days, and milder symptoms.
Bacillary dysentery [Shigellosis] caused by different *Shigella* species, which multiply in the gut-lining cells.	Transmission by direct *faecal* infection in *overcrowded* families and institutions. Spreads to food by flies and food-handlers. Prevented by improved water supply, sanitation and lavatory cleaning, reduction of overcrowding and exclusion of infected food-handlers.	2–3 days. Fever, watery diarrhoea, with blood and abdominal pain. Short duration.
Cholera caused by *Vibrio cholerae* toxin.	Transmitted by faeces-contaminated water or food from a patient or a *carrier*. Shellfish often infected. Person to person contact and houseflies transmit from faeces to food. Prevention by *pure water supply*, careful personal hygiene. Vaccination protects for up to 6 months.	6 hours to 5 days. Vomiting and profuse watery diarrhoea every few minutes, leading to *dehydration* (see Section 8.19).
Undulant fever caused by different *Brucella* species which penetrate body cells.	Transmitted from animals – pigs, goats and cows – *direct* to slaughterhouse, and dairy workers, veterinary surgeons and farmers. Also by infected *raw milk* and cheese. Prevented by milk *pasteurisation* and vaccination of cattle, or slaughter of infected animals.	Long incubation, up to 4 weeks. Fever, sweating, backache, headache and fever of prolonged duration occurring in waves.
Campylobacteriosis caused by *Campylobacter* species.	Transmitted mainly from animal sources mainly poultry, also cats and dogs. Contaminated water and raw *milk* are sometimes a means of transmission.	3–5 days. Fever, vomiting, abdominal pain and watery diarrhoea.

Escherichia coli infections. This is a *normal* inhabitant of the human gut. Some types of it are pathogenic.	Transmitted by contaminated drinking *water*. The presence of *Escherichia coli* in the water shows it is contaminated with faeces. Purified sewage water is tested by trying to cultivate *E. Coli* – if it is *absent* the water is not faecal-contaminated.	May be *one* cause of infantile gastro-enteritis, and travellers' diarrhoea.
Tuberculosis *Mycobacterium tuberculosis*	Transmitted from infected cows in raw *milk*, or by droplet infection from infected patients. Prevention is by *pasteurisation* of milk, elimination of TB infected milk-cattle, improved personal hygiene and nutrition. Immunisation of non-immune young people with BCG vaccine.	Between 1 and 2 million in the world die of tuberculosis. Fever, night sweats, weight loss.

Table 11.5 *Short-term food storage*

Food	*Preparation*	*Storage time*	
Meat and Poultry	Cover loosely	Larder, cupboard Refrigerator	1–2 days 2–5 days
Cooked meat	Cool quickly and cover loosely – keep away from *raw* meat, poultry, fish.	Larder, cupboard Refrigerator	1–2 days 2–4 days
Fish	Cover loosely	Larder, cupboard Refrigerator	eat same day 1–2 days
Milk and Cream	Keep in original bottle, away from sunlight.	Larder, cupboard Refrigerator	1 day 3–4 days
Eggs	Store in dark, small end down, away from strong smelling foods.	Larder, cupboard Refrigerator	7 days 3 weeks
Cheese	Wrap firm cheese	Larder, cupboard Refrigerator	7 days 2 weeks
Butter	Turn rancid in bright light and exposed to air. Keep in original light proof wrapper or covered dish.	Larder, cupboard Refrigerator	1 week 2–3 weeks
Margarine		Larder, cupboard Refrigerator	2 weeks 6 weeks
White fats		Larder, cupboard Refrigerator	3 months 6 months

Oils		Keep indefinitely because of natural and added antioxidants.	
Fruits and Vegetables	Remove damaged parts and wrap loosely.	Larder rack in cool dark conditions with ventilation.	
Green vegetables		EAT same day	
Salad vegetables		Refrigerator	3 days
	Fruits should not be damaged.	Larder rack with ventilation. Eat as near to date of purchase as possible.	
Bread	Wrap loosely	Ventilated bin.	
Dry goods Sugar, rice and flour	Store in packet or container.	Larder cupboard, cool, dry, well-ventilated	2–3 months

Table 11.6 *Food preservation methods*

Principle	*Methods*	*Application*
Heating Denatures micro-organism proteins. [Spores are heat resistant]	*Pasteurisation* (Section 7.12). Temperatures of 62–80°C for various times destroy most pathogenic bacteria	Milk, eggs, ice cream, fruit juices
	Cooking by boiling, roasting, grilling and baking are forms of *heat sterilisation* (Section 7.8)	Most high-temperature cooking methods
	Canning – Bottling involves *pre-treatment* by peeling, blanching and addition of liquor, followed by *sterilisation* involving cooking at 115–125°C in pressure-cooking vessels. High acid (pH 3) citrus fruits require 100°C for few minutes. Low acid (pH 5 and over) meat, fish, milk and certain vegetables need 115°C and over. Foods are sealed into containers entirely free of air and oxygen.	Most foods. Shelf-life 1–4 years. 'Blown cans' or 'Swells' caused by hydrogen H_2 from acid action on metal can, and carbon dioxide (CO_2) gases from *clostridium* species activity, contents spoiled and discarded.
Low-temperature cooling Below −20°C. Food poisoning and food spoilage micro-organisms are *dormant*. Cell *enzyme* activity is reduced	*Domestic deep-freezing* – food frozen and stored at −20°C for up to 3 months.	Mainly meat, fish, poultry, vegetables, fruits and *pre-cooked convenience* foods
	Commercial freezing – food frozen by different methods at −30°C to −40°C by *plate-*, *blast-*, *cryogenic-* or *spray*-freezing. Foods stored for very long periods.	
Dehydration (a) Water removal from food (b) Water removal from micro-organisms by osmosis	*Sun*-drying – food liable to contamination.	Fruits, vegetables and fish
	Commercial dehydration by fluidised bed, spray-, roller-, vacuum- or accelerated freeze-drying	Fruits, vegetables, eggs, milk, coffee, soup, potatoes and meat
	Sugar – syrups and preserves, jams and sugar crystallisation.	Fruits

	Salt (sodium chloride) – salt curing and sweet curing. (High levels of sugar and salt in foods should be indicated on *labels*.) (Sections 8.19 and 9.6). Sodium nitrate and sodium nitrite used in pickled meats can form carcinogenic nitrosamines	Vegetables, fish, bacon and ham
Acidity - pH (Section 2.11). Strong acid solutions above pH 4 destroy most but not all bacteria	*Pickle* using vinegar – ethanoic (acetic) acid.	Pickles and sauces.
	Acid preservatives Sulphur dioxide gas Benzene carboxylic – (Benzoic) acid Propanoic (propionic) acid	Beer, dried fruits, dried potatoes and peas, jams, pickles, sausage, fruit juices and cordials. Artificial creams, fruit juices, pickles, sauce. Bread and cakes
Gases Inert gases	*Carbon dioxide* slows down fruit-ripening in fruit gas stores.	Apples, bananas
	Nitrogen gas displaces air and oxygen in containers.	Coffee extract
Smoke gases	Phenols , methanal (formaldehyde) and volatile acids from oak wood-smoke give flavours and are mild preservatives	Kippers and fish-smoking
Irradiation [Fig 7.2] (1) Rays similar to *X-rays* and *Gamma* rays destroy bacteria. Exposure to different dose levels produces different degrees of sterilisation	*High dose* produces almost complete sterilisation. *Medium dose* destroys most pathogenic bacteria. *Low dose* produces a state somewhat similar to pasteurisation	This method is *not* used universally and is not permitted in certain countries e.g. UK. In the USA it is used for bacon, and preventing wheat infestation
(2) Ultra-violet rays	From ultra-violet ray tubes and lamps	Helps to provide modest sterilisation for bread and cakes in shops, and air purification
(3) Microwaves	From microwave cookers	Provides sterilisation similar to cooking

when administered in large amounts to laboratory animals, over several generations. In this way it has been shown that certain substances are *carcinogenic* and the cause of certain cancers in animals, and their use is *not* permitted in foods.

Those substances which are proved to be safe are then *permitted* for use as food additives and are only used in extremely small amounts, for example 10mg of *antioxidant* to every 100g of cooking fat or lard – a concentration of about 0.01 per cent.

The UK, European Common Market countries and the USA have their own food laws. The developing countries are associated with the Food and Agriculture Organisation (FAO) and the World Health Organisation's (WHO) manual called the '*Codex Alimentarius*' which is concerned with food additives as well as hygiene and composition of about 200 major foods.

The European Economic Community (EEC) food-labelling regulations provide a list of *chemical names* for additives and also give each a *serial number*. For example, tartrazine, (food colouring) is E102; benzoic acid (food preservative) E210; butylated hydroxyanisole (antioxidant) E320.

Table 11.7 summarises some of the more important additives used in food under the main categories of food quality improvers, preservatives and antioxidants, and nutritional additives or fortifying agents.

11.16 **CANCER AND FOOD**

Cancer is a harmful growth or tumour found occurring on the skin and in most parts of gut and mouth and liver. The tumour is the result of *uncontrolled division* of body cells under the influence of an *initiator* which may be *radiation*, sunlight of X-rays causing skin cancer, or *chemicals* called *carcinogens* found in small amounts in tobacco smoke tars, coal tar, aflatoxins (Section 10.3), nitrosamines (Table 11.6) packaging material plastics – vinyl chloride and acrilonitrite (Section 11.17) and coaltar dyes – butter yellow, and cyclamate sweeteners are both now *banned* for use as food additives.

In addition certain *viruses* (Section 11.3) are known to cause cancer in certain animals; it is also possible that the tendency to cancer is *inheritable*.

It is important to note that cancer is not an *infectious* disease such as bacterial food poisoning, neither is it a *deficiency* disease like scurvy.

Cancer cells require a special *promotor* substance which may be a component of the blood to promote tumour growth; in addition the tumour requires nutrients from the *diet* leading to the *emaciation* and weight loss of the body. More than one risk factor is responsible for most cancers, in the same way as more than one risk factor is responsible for heart disease (Section 9.6). Some of these factors are similar to those associated as risk factors in heart disease.

1. *Smoking* is a proved cause of lung cancer.
2. *High saturated or animal origin lipid* intake causes a need to secrete *more* bile juice (Section 8.9) whose *breakdown* products may become carcinogenic products and components of the faeces resulting in bowel cancers. Excessive fat intake may also be related to breast and prostate cancers. The overall lipid fat intake should be reduced to 30 per cent of the daily energy intake.
3. *Dietary fibre* if *absent* from the diet causes the faeces to become more *concentrated* and remain in contact with the bowel lining for *longer* periods of time. If there is a *high* fibre intake, the faeces are *less* concentrated, being loose and bulky and move *quickly* through the bowel *reducing* the time of contact with the bowel-lining and inhibiting the initiation of cancer growth.
4. *Obesity* (Section 9.5) may also be linked with cancer of the gall-bladder and womb.
5. *Alcohol* consumed in excess has links with cancer of the throat and oesophagus, more so in people who smoke.
6. *Salt* (sodium chloride) in cured, pickled and smoked foods may also be contaminated with nitrosamines known to cause cancer in animals. Consumption of these foods should be reduced.

The *preventative* measures given for obesity and heart disease may well apply to avoidance of cancer by non-smoking, reduced lipid intake, increase in dietary fibre intake and moderate alcohol consumption.

In addition to tobacco smoking, alcohol and diet, other suggested factors include: pollution, industrial occupation, medicines and medical treatments, sex and reproduction and the effect of the surrounding soils, rocks or external environment.

11.17 FOOD PACKAGING

Packaging is used to:

(a) *protect* food from exposure to light, oxygen, moisture and physical damage;
(b) *preserve* food in vacuum-sealed metal *cans*, glass bottles, *plastic bags*, or in combined metal and plastic sterilisable or *retortable pouches*;
(c) *present* food in an *attractive* way together with a *label* which includes such *information* as food name, ingredients, net quantity, datemark,

Table 11.7 *Major permitted food additives*

Food additive category and type	*Examples and use*
Quality improvers	
A. *Flavourings*	
Natural	Unprocessed *dried* and ground herbs, spices, often contaminated by micro-organisms. *Natural essences* or ethanol extracts of essential oils of lemon, vanilla, etc.; concentrated *oleoresin* extracts in dispensed or encapsulated forms, are all processed and more hygienic.
Synthetic	Mainly *esters*, or complex *hydrocarbons* in ethanol, dispensed or encapsulated. Main solvent is ethanol, the flavour *carriers* are gums, starches or salt
B. *Colourings* (E100+)	
Natural from plants, fruits and vegetables, or animals	Chlorophyll (green), carotenes (yellow/orange), annatto (yellow), alkanet (red), cochineal – insect (dark red), saffron (yellow), turmeric (yellow), paprika (yellow orange). Many *untested* for harmful effects in large doses.
Synthetic dyes all man-made chemicals	Tartrazine (orange yellow) (this may cause allergy in certain people), amaranth (red), black BN (black), brown FK (for kippers). Extensively tested for safety.
C. *Sweeteners*	
Nutritive These have an *energy* or nutritive value	Glucose. Sorbitol, is poorly absorbed and tolerated by diabetics *Aspartame*, 180 times sweeter than sucrose, is a *di*peptide of *two* amino-acids – aspartic acid and phenylalanine. Both amino-acids can be used by the body
Non-nutritive have *no* energy or nutritional value	Mainly saccharin. (*Cyclamate* is banned since it was found to be harmful when tested on laboratory animals)

D. *Textural aids* (E400+)	
Emulsifiers or creaming agents	Modified lipids, glyceryl monostearate (GMS) gelatin and lecithin.
Stabilisers or thickening agents	Gums, waxy starches and cellulose derivatives.
Humectants or moisturisers	Prevent drying of cakes and dried fruits. Propanetriol (glycerine) and sorbitol.
Anti-spattering agents	Added to cooking fats and oils. Mainly lecithin.
Lubricants	Food quality liquid paraffin, prevents clumping of dried fruits.
Preservatives	
Antimicrobial (E200+)	Antibiotic nisin in canned foods, cheeses and cream.
Prevent growth of micro-organisms	*Nitrates* and *nitrites* in cured bacon, ham, canned meats, drinking water, vegetables. Can be changed into harmful carcinogenic *nitrosamines* by interaction in food or the human body
Antioxidants (E300+) Prevent chemical damage to lipid-containing food – rancidity.	Gallic acid and butylated hydroxy-anisole, BHA, and butylated hydroxy-toluene BHT. Also vitamin C (ascorbic acid) and vitamin E (tocopherols). In edible cooking oils and margarines
Nutritional additives	
Vitamins	'A and D' to margarine; 'B group' to bread, breakfast cereals and TVP; 'C' to fruit drinks and bread
Minerals	Ca, Fe to bread flour. Iodides to table salt.
Amino-acids	Textured vegetable protein (TVP) – methionine.

instructions for use, and storage conditions, the *proportion* of recommended daily amounts (RDA) of nutrients and energy could also be included.

Glass, metals, paper and cardboard are mainly *recyclable* materials, able to be processed and *remade* again into packaging materials.

Plastic *polymer* materials such as cellulose (Cellophane), polythene, polypropylene, polyvinyl chloride (PVC) (Vitafilm), polyvinylidene chloride (Saran), polyester (Melinex – shrink wrapping) are *non-recyclable* and the cause of waste as non-degradable plastics.

Meats and other foods can be vacuum- or heat-sealed into plastic packages together with or without an *inert* oxygen-free atmosphere of nitrogen or carbon dioxide.

Laminates are made by joining sheets of different plastic, metal foil or paper together.

Certain plastic packaging films are *porous* to air, moisture and odours – for example, cellulose film; others are *non-porous* and a complete barrier to moisture as in 'boil-in-the-bag' polythene.

Certain laminates and aluminium foil are opaque and provide a barrier to *light* in addition to moisture and air for packaging butter, margarine, freeze-dried soups, biscuits and cheeses.

11.18 QUESTIONS

1. What are the main causes of food spoilage? What methods can be used to prevent this occurring in food stored for a short period of up to seven days?
2. What are the main methods of long term food storage of up to three and six months?
3. What are the main harmful *infectious* diseases which can be obtained from infected food?
4. What measures can be taken to prevent infectious food poisoning?
5. Describe the importance of a pure water supply in preventing disease.
6. Name and briefly describe four diseases transmitted by low standards of food care.

CHAPTER 12

WORLD FOOD

12.1 WORLD PEOPLE

The planet *Earth* came into being about 5000m years ago and human beings arose as a species called *Homo sapiens* or 'Wise man', some 40 000 years ago, to produce the different *races* which form the Earth's human *population* unevenly distributed today over the Earth's surface. A *population* is defined as a group of individuals of the same species within a *community*. The other members of the community include other living *organisms* namely all plants and animals; together they *share* the same *external environment* providing all their needs for *life* by food, water, warmth, climate, air and *space* in which to live.

About 70 per cent of the Earth's surface is *water* – seas, lakes and rivers – the remaining 30 per cent is land forming the main *regions* in which human beings live. Asia forms 34 per cent of the land surface, Africa 22 per cent, North America 14 per cent, Latin America 13 per cent, Oceania (Australia, New Zealand and Polynesia) 10 per cent and Europe 7 per cent.

Primitive human beings or *palaeolithic* people, were hunters, trappers and gatherers of 'free' food, were followed by *mesolithic* people who lived together in communities close to lakes and were the pioneers of simple *agriculture.* Their total number in the world, 10 000 years ago, has been estimated at 50m.

The neolithic people with established agricultural communities, were followed by the Bronze Age people who introduced *money* and began to live in *cities.*

The *Iron* Age of over 2000 years ago, passed into the *Middle* Ages and thence into the *Industrial* age of *Modern* times, with its advancement of machinery, energy use and development of science and medicine. Throughout all these times there was a *small* net increase in the world population limited by food *famine*, *malnutrition*, *wars*, *earthquakes* and *infectious disease* - for example, Black death in Britain in the 1300s reduced the population by 25 per cent from 3.7m to 2.8m; two world wars killed over 60m, and the potato crop failure in Ireland in 1845 caused the death of 1m by starvation, whilst 10m died of starvation in the 1769 famine in India.

12.2 POPULATION CHARACTERISTICS

Populations of human beings share the following population *characteristics* with populations of all other living organisms; this has already been described with reference to *bacteria* populations (Section 11.4 and Figure 11.3). The numerical study of human populations is called *demography*, and is determined by census or counting, undertaken in most countries on a periodic basis. The world population in 1983 was estimated as 4677m.

(a) *Birth rate* is the number of live births per 1000 of a human population per year, currently 29 for the whole world.
(b) *Death rate* is the number of deaths per 1000 population per year, and currently 11 for the whole world.
(c) *Growth* or rate of natural increase is equal to the birth rate *minus* the death rate divided by ten as an annual percentage.

For example the world rate of growth is: birth rate 29 minus death rate 11,

$$\text{Growth rate for world} = \frac{29 - 11}{10} = 1.8 \text{ per cent}$$

Graphs can be used to show growth in populations. The graph curve has the same S-shape for *all* living organisms, and is shown in Figure 11.3 for bacteria and applies equally to human populations. This graph is used to forecast or *project* population estimates in future years.

(d) *Doubling-time* is the number of years to *double* present populations; it is based on an *unchanged* growth rate. The current world doubling time is 39 years, meaning the world population will double itself from 4677m to 9354m by the year 2022.
(e) *Infant Mortality Rate* is the annual number of deaths per 1000 amongst children under *one* year old and is currently 84 for the world
(f) *Age distribution* is a measure of the population percentage aged *15 years* and under, currently 34 per cent for the world; and the population percentage aged *64 years* and over, currently 6 per cent for the World.

(g) *Life expectancy* is the average number of years a newborn child can expect to live if current death rate does not alter. At present this is 62 years for the world.
(h) *Distribution* is an indication of the percentage of the population living in towns, and is currently 39 per cent for the world, with 61 per cent living in the country.
(i) *Density of populations* is the number of people in a square kilometre or km^2 of cultivated *arable* land, and is currently about $98/km^2$ for the whole world.

12.3 **WORLD ECONOMIC ZONES**

There are more than 150 different countries in the world. They are divided into two main economic zones called the *developed* or *more developed* countries and the *developing* or *less developed* countries. This classification is by the Food and Agriculture Organisation (FAO) of the United Nations.

(a) The *developed* countries include: Europe, North America, United States, Australia, New Zealand, Japan and the USSR. These are countries which have fully used their resources of minerals, fossil fuels for industry and have *advanced* agriculture methods.
(b) *Developing countries* comprise all other countries of the world who have not as yet fully used their natural resources and in many cases have *primitive* agricultural methods.

A *general* comparison of developed and developing countries is given in Table 12.1. It is very important to note that *variation* exists within regions, countries and also in towns and villages. Exceptions are more often the rule, and extreme exceptions are quoted in the table for highest and lowest values. Of greater importance is the variation which exists between *individual human beings* within a country.

12.4 **THE POPULATION EXPLOSION**

The world population in 1983 was estimated at 4677m; this is *double* the population of fifty years ago, *four* times that of 200 years ago and almost 90 times the estimated population of the Stone Age 10 000 years ago (see Figure 12.1).

The *projected* or *estimated* world population for the year 2000 is between 4880m and 6900m, whilst the present population is estimated at current increase rate to *double* again to 9354m by the year 2022! The projected population in 2020 is estimated at 7810m.

One of the main reasons for the population explosion in the UK is the

Table 12.1 *general comparison of developed and developing countries*

Countries	*Developed countries* Europe, North America, Australia, New Zealand, Japan, Israel and USSR	*Developing countries* Rest of world	*Exceptions* Certain Eastern European countries; China and South East Asian countries
Population (1983)	1158m - 25%	3519m - 75%	
Population 2000 (Estimate)	1273m -20%	4857m - 80%	
Birth rate	15	33 (i.e. double)	53 Kenya 10 West Germany
Infant mortality rate	19	93 (4.9 times)	Sweden 7 Finland 211 East Timor Japan
Death rate	10	12 (i.e. 1.2 times)	29 Gambia 4 Cost Rica and Fiji Fiji
Growth rate	0.6%	2.1% (i.e. 3.5 times)	4.1 Kenya –0.2 West Germany
Doubling times	118 yrs (i.e. 3.6 times)	32 yrs	3465 yrs Sweden, Austria 18 yrs Kenya
Population under 15 yrs	23	38 (1.6 times)	50 Botswana 18 Luxembourg
Population over 64 yrs	11	4	16 Sweden 2 Several countries

Life expectancy	73 yrs	58 yrs	40 Ethiopia 76 Japan and Iceland
Main cause of death	Heart, stroke and circulation diseases, and cancer	Infectious diseases, parasites and malnutrition	Variation within countries
Population density per km^2	$59/km^2$	$128/km^2$	Honk Kong 62 675/km^2 Holland 694/km^2 Australia 3/km^2 Mongolia 1/km^2
Urban population as %	70%	30%	Singapore 100% Burundi 2%
Wealth as national income per head	8657$ US (i.e. 11.9 times)	728$ US	Qatar $27 790 Ethiopia $142
Share of world trade	80%	20%	Varied
Share of expenditure on arms	75%	25%	China 10%
Education	High standards of literacy	Low standards of literacy	

SOURCE Abstracted from 1983 *World Population Data Sheet* (Population Concern, 1983)

fig 12.1 *the population explosion: estimated population of the world from origin of human beings to a projected estimate of 6000–6900m in AD 2000*

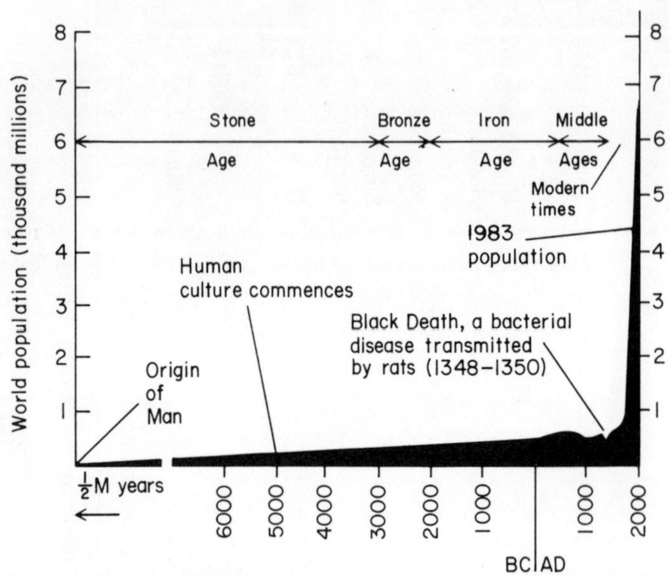

reduction in the *infant mortality rate.* In the UK in 1840 the rate was 145 per 1000, in 1981 it was 12 per 1000, a reduction of almost 90 per cent, achieved mainly by:

1. *Conquest of infectious diseases* through medicine and improved public, personal and food hygiene.
2. *Clean water* supply.
3. *Improved nutrition.*
4. *Welfare* services for mother and child.

These measures allowed *more* people to survive and reproduce.

12.5 FOOD AND THE WORLD POPULATION

The growth of the human population is similar to the growth of a bacteria population as described in Section 11.4, Figure 11.3. The comparable position of the present human population is shown on the graph in Figure 11.3, and is located in the region of *rapid* growth, also called *exponential increase*. Continued increased growth along this graph will result in the following effects:

(a) *Overcrowding* of cities.
(b) *Pollution* of water, air and land.
(c) *Food* resources being decreased.
(d) *Death rate* will increase because of decreased food supplies and medical services.

This is expected to occur about the year 2050 when the present world population will have more than doubled. Plate 12.1 shows the increased pollution resulting from an increasing population.

Plate 12.1 *an increasing population in Europe leads to water pollution from industrial waste and human sewage; requires frequent checks on the water as shown on the river Rhine, one of the most polluted waters in Europe (WHO)*

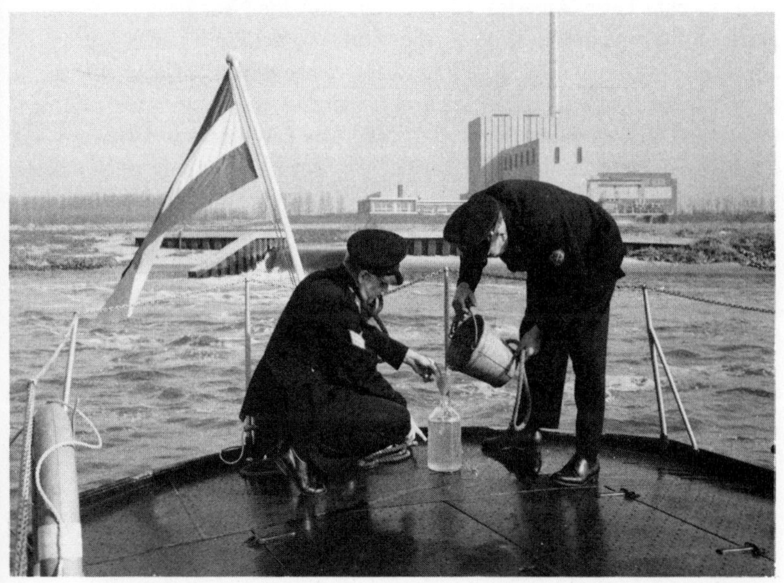

Under-nutrition in the world

World-edible energy intake
The *average* intake of edible or food energy needed to maintain *moderate* activity per head of the world population is 10.0MJ daily. (See Section 10.5).

(a) The *more developed* countries have a general energy intake 34 per cent *greater* than the average. In Luxembourg it is 49 per cent more and in Sweden 17 per cent more than average.
(b) Some *less developed* countries have an energy intake 1 per cent more than the average, whilst it can be 10–25 per cent less in many African and Asian countries, whilst in areas where hunger is prevalent it can be 50 per cent below the average intake or 5MJ instead of 10MJ daily.

The Food and Agriculture Organisation of the United Nations has estimated that 10 per cent or 435m of the world's population are *under-nourished* because of an inadequate intake of food. These under-nourished people do not have a *healthful* or balanced diet, and this lack results in the *dietary deficiency disorders* described in Sections 9.2 and 9.3, mainly protein energy malnutrition or PEM.

These people live mainly in the *developing countries*; Far East countries have an estimated 28 per cent of the population under-nourished, Africa 23 per cent, Latin America 13 per cent and the Near East 10 per cent. Most of the under-nourished in the world are *children* under 5 years of age, and 10–15m or 0.25–0.37 per cent of the world are near *starvation* with an energy intake insufficient to maintain the *basic metabolic rate* (Section 5.13), at a level of 1.2 × BMR. The FAO estimates that 15 000 die daily of hunger – that is, 5.5m per year, or 0.13 per cent of the world population.

Table 12.2 makes a *general* comparison of the nutrition of people in the developed and developing countries; it must be indicated that there are many exceptions – for example, the Eskimos consume a diet of 47 per cent lipid, 45 per cent protein and 8 per cent carbohydrates.

Between the extremes indicated in the table are a wide range of variations from the wealthiest to the poorest countries. Poor and bad nutrition can also be found in individual wealthy countries to different extents.

12.6 FOOD AND INCOME

An increasing world population, with people living together in communities, led to food being only obtainable by *barter* or for *money*. The 'free' food of the early Stone Age was no longer sufficient to support the greatly increased world population. Today food for a healthful diet can only be *purchased*, and *low income* or *poverty* is equated with *under-nutrition*, whilst a *high income* or *affluence* is equated with *over-nutrition*.

The personal income per head of the developing countries averages only 8 per cent or less than *one-tenth* of the developed countries average income – the association of poverty with food shortage, malnutrition and illiteracy is obvious.

Table 12.2 *general comparison of nutrition in developed and developing countries*

	Developed countries (25% world population)	*Developing countries (75% world population)*
Total world food production	55% by advanced agricultural and food technology. OVER–production – grain, beef, cheese and butter mountains well-stored. *Livestock* fed on grain sufficient to feed 35% of world population	45% mainly by primitive agriculture. UNDER-production – losses caused by drought, pests and disasters. Losses in storage considerable because of pests and climate. Little fed to livestock
Water	Almost all have access to adequate *pure*, clean, *disease-free* supply. Effective sewage disposal. Good land irrigation	Impure, inadequate, supply to up to 50% population. Waterborne diseases. Little or no sewage disposal. Poor land irrigation
General diet	OVER-nutrition. Varied healthful diet, ample energy supplies for cooking	UNDER-nutrition in 25%. Monotonous staple diet, with shortage of wood-fuel for cooking
Energy daily intake per head	Exceeds 10MJ per head by 34%	Below 10MJ in most countries by 1%
Protein Intake usually about 10% of total energy intake in all countries	HIGH general intake. Approximately 90g or more daily. 60% from animal sources. 40% from plant sources	LOW general intake. Approximately 50g daily, and often less. 80% from plant sources. 20% from animal sources
Carbohydrate	Forms about 50% of energy intake, composed of: Sucrose, greater than 15% HIGH Cereals 45% Starches 40% *Low* dietary fibre	Forms more than 70% of energy intake, composed of: Sucrose, less than 4% LOW Cereals 43% Starches 53% *High* dietary fibre
Lipids	Forms about 40% of energy intake from mainly animal sources with high *saturated* alkanoic (fatty) acid and cholesterol	Less than 20% of energy intake mainly from *plant* sources with corresponding higher *polyunsaturated* alkanoic (fatty) acid (PUFA) content
Mineral intake	Seldom deficient	Frequently deficient in iron and iodine
Vitamin intake	Seldom deficient	Frequently deficient in vitamins A, B_1, B_{12} and nicotinic acid, C and D

Food value for money

Foods from *plant* sources, cereals, pulses, vegetables and fruits are usually cheaper on a unit weight basis, than foods from *animal* sources, meat, fish, eggs and dairy products.

Proteins, particularly from animal sources, are more expensive compared with other nutrients, and consequently the food purchaser seeks the most protein for a penny or other unit of money denomination.

The amount of *nutrient* bought for a penny can be calculated from the following:

Stage one Food *item* for a penny:

Food item costs A pence for B grammes

Therefore, 1 penny buys $\frac{1 \times B}{A}$

1 penny buys = C grammes.

Stage two Food *nutrient* for a penny.

Refer to the food composition tables (Appendix A) to find the *food items composition.*

Multiply the value for each nutrient by C (grammes) and divide by 100 to obtain nutrient for a penny.

Example One can (198g) of Corned beef costs 59p in 1983. Calculate the amount of protein and nicotinic acid for one penny.

Stage one

Corned beef costs 59p for 198g

One peny buys $\frac{1 \times 198}{59} = 3.36\text{g}$

Stage two

Referring to Appendix A, food composition tables (Appendix), corned beef contains 25.3g protein and 3.4mg nicotinic acid per 100g.

(a) Protein for a penny in corned beef $= \frac{25.3 \times 3.36}{100}$

Protein for a penny $= 0.85$ g

(b) Nicotinic acid for a penny in corned beef $= \frac{3.4 \times 3.36}{100}$

Nicotinic acid for a penny $= 0.114$ mg

See Appendix B.

Food costing

The economic planning of meals is related to the:

(a) *Nutrient content* of each food item as indicated in food composition tables (Table 9.1, Section 9.1).
(b) *Nutrient costs* as calculated previously; two important factors to be considered are whether the foods are (i) *raw* and *uncooked* or (ii) *pre-cooked*, ready to eat as in most 'convenience' foods.
(c) *Cooking*, to make raw foods palatable, requires *energy* from mainly *fossil fuels* - oil, coal, gas or electricity. People in developed countries use forty times the *irreplaceable* fossil fuel energy as the rest of the world. The amount of energy used in cooking *adds* to food costs; this can be between 4 and 20 per cent of the cost of the total energy used in the home.

Fuel wood

Developed countries use 40 per cent of all the world's wood production for *industrial* purposes; paper-making, furniture, building and veneers, whilst developing countries use 45 per cent of the world's wood as fuel for *cooking* and *heating* purposes. *One third* of the population of developing countries using fuel wood are experiencing serious *shortages* of fuel wood and this is expected to increase by the year 2000 when *half* the developing countries' population will have inadequate fuel wood supplies to cook *diminishing* world food supplies.

Basic cheap foods

The cheapest sources of nutrients in the UK are summarised in Table 12.3 (see also Appendix B). A cheap healthful diet can be constructed from these sources using the daily recommended intakes in Table 10.1 and Table 10.11. It is interesting to note that some: skimmed milk powder, canned fish, mung and soya beans, dried egg, and wheat and maize flours are important *famine relief* foods, being cheap sources of energy and protein, minerals and vitamins. Plate 12.2 illustrates the mung bean, a high protein food and the noodles made from it.

12.7 CORRECTING WORLD FOOD IMBALANCE

All populations of living organisms, whether human beings or bacteria (Section 11.4), interact with the surrounding environment and are affected by changes in its supplies of food, water and material resources.

At present a state of *imbalance* exists where part of the human population has a *surplus* of food, wealth and medical supplies, and another part

Plate 12.2 *the mung bean, composed of 22 per cent protein, 1 per cent lipid, 35 per cent carbohydrate and useful amounts of iron, calcium, Vitamins B_1, B_2, nicotinic and folic acids is made into noodles. In this form, it is a valuable low-cost, high-protein food used in developing countries of South-east Asia (FAO, UN)*

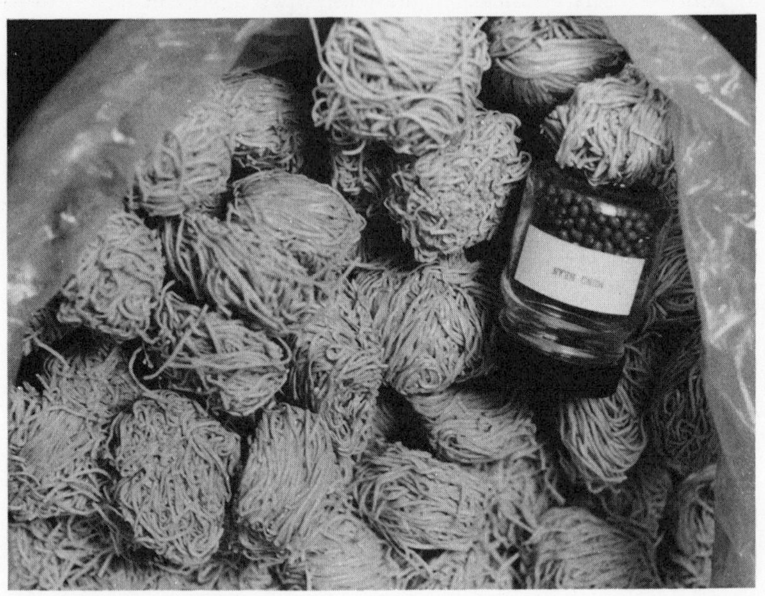

has a *deficit* of these components forming part of the environment of human beings on Earth.

Food shortage, under-nutrition, infectious disease, poverty and illiteracy *coexist* in the world with food surplus, over-nutrition, wealth and literacy. The mid-way position of *equilibrium*, or a state of *human homeostasis* (Section 1.3 and 8.14) where the human population exists in a *steady* environment with sufficient food, water and material resources for a *healthful life*, is yet to be achieved.

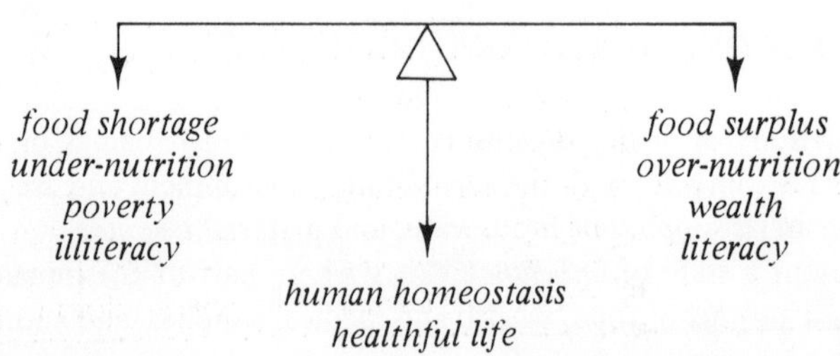

Table 12.3 *some cheap sources of nutrients in the UK diet*

Nutrient	*Plant source*	*Animal source*
Energy		
(a) Lipids	Margarine, cooking oils	Lard, dripping, suet, butter
(b) Carbohydrates	Sugar, bread, potatoes, some biscuits, breakfast cereals	NONE
Protein	Bread, pulses, potatoes, baked beans, some breakfast cereals, peanuts, textured vegetable protein	Canned fish, pilchards, tuna, mackerel – skimmed milk, eggs, Cheddar cheese ox liver, ox kidney, evaporated milk, fresh milk
Vitamin B_1 thiamine	Wheatgerm, certain fortified breakfast cereals, wholemeal bread, yeast extract, potatoes	Cod roes, milk, bacon, cheese
Vitamin B_2 riboflavin	Yeast extract, certain fortified breakfast cereals, wheatgerm, bran, potatoes	Liver, skimmed milk powder, eggs, cheese
Nicotinic acid	Bran, yeast extract, certain fortified breakfast cereals, peanuts, potatoes and bread	Ox liver, meat extract, ox kidney, chicken, skimmed milk powder
Vitamin C ascorbic acid	Rosehip and blackcurrant syrups, orange juice, fresh cabbage, new potatoes	NONE
Vitamin A retinol/carotenes	Carrots, fortified margarine	Ox liver, butter, cheese, skimmed milk powder
Vitamin D cholecalciferols	Fortified margarine	Fatty fish, butter, eggs
Calcium	Molasses treacle, green vegetables, bread, dried figs	Skimmed milk powder, evaporated milk, Cheddar cheese, fresh milk, ice cream, tinned fish
Iron	Treacle molasses, wholemeal bread, soya beans, wheatgerm, cocoa powder (curry powder)	Ox liver, ox kidney, corned beef
Cheapest sources of at least *four* nutrients	Bread, fortified cornflakes, flour, lentils, peas, soya beans, wheatgerm, yeast extract, bran, potatoes	Cheddar cheese, skimmed milk powder, eggs, evaporated milk, beef extract, canned pilchards, mackerel

Periodically the imbalance is upset further by *famine* caused by drought, floods, earthquakes, wars or crop destruction by pests and diseases.

Methods for correcting the world food imbalance include the following:

1. Food organisation

A. International level

Long-term international measures are through the United Nations, *Food and Agriculture Organisation* set up in 1945, with 152 countries as members, which serves to *advise* and *recommend* member countries on how to:

1. raise standards of *nutrition*,
2. improve *food* distribution and production,
3. improve condition of life in rural populations.

For example Table 10.1 of recommended daily intake of nutrients was prepared by FAO.

The *World Health Organisation* (WHO) formed in 1948, *advises* and provides *practical* assistance to its 138 member countries in methods aimed at raising health standards through *nutrition*, disease control and family planning.

The *United Nations Children's Fund* (*UNICEF*) provides material aid of every kind exclusively to children in conjunction with WHO and FAO. United Nations Children's Fund depends entirely on voluntary contributions.

Short-term international famine relief organisations serve to provide rapid *practical* assistance by providing *food* and *medical* supplies and services through many charitable organisations such as: Save the Children Fund, Oxfam, Help the Aged, Children's Relief International, International Red Cross Society, Christian Aid and the International Handicapped Organisation. Famine relief is also supported by donations of food, money and materials from governments of various developed countries from their *surpluses*.

B. National food organisation

Governments of different countries have departments or ministries concerned with health or agriculture whose responsibility also includes nutrition. In the UK it is the concern of the Department of Health and Social Security, who amongst other functions prepare tables of recommended daily intakes of energy and nutrients (Report no. 15, 1979). Other important reports include 'Diet and Coronary Heart Disease' - no. 7, 1974, and 'Present-day Practice in Infant Feeding' - no. 9, 1974.

2. Education and birth control

Knowledge gained by literacy and general education is not available to one third of the children between 6 and 11 in the world. *Nutrition education* by teachers, nurses, doctors, home economists, media writers for magazines, radio and television, provide the means to inform on all aspects of a healthful diet and an understanding of nutrition problems in the world.

Birth control or family planning by legalised abortion or different contraceptive techniques is used by 30 per cent of the world's family couples in developed and in certain developing countries. Contraception as a means of reducing the world population birth rate is *not* used by more than 50 per cent of the world's family couples. Family planning, birth control, later marriages, literacy and education, are important *factors* for reducing the world birth rate (See Plate 12.3).

3. Agriculture and fisheries

Only 11 per cent of all the land in the world is actually cultivated whilst another 22 per cent is potentially *usable*; the remainder is unsuitable for cultivation, being too dry, cold or mountainous.

Methods to increase food production in developing countries require improved techniques, seeds and livestock, equipment, irrigation methods, fertilisers and pesticides - which in turn involve *money* and *education*. Loans are available through the *World Bank*, and the *International Development Association* promotes economic development in developing countries.

4. Work

There are 17m unemployed in developed countries and more than eighteen times this number - or 298m - unemployed in the developing countries. Improved agriculture could provide work for many more in developing countries. Work provides the *means* to buy or obtain food.

World Food Programme, WFP, started by the UN and FAO in 1962 operates a 'food for work' project in seriously-affected developing countries. The food is payment to people working planting trees, building houses and roads, or digging irrigation canals. WFP also provides food in international emergencies to feed victims of natural disasters and political disorders in over 95 developing countries (see Plate 7.1).

Conclusion - food for thought

In November 1983 when famine threatened several African countries because of drought, an international relief organisation issued an urgent appeal for 8000 tonnes of food, and one million US dollars cash - that is one *thousandth* part of what is spent on *arms daily* in the world.

Plate 12.3 *India was the first developing country to introduce government-supported family planning, mainly by use of intra-uterine contraceptive loops (WHO)*

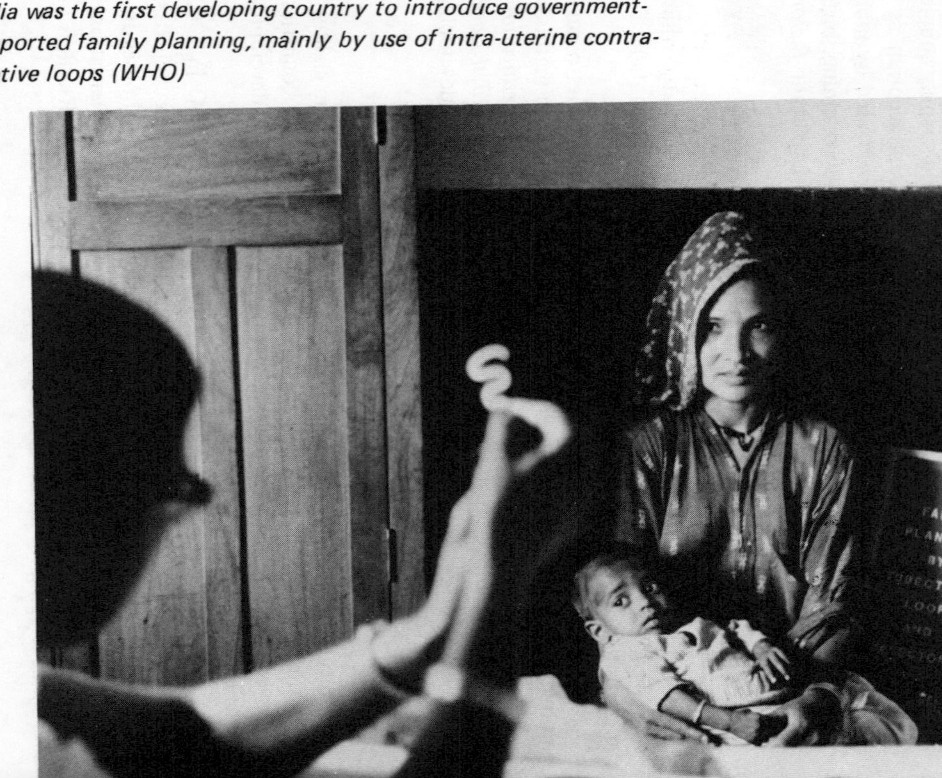

12.8 QUESTIONS

1. What organisations help developing countries where there are food shortages? Desribe in some detail how a *named* organisation works in famine relief.
2. What foods are imported into the UK? Is it possible for the UK to be self-supporting with respect to its food needs?
3. Name and describe the nutrient composition of two food items that can be used in famine relief. Suggest ways of preparing these items in an attractive way.
4. Summarise the main features of dietary imbalance between the diet of a wealthy developed country and one of the poorest developing countries.
5. What important factors can help to *reduce* the world birth rate?
6. What are the main causes of food shortage in developing countries?
7. Comment on the way in which human nutritional requirements are met in a technologically advanced society and in one which is technologically less advanced.

APPENDIX A

COMPOSITION OF FOODS

Food 100g edible portion raw uncooked unless stated otherwise	Energy						Fat-soluble vitamins		Water-soluble vitamins						Mineral elements	
	Water	Kilojoule	Kilocalorie	Protein	Total lipid fat	Total carbohydrate	A retinol equivalents	D cholecalciferol	B_1 Thiamin	B_2 Riboflavin	Nicotinic acid equivalents	Free folic acid	B_{12} cyanocobalamin	C ascorbic acid	Ca calcium	Fe iron
	(g)	(kJ)	(kcal)	(g)	(g)	(g)	(μg)	(μg)	(mg)	(mg)	(mg)	(μg)	(μg)	(mg)	(mg)	(mg)
FRUIT																
Apples – sweet eating	84	240	58	0.3	0.6	15.0	9	0	0.04	0.02	0.1	3	0	5	7	0.3
Apricots	85.3	214	51	0.9	0	12.8	270	0	0.03	0.05	0.7	–	0	7	17	0.5
Avocado Pears	73.6	720	171	2.2	17.0	6.0	29	0	0.11	0.20	1.6	31	0	14	10	0.6
Bananas	75.7	360	85	1.1	0.2	22.2	19	0	0.05	0.06	0.6	12	0	10	8	0.7
Black currants – stewed with sugar	82	260	62	1.0	0.1	16.1	22	0	0.05	0.03	0.3	–	0	136	17	0.9
Dates – dried	22.5	1150	274	2.2	0.5	72.9	5	0	0.09	0.10	2.2	14	0	0	59	3.0
Figs – dried	23.0	1150	274	4.3	1.3	69.1	8	0	0.10	0.10	1.7	3	0	0	126	0.35
Gooseberries	88.9	160	39	0.8	0.2	9.7	29	0	0.15	0.03	0.3	–	0	25	9	0.08
Grapefruit	88.4	160	39	0.6	0.1	9.8	8	0	0.04	0.02	0.2	7	0	40	17	0.3
Guava	82.2	268	64	1.1	0.4	15.7	50	0	0.06	0.04	1.3	–	0	326	24	1.3
Lemons	90.1	110	27	1.1	0.3	8.2	2	0	0.04	0.02	0.1	7	0	80	26	0.6
Mango	81.7	280	66	0.7	0.4	16.8	480	0	0.05	0.05	1.1	–	0	35	10	0.4
Olives – green in brine	78.2	490	116	1.4	12.7	1.3	30	0	0.03	0.08	0.5	–	0	0	61	1.6
Oranges	86.0	210	49	1.0	0.2	12.2	20	0	0.10	0.03	0.2	13	0	50	41	0.4
Papaya (Pawpaw)	90.8	135	32	0.4	0.1	8.3	160	0	0.03	0.03	0.4	–	0	52	21	0.6
Peaches	86.6	190	46	0.6	0.1	11.8	133	0	0.02	0.05	1.0	2	0	7	9	0.5
Pears	83.2	260	61	0.5	0.4	15.5	0.2	0	0.02	0.04	0.1	4	0	4	8	0.3
Pineapple	86.7	200	47	0.4	0.2	12.2	7	0	0.08	0.03	0.2	9	0	17	17	0.5
Plums	85.7	210	50	0.7	0.1	12.3	25	0	0.07	0.04	0.5	1	0	6	13	0.4
Prunes – (dried plums)	28.0	1070	255	2.1	0.6	67.4	160	0	0.1	0.17	1.6	0.7	0	3	51	3.9
Raisins – (dried grapes)	18.0	1210	289	2.5	0.2	77.4	2	0	0.1	0.08	0.5	4	0	1	62	3.5
Raspberries	84.2	240	57	1.2	0.5	13.6	13	0	0.03	0.09	0.9	–	0	25	41	1.0
Rhubarb	94.9	70	16	0.5	0.1	3.8	10	0	0.01	0.03	0.3	9	0	9	96	0.8
Strawberries	89.9	150	37	0.7	0.5	8.4	6	0	0.03	0.07	0.6	15	0	60	21	1.0
Watermelon	92.6	110	26	0.5	0.2	6.4	59	0	0.03	0.03	0.2	2	0	7	7	0.5

Table A.1 (*continued*)

Food 100g edible portion raw uncooked unless stated otherwise	Water (g)	Energy: Kilojoule (kJ)	Energy: Kilocalorie (kcal)	Protein (g)	Total lipid fat (g)	Total carbohydrate (g)	Fat-soluble vitamins: A retinol equivalents (μg)	Fat-soluble vitamins: D cholecalciferol (μg)	Water-soluble vitamins: B_1 Thiamin (mg)	B_2 Riboflavin (mg)	Nicotinic acid equivalents (mg)	Free folic acid (μg)	B_{12} cyanocobalamin (μg)	C ascorbic acid (mg)	Mineral elements: Ca calcium (mg)	Fe iron (mg)
VEGETABLES																
Bread Fruit	72.0	457	109	1.5	0.3	25.4	10	0	0.08	0.05	0.7	–	0	31	28	2.0
Broad bean – dry seeds	12.6	1420	339	24.0	2.2	58.2	3	0	0.53	0.30	2.5	–	0	6	77	6.3
Baked lima beans, canned	74.7	400	96	5.4	0.3	18.3	19	0	0.03	0.05	0.5	–	0	6	28	2.4
Beans – runner or string	90.1	130	32	1.9	0.2	7.1	60	0	0.07	0.11	0.5	39	0	19	56	0.8
Brussels sprouts	84.8	200	47	4.7	0.4	8.7	55	0	0.10	0.16	0.9	45	0	90	32	1.5
Cabbage, savoy	90.0	130	31	3.0	0.4	5.6	20	0	0.05	0.06	0.3	60	0	45	47	0.9
Carrots	88.6	170	40	1.1	0.2	9.1	1100	0	0.06	0.12	0.6	15	0	8	37	0.7
Cassava (manioc) cooked	69.0	520	124	0.9	0.1	30.0	–	0	0.06	0.05	0.9	–	0	26	12	1.0
Cauliflower	91.0	110	27	2.7	0.2	5.2	6	0	0.11	0.10	0.6	32	0	78	25	1.1
Celery stalks	94.1	70	17	0.9	0.1	3.9	24	0	0.05	0.03	0.4	–	0	9	39	0.5
Cowpea (Kaffai bean)	10.8	1436	342	23.1	1.4	61.4	20	0	0.75	0.18	2.5	–	0	1	100	7.6
Cucumber	95.6	50	13	0.8	0.1	3.0	30	0	0.04	0.05	0.2	10	0	8	25	1.1
Egg plant (Aubergine)	92.4	100	25	1.2	0.2	5.6	1	0	0.05	0.05	0.6	8	0	5	12	0.4
Lentils, dried	11.1	1420	340	24.7	1.1	60.1	6	0	0.25	0.49	2.0	25	0	0	79	8.6
Lettuce	95.1	60	14	1.3	0.2	2.5	97	0	0.06	0.07	0.3	24	0	8	35	2.0
Locust bean, African (Cake)	14.8	1814	432	36.5	28.3	15.8	–	0	0.04	0.61	1.9	–	0	2	378	36.5
Maize (sweet corn)	72.7	400	96	3.5	1.0	22.1	40	0	0.15	0.12	1.7	27	0	12	3	0.7
Mushrooms	90.8	90	22	2.8	0.2	3.7	0	0	0.1	0.44	6.2	20	0	5	9	0.8
Okra	88.9	150	36	2.4	0.3	7.6	52	0	0.17	0.21	1.0	25	0	31	70	1.0
Onions	89.1	160	38	1.5	0.1	8.7	4	0	0.03	0.04	0.2	15	0	10	27	0.5
Peas, green, canned	82.3	280	67	3.4	0.4	12.7	45	0	0.11	0.06	0.9	8	0	9	25	1.6
Peppers, green, chillies	92.8	100	24	1.2	0.2	5.3	21	0	0.08	0.22	0.5	8	0	128	9	0.4

Plantain ripe	65.4	570	135	1.2	0.3	32.1	130	0	0.08	0.04	0.6	–	0	20	0.8	1.3
Potatoes, fried chips	1.8	2412	570	5.3	39.8	50.0	trace	0	0.21	0.07	4.8	4	0	16	40	1.8
Potatoes	79.8	320	76	2.1	0.1	17.7	trace	0	0.11	0.04	1.2	9	0	20	8	0.8
Soybean, dried	10.0	1690	403	34.1	17.7	33.5	8	0	1.10	0.31	2.1	–	0	trace	226	8.4
Spinach	90.7	110	26	3.2	0.3	4.3	810	0	0.10	0.20	0.6	176	0	51	106	3.1
Sweet potatoes	70.6	480	114	1.7	0.4	26.3	880	0	0.10	0.06	0.6	35	0	21	32	0.7
Taro (cocoyan)	73.1	430	102	1.8	0.1	24.0	trace	0	0.10	0.03	0.8	–	0	8	51	1.2
Tomatoes	93.5	90	22	1.1	0.2	4.7	90	0	0.06	0.04	0.7	4	0	23	13	0.6
Turnips, roots	91.5	130	30	1.0	0.2	6.6	trace	0	0.04	0.07	0.6	17	0	36	39	0.5
Waterleaf (Fameflower, potherb)	90.8	105	25	2.4	0.4	4.4	trace	0	0.08	0.18	0.3	–	0	31	28	2.0
Watercress	93.3	80	19	2.2	0.3	3.0	400	0	0.10	0.27	0.9	200	0	75	151	2.0
Yams	69.0	500	119	1.9	0.2	27.8	trace	0	0.11	0.02	0.3	–	0	6	52	0.8
Yeast, bakers' compressed	71.0	360	86	12.1	0.4	11.0	trace	0	0.71	1.65	11.2	40	trace	trace	13	4.9
CEREALS AND GRAIN PRODUCTS																
Barley, pearled	12.0	1450	346	9.0	1.4	76.5	0	0	0.12	0.05	3.1	9	0	0	16	2.0
Maize – cornflakes	3.8	1610	385	7.9	0.4	85.3	0	0	0.43	0.1	2.1	14	0	0	3	1.4
Maize – meal flour	12.0	1540	368	7.8	2.6	76.8	34	0	0.20	0.06	1.4	17	0	0	6	1.8
Maize – ground hominy	11.0	1530	365	8.8	1.1	78.0	44	0	0.15	0.05	0.5	15	0	0	4	1.0
Millet, peeled	11.8	1370	327	9.9	2.9	72.9	0	0	0.73	0.38	2.8	–	0	0	20	6.8
Oatmeal	10.3	1620	387	13.8	6.6	67.7	–	0	0.60	0.14	1.1	–	0	0	53	3.6
Pasta – macaroni, spaghetti	10.4	1540	369	12.5	1.2	75.2	0	0	0.10	0.06	2.0	4	0	0	23	1.2
Rice – polished, cooked	72.6	460	109	2.0	0.1	24.2	0	0	0.02	0.01	0.4	3	0	0	10	0.2
Sorghum (all species) grain	10.1	1450	347	10.7	3.2	74.1	10	0	0.34	0.15	3.3	–	0	0	26	10.6
Soybean – full fat flour	8.0	1450	347	36.7	20.3	30.4	11	0	0.85	0.31	2.1	–	0	0	199	8.4
Wheat – whole or wholemeal flour	12.6	1390	331	12.1	2.1	71.5	40	0	0.55	0.12	4.3	25	0	0	41	3.3
Wheat – bran	8.0	850	202	14.0	5.5	71.0	0	0	0.90	0.40	30.0	130	0	0	110	13.0
Wheat – germ	11.5	1520	363	26.6	10.9	46.7	65	0	2.0	0.68	4.2	257	0	0	72	9.4
Wheat – white bread	39.0	1050	251	7.8	1.7	49.7	0	0	0.18	0.03	1.4	6	0	0	100	1.7
Wheat – wholemeal bread	36.4	1010	241	9.1	2.6	49.3	0	0	0.30	0.10	2.8	22	0	0	23	2.5
SUGAR AND SWEETS																
Caramel, full cream toffee	7.6	1670	399	4.0	10.2	76.6	1	0	0.03	0.17	0.2	–	0	0	148	1.4
Chocolate, milk sweet	0.9	2180	520	7.7	32.3	56.9	27	0	0.06	0.34	0.3	21	0	0	220	1.1
Chocolate, plain sweet	0.9	2210	528	4.4	35.1	57.9	trace	0	0.02	0.14	0.3	–	0	0	63	1.4
Honey	17.2	1270	304	0.3	0	82.3	0	0	trace	0.04	0.3	–	0	0.06	5	0.5
Jams – various	29.0	1140	272	0.6	0.1	70.0	1	0	0.01	0.03	0.2	5	0	2	12	1.0
Molasses – treacle	24.0	970	232	–	–	60.0	–	0	0.08	0.16	2.8	7	0	0	273	6.7
Sugar, brown	2.1	1560	373	0	0	96.4	0	0	0.01	0.03	0.2	–	0	0	85	3.4
Sugar, white	trace	1610	385	0	0	99.5	0	0	0	0	0	0	0	0	0	trace

Table A.1 (*continued*)

Food 100g edible portion raw uncooked unless stated otherwise		Energy					Fat-soluble vitamins		Water-soluble vitamins						Mineral elements	
	Water	Kilojoule	Kilocalorie	Protein	Total lipid fat	Total carbohydrate	A retinol equivalents	D cholecalciferol	B_1 Thiamin	B_2 Riboflavin	Nicotinic acid equivalents	Free folic acid	B_{12} cyanocobalanin	C ascorbic acid	Ca calcium	Fe iron
	(g)	(kJ)	(kcal)	(g)	(g)	(g)	(μg)	(μg)	(mg)	(mg)	(mg)	(μg)	(μg)	(mg)	(mg)	(mg)
NUTS																
Cashew nuts	5.2	2350	561	17.2	45.7	29.3	10	0	0.45	0.25	1.8	8	0	0	38	3.8
Coconuts, dried	3.5	2770	662	7.2	64.9	23.0	0	0	0.06	0.04	0.6	0	0	0	26	3.3
Peanuts, roasted	1.8	2440	582	26.2	48.7	20.6	36	0	0.33	0.13	17.1	28	0	0	74	2.2
Pine nuts (seeds)	3.1	2660	635	13.0	60.5	20.5	3	0	1.28	0.23	4.5	–	0	0	12	5.2
Sunflower seeds	4.8	2340	560	24.0	47.3	19.9	5	0	1.96	0.23	5.4	–	0	0	120	7.1
OILS AND FATS																
Butter	17.4	3000	716	0.6	81.0	0.7	990	0.75	trace	0.01	0.1	0	trace	trace	16	0.2
Margarine, salted	19.7	2920	698	0.5	78.4	0.4	990	8.00	–	–	–	3	trace	–	13	0.05
Peanut butter	1.8	2430	581	27.8	49.4	17.2	0	0	0.13	0.13	15.7	20	0	0	63	2.0
Cooking oil – corn oil	–	3700	883	–	99.9	–	–	–	–	–	–	–	–	–	–	–
Cooking oil – palm oil	–	360	860	–	98.9	0.3	25000 (in unrefined oil)	–	–	–	–	–	–	–	6	–
Lard (pork fat)	1.0	3740	893	trace	99.0	0	trace	–	trace	trace	trace	–	–	–	1	0.1
Cod-liver oil	0	3770	901	0	99.9	0	25500	213	0	0	0	0	0	0	0	0
FISH AND SEA FOODS																
Fish: Blue fish (elfi)	76.0	445	106	18.6	3.0	0	trace	trace	0.15	0.15	8.0	–	–	–	59	5.2
Cod	81.2	330	78	17.6	0.3	0	trace	trace	0.06	0.07	2.2	6	2	2	11	0.5
Croaker (cassava fish)	76.3	370	88	17.4	1.5	0	–	–	0.09	0.07	4.8	–	–	–	12	0.7

Herring	62.8	1020	243	17.3	18.8	0	40	23	0.06	0.24	4.3	3	10	0.5	57	1.1
Hake, South African (stock fish)	69.8	600	142	21.8	5.4	0	–	–	–	–	–	–	–	–	–	–
Mackerel	67.2	800	191	19.0	12.2	0	135	18	0.15	0.35	7.7	–	10	0	5	1.0
Salmon, canned	64.2	850	203	21.7	12.2	0	18	13	0.03	0.18	6.5	4	4	trace	93	1.4
Sardines, canned in oil	50.6	1300	311	50.6	24.4 (50g = canning oil)	0.6	55	7	0.02	0.16	4.4	6	23	0	354 [edible from bones]	3.5
Snapper	77.4	380	90	19.8	0.6	0	–	–	–	–	–	–	–	–	–	–
Tunny (tuna) (canned in oil)	52.5	1210	290	23.8	20.9 [15g = canning oil]	0	27	6	0.05	0.06	10.8	7	4.6	0	7	1.2
Crustaceans: Crab, canned	77.2	420	110	17.4	2.5	1.1	trace	trace	0.08	0.08	2.5	3	trace	trace	45	0.8
Lobster	78.5	380	91	16.9	1.9	0.5	trace	trace	0.15	0.13	1.5	7	trace	5	29	0.6
Shrimps	78.2	490	116	18.7	2.2	0.7	18	2.6	0.07	0.05	1.25	8	2	2	115	3.1
Molluscs: Mussels	82.5	320	76	12.0	1.7	2.2	54	trace	0.16	0.22	1.6	–	–	trace	88	5.8
Octopus	82.2	310	73	15.3	0.8	0	–	–	0.02	0.06	1.8	–	–	–	29	0.2
Snails	82.0	310	75	15.0	0.8	2.0	–	–	–	–	–	–	–	–	170	3.5
MEAT, POULTRY AND INSECTS																
Meat: Bacon, medium fat	20.0	2620	625	9.1	65.0	trace	0	0	0.36	0.11	1.8	trace	trace	0	13	1.2
Beef, round	69.0	820	196	19.5	12.5	–	trace	trace	0.08	0.17	4.7	4	2	–	11	2.9
Beef, corned canned	59.3	900	216	25.3	12.0	0	0	trace	0.02	0.23	3.4	1	1.7	0	14	4.3
Camel meat	59.1	1125	267	19.6	20.3	0	–	–	–	–	–	–	–	–	–	–
Ham, boiled	57.0	1130	269	19.5	20.6	0	trace	trace	0.54	0.26	4.2	1	0.3	0	10	2.5
Lamb chops, medium fat	52.0	1480	352	14.9	32.0	0	trace	trace	0.13	0.18	4.3	1	2	0	9	2.2
Pork cutlets	53.9	1430	341	15.2	30.6	0	trace	trace	0.80	0.19	4.3	4	1	0	9	2.3
Rabbit	70.4	670	159	20.4	8.0	0	trace	trace	0.04	0.18	12.8	4	10	0	18	2.4
Offal: Heart, average	76.8	516	123	15.3	6.1	0.6	trace	trace	0.53	1.05	6.6	1	3	3	10	2.4
Kidney, average	76.6	507	120	16.3	5.4	0.85	95	trace	0.37	2.21	7.5	30	31	12	11	5.7
Liver, average	70.7	570	136	20.1	4.3	3.88 [glycogen]	9600	0.75	0.35	2.90	16.0	155	80	30	10	10.5
Sausage (beef, pork average)	45.0	1640	390	10.0	35.0	10.0 [starches]	trace	trace	0.16	0.14	3.3	2	trace	0	30	1.3
Tongue, average	70.0	770	184	16.8	12.0	0.6	trace	trace	0.15	0.28	10.0	2	5	trace	8	2.5
Poultry: Chicken (roasted fresh/skin)	67.0	1050	251	19.5	12.6	0	400	trace	0.08	0.12	7.4	–	–	–	11	1.5
Duck (medium fat)	54.0	1360	326	16.0	28.6	0	–	–	0.10	0.24	5.6	–	–	–	15	0.4

Table A.1 (*continued*)

Food 100g edible portion raw uncooked unless stated otherwise	*Energy*						*Fat-soluble vitamins*		*Water-soluble vitamins*						*Mineral elements*	
	Water	*Kilojoule*	*Kilocalorie*	*Protein*	*Total lipid fat*	*Total carbohydrate*	*A retinol equivalents*	*D cholecalciferol*	B_1 *Thiamin*	B_2 *Riboflavin*	*Nicotinic acid equivalents*	*Free folic acid*	B_{12} *cyanocobalamin*	*C ascorbic acid*	*Ca calcium*	*Fe iron*
	(g)	(kJ)	(kcal)	(g)	(g)	(g)	(μg)	(μg)	(mg)	(mg)	(mg)	(μg)	(μg)	(mg)	(mg)	(mg)
Goose (medium fat)	51.0	1480	354	16.4	31.5	0	–	–	0.10	0.24	5.6	–	–	–	15	1.8
Turkey, roasted	64.2	2180	910	20.1	15.0	0.4	trace	trace	0.13	0.14	7.9	2	–	–	8	1.5
Insects: Caterpillars (palm weevil larvae – smoked)	20.4	1400	333	62.3	4.6	6.5	0	–	0.10	0.12	4.2	–	–	0	513	7.0
Crickets	76.0	490	117	13.7	5.3	2.9	–	–	–	–	–	–	–	–	18	13.0
Grasshoppers (floured and gulled)	7.0	1764	420	62.2	10.4	15.8	–	–	–	–	–	–	–	–	177	–
Locusts, fried	48.0	900	215	30.0	10.0	–	–	–	–	–	–	–	–	–	150	5.0
MILK, MILK PRODUCTS AND EGGS																
Cows milk, pasteurised whole	88.5	270	64	3.2	3.7	4.6	42	0.15	0.04	0.15	0.07	5	0.3	1	116	0.04
Cows milk, skimmed	90.9	140	34	3.5	0.07	4.8	trace	trace	0.04	0.17	0.1	4	0.3	2	123	0.1
Goats' milk	86.6	300	71	3.6	4.2	4.8	40	0.05	0.05	0.12	0.2	0.7	trace	2	129	0.1
Cream, whipping	64.1	1200	288	2.2	30.4	2.9	250	0.75	0.02	0.17	0.07	2	0.2	1	75	0.1
Yoghurt	86.1	300	71	4.8	3.8	4.5	44	trace	0.04	0.02	0.18	1	0.2	2	150	0.2
Ice cream	62.1	870	207	4.0	12.5	20.6	155	trace	0.04	0.19	0.1	trace	0.4	1	123	0.1
Hard cheese – Cheddar	37	1670	398	35.0	32.2	2.1	390	0.25	0.03	0.46	0.1	6	1.5	0	750	1.0
Semi-hard cheese – Edam	43.4	1350	325	26.1	23.6	3.5	180	0.18	0.06	0.35	0.07	–	1.4	0	765	0.7
Soft cheese – Camembert	51.3	1200	287	18.7	22.8	1.8	303	0.18	0.05	0.45	1.45	–	1.2	0	382	0.5
Cottage cheese – non-cream	79.4	360	86	17.2	0.6	1.8	10	0.02	0.04	0.31	0.1	–	0.5	1	90	0.4
Hen-egg – white	87.6	210	51	10.9	0.2	0.8	0	0	0.02	0.23	0.1	2	0.1	0	9	0.2
Hen-egg – yolk	50.0	1510	360	16.1	31.9	0.6	1020	8.75	0.32	0.52	0.02	47	5.0	0	140	7.2

MISCELLANEOUS																
Apple sauce	75.7	380	91	0.2	0.1	23.8	18	0	0.01	0.01	0.1	2	0	1	4	0.5
Curry powder	–	840	200	10	10	25	–	–	–	–	–	–	–	–	650	75
Gelatin, dry	13	1420	340	85.6	0.1	0	0	0	0	0	0	0	0	0	–	–
Mayonnaise	15.1	3000	718	1.1	78.9	3.0	84	3	0.02	0.04	trace	14	0	0	18	0.5
Mustard	78.1	380	91	5.9	6.3	5.3	–	–	–	–	–	–	0	–	124	1.8
Ovaltine powder	2.0	1660	397	15.2	5.0	73.5	1500	12	2.0	3.0	19.0	80	0	15	360	23
Tomato ketchup	68.6	440	106	2.0	0.4	25.4	420	0	0.09	0.07	1.6	–	0	15	22	0.8

SOURCE Abstraced from and reproduced by permission of Ciba-Geigy from the *Geigy Scientific Tables*, vol. 1, 8th Edn, 1981, and from the Food and Agriculture Organisation of United Nations, *Food Composition Tables For Use in Africa*, 1968.

APPENDIX B

COST OF FOOD ENERGY AND NUTRIENTS

Tables B.1–B.7 summarise by analysis the *quantity* of energy and certain nutrients which could be purchased for *one UK penny* based on the *average* food prices of selected items during *December 1983*.

Food prices will show variation from season to season within a year and usually show a general increase from year to year. For example the amount of protein bought for one UK penny has *decreased* by 50 to 60 per cent from what could be bought eight years ago; an average annual decrease in quantity per penny of 6 to 7 per cent.

The cheapest sources of food items and nutrients are indicated by a *. The method of calculation is described in Section 12.6. Also included in certain tables for *comparison* are the quantities of pure glucose, vitamin C tablets, etc., bought for one penny.

Table B.1 *value for money: vegetables*

		Energy or nutrient for one UK penny		
Food Item	*Price per 100g*	*Protein g/p*	*Energy kJ/p*	*Vitamin C mg/p*
Baked beans	8.0	0.67	50	–
Brussels sprouts	5.3	0.75	21	17*
Cabbage white	4.6	0.43	20	5
Carrots	2.6	0.26	38	2
Cauliflower	12.1	0.15	4	5
Leeks	8.2	0.23	15	2
Onions	3.5	0.25	28	3
Parsnips	4.6	0.36	46	3
Potatoes	2.7	0.76*	135*	5
Potato crisps	22.0	0.29	101	1
Tomatoes	7.1	0.12	9	3
Turnips	2.2*	0.36	39	16
Vitamin C tablets	750.0	–	–	14

Table B.2 *value for money: fruit*

Food item	*Price per 100g*	*Energy kJ/p*	*Vitamin C mg/p*
Apples	7.1	27	0.41
Bananas	7.1	47*	1.39
Grapefruit	5.2	18	7.60*
Pears	6.6	27	0.45
Grapes	8.15	32	0.49
Tangerines	5.15	27	5.45
Glucose powder	12.0	139	–
Vitamin C tablets	750.0	–	14.0

Table B.3 *value for money cereals and products*

Food item	*Price per 100g*	*Energy and nutrients for one UK penny*					
		Energy kJ/p	*Protein g/p*	*Iron mg/p*	B_1 *mg/p*	B_2 *mg/p*	*Nicotinic acid mg/p*
Bread, white	6.9	143	1.15	0.24	0.02	0.004	0.20
Biscuits, water	21.9	84	0.5	0.07	0.005	0.001	0.13
Rice, brown	8.8	171	0.8	0.05	0.09*	0.003	0.34
Oatmeal	6.8*	238*	2.1*	0.60*	0.07	0.015*	0.56*
Nicotinic acid tablets	1440.0	–	–	–	–	–	69.0
Yeast, iron and B_1 tablets		–	–	6.6	2.5	–	–

Table B.4 *value for money: meat and meat products*

Food item	*Price per 100g* 100g/p	*Energy or nutrient for one UK penny* *Protein* g/p	*Energy* kJ/p	*Iron* mg/p	*Thiamin* mg/p	*Riboflavin* mg/p	*Nicotinic* mg/p
Beef, topside	46.9	0.42	16	0.04	0.001	0.004	0.17
Beef, sirloin	71.6	0.23	16	0.02	0.0005	0.002	0.10
Beef, fillet	86.8	0.21	10	0.03	0.0009	0.003	0.09
Beef, stewing	32.0	0.62	23	0.06	0.001	0.007	0.13
Beef, mince	25.0	0.75*	37	0.10*	0.002	0.013*	0.32
Pork, fillet of leg	26.6	0.63	42	0.03	0.02*	0.005	0.30
Pork, loin chops	28.0	0.57	49*	0.024	0.02*	0.005	0.25
Lamb, loin chops	35.5	0.42	44	0.03	0.002	0.004	0.28
Lamb, leg	31.9	0.56	31	0.05	0.004	0.008	0.30
Bacon	14.0	0.63	79	0.10	0.03*	0.018*	0.80*
Sausages (beef and pork)	11.0*	0.90*	122*	0.12*	0.003	0.011	0.54*
Nicotinic acid tablets		–	–	–	–	–	69.0
Yeast, iron and thiamine tablets		–	–	6.6	2.5	–	–

Table B.5 *value for money; dairy and oil products*

Food item	*Price per 100g*	*Protein g/p*	*Energy kJ/p*	*Energy or nutrient for one UK penny*					
				Vitamins mg/p	*D mg/p*	B_1 *mg/p*	B_2 *mg/p*	*Nicotinic mg/p*	*Calcium mg/p*
Milk, cows'	3.7	0.86	73	37	0.47	0.01*	0.05*	0.21	32.0*
Butter	20.0	0.03	150	37	0.04	—	—	—	0.75
Margarine	10.0	0.05	290*	90	0.80	—	—	—	0.40
Cheese, Cheshire	26.0	1.30*	65	12	0.01	0.001	0.02	0.23*	30.0
Cream, double	27.8	0.05	68	12	0.006	0.0007	0.002	0.04	1.7
Eggs	17.0	0.75	40	8	0.10	0.005	0.02	0.22	3.0
Cod liver oil	45.0	—	84	400*	4.70*	—	—	—	—

Table B.6 *value for money: fish*

Food item	*Price per 100g*	*Energy or nutrient for one UK penny*								
		Protein g/p	*Energy kJ/p*	*Vitamin A μg/p*	*Vitamin D μg/p*	B_1 *mg/p*	B_2 *mg/p*	*Nicotinic acid mg/p*	*Calcium mg/p*	*Iron mg/p*
Mackerel	10.3	1.83*	89*	4.3*	1.7*	–	0.01*	0.44	3.0	0.09*
Herring	15.2	1.10	64	3.0	1.5	–	0.01	0.46*	2.2	0.05
Coley (Saithe)	17.6	1.02	19	–	–	0.005*	0.01	0.18	0.8	0.01
Lemon sole	19.8	0.85	18	–	–	0.003	0.004	0.33	2.6	0.01
Whiting	20.9	0.84	15	–	–	–	–	–	2.4	0.03
Trout	24.6	0.77	15	–	–	–	–	–	1.4	0.04
Cod	28.4	0.61	11	–	–	0.003	0.003	0.11	0.5	0.01
Haddock	28.8	0.58	11	–	–	0.002	0.002	0.24	0.6	0.02
Plaice	33.2	0.53	12	–	–	0.002	0.002	0.15	0.4	0.004
Salmon tinned	45.0	0.44	19	2.0	0.3	0.001	0.004	0.22	2.0	0.03
Sardines tinned	33.6	0.7	32	–	0.2	0.001	0.010	0.39	16.1*	0.08

Table B.7 *value for money: miscellaneous*

Item	*Price per 100g*	*Energy kJ/p*	*Protein g/p*
Sucrose, white sugar	4.5	360*	–
Glucose powder	12.1	140	–
Starch, cornflour	12.8	120	–
Minced meat	8.4	140	0.07
Chocolates, fancy mixed	43.0	45	0.09
Mineral waters carbonated	3.0	55	–
Beers	10.0	13	0.03
Wines	29.2	12	–
Sherry	26.5	18	0.004
Whisky	93.0	11	–

ADDRESSES

BNF	British Nutriton Foundation, 15 Belgrave Square, London, SW1X 8PS
Ciba-Geigy Ltd	Geigy Pharmaceuticals, Publicity Department, Horsham, West Sussex, RH12 4AB.
College of Health	College of Health, 18 Victoria Park Square, London, E2 9PF.
FAO	Food and Agriculture Organisation of United Nations, Via Delle Terme di Caracalla, 00100 Rome, Italy.
HMSO	Her Majesty's Stationery Office, PO Box 569, London, SE1 9NH.
Holtain Ltd	Holtain Ltd, Crosswell, Crymych, Dyfed, SA41 3UF.
MAFF	Ministry of Agriculture, Fisheries and Food, Publications Unit, Lion House, Willowburn Trading Estate, Alnwick, Northumberland, NE66 22PF.

WHO	World Health Organisation, 1211 Geneva 27, Switzerland.

BIBLIOGRAPHY

Bender, A. E., *Dictionary of Nutrition and Food Technology* (London: Butterworths, 1982).

Bender, A. E. and D. A. Bender, *Nutrition for Medical Students* (Chichester: John Wiley & Son, Inc., 1982).

Bingham, S., *Dictionary of Nutrition* (London: Barrie & Jenkins, 1977).

British Nutrition Foundation, *Nutrition Bulletins.*

Ciba-Geigy, *Geigy Scientific Tables, vol. I – Body Fluids, Body Composition and Nutrition* (Basle: Ciba-Geigy, 1981).

College of Health, *Self-Health*, Quarterly Journal.

Davidson, Sir Stanley, R. Passmore, J. F. Brock and A. S. Truswell, *Human Nutrition and Dietetics* (Edinburgh, London, New York: Churchill Livingstone, 1981).

Department of Health and Social Security, *Recommended Daily Amounts of Food Energy and Nutrients for Groups of People in the UK*. Report no. 15 (London: HMSO, 1979).

Department of Health and Social Security, *Eating for Health* (London: HMSO, 1982).

Food and Agriculture Organisation, *Handbook on Human Nutritional Requirements* (Rome: FAO, United Nations, 1974).

Health Education Council, *Proposals for Nutritional Guidelines for Health Education in Britain*, 1983, from Health Education Council, 78 New Oxford Street, London, WC1A 1AH.

Kilgour, O. F. G., *Shopping Science* (London: Heinemann, 1976).

Kilgour, O. F. G., *An Introduction to Science for Catering and Homecraft Students* (London: Heinemann, 1980).

Kilgour, O. F. G., *Multiple Choice Questions in Food and Nutrition* (London: Heinemann, 1980).

Kilgour, O. F. G. and A. L'Amie, *Experimental Science for Catering and Homecraft Students* (London: Heinemann, 1976).

Ministry of Agriculture, Fisheries and Food, *Look at the Label*, List of serial numbers as alternatives for specific names of additives (London: HMSO, 1983).

Paul, A. A. and D. A. T. Southgate, *The Composition of Foods* (London: HMSO, 1979).

Paul, P. C. and H. H. Palmer, *Food Theory and Applications* (Chichester: John Wiley & Son, Inc. 1972).

Population Concern, *World Population Data Sheet, 1983*, from Population Concern, 27/35 Mortimer Street, London, W1N 7RJ.
Robins, G. V., *Food Science in Catering* (London: Heinemann, 1980).
Taylor, T. G., *Principles of Human Nutrition*, Studies in Biology, no. 94 (London: Edward Arnold, 1978).
Taylor, T. G., *Nutrition and Health*, Studies in Biology, no. 141 (London: Edward Arnold, 1982).

INDEX

Alternative terms and spellings are given in brackets. Page numbers in italics refer to illustrations.

This book has extensive *contents* pages (pp. vii–xii), composed of chapter titles and metricated sections, together with a *glossary* (pp. xxii–xxiv). These should be referred to *before* the index.